WAKING THE WARRIOR GODDESS

Dr. Horner has assembled a great deal of useful information about the prevention and treatment of breast cancer. I will recommend this book to patients and families of all people concerned with this dreadful disease and its increasing frequency.

> —Andrew Weil, M.D., Founder and Director of the Program for Integrative Medicine, and Clinical Professor of Internal Medicine University of Arizona; Best-selling author of *Spontaneous Healing, 8 Weeks to Optimum Health, Eating Well for Optimum Health,* and *The Healthy Kitchen*

This book is a significant resource for women who feel inspired and desire to participate in their life and health. When you combine inspiration with information you have the potential to alter the physical world, health, your life, and derive the associated physical benefits. Without information, women have no choice about their health.

> —Bernie Siegel, M.D., Founder of Exceptional Cancer Patients; Best-selling author of *Love, Medicine, and Miracles: Lessons Learned about Self-Healing from a Surgeon's Experience with Exceptional Patients; 365 Prescriptions for the Soul: Daily Messages of Inspiration, Hope, and Love* and *Help Me to Heal*

Christine Horner, M.D., presents a powerful and comprehensive approach to achieving the very best of health. This is a prescription every doctor should write.

> —Neal Barnard, M.D., President of Physicians Committee for Responsible Medicine; Adjunct Associate Professor at the George Washington University School of Medicine; Author of *Breaking The Food Seduction; Turn Off the Fat Gene; Eat Right, Live Longer;* and *Food for Life: How the New Four Food Groups Can Save Your Life*

Dr. Christine Horner has done every woman a great favor by compiling under one cover all the essential knowledge for achieving breast health naturally. *Waking the Warrior Goddess* is enchantingly scripted, rich in practical tips and profoundly empowering. Read this book and follow its recommendations now, and you will create not only healthy breasts, but a healthy, fulfilling life!

> —Nancy Lonsdorf, M.D., Medical Director of The Raj Ayurveda
> Health Center; Author of *A Woman's Best Medicine* and *A Woman's*
> *Best Medicine for Menopause*

For most women, breast cancer remains the most threatening disease possible. Christine Horner's book offers the best available knowledge to prevent this dreaded illness. All women and their husbands should heed this advice.

> —C. Norman Shealy, M.D., Ph.D., President of Holos University
> Graduate Seminary; Founding President of American Holistic
> Medical Association; Author of *Miracles Do Happen, 90 Days*
> *to Stress-Free Living,* and *The Creation of Health*

This book is a paradigm shifter! I recommend that all women read it. You'll never think the same about your body or your health again.

> —Marci Shimoff, Coauthor of *Chicken Soup for a Woman's Soul*

This may be one of the most important books of our time for women. The information in this book can help stop the epidemic of breast cancer.

> —Jennifer Read Hawthorne, Coauthor of *Chicken Soup for the Woman's*
> *Soul;* Author of *The Soul of Success: A Woman's Guide to Authentic Power*

An important contribution to understanding and preventing breast cancer. Dr. Horner's sensitivity to ancient healing sciences is particularly valuable to patients and practitioners alike.

> —Tom Newmark, President of New Chapter Herbs; Coauthor of
> *Beyond Aspirin* and *Life Bridge*

WAKING
THE
WARRIOR
GODDESS

DR. CHRISTINE HORNER'S PROGRAM TO
PROTECT AGAINST & FIGHT BREAST CANCER

Christine Horner, M.D., F.A.C.S.

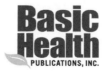

**Basic
Health**
PUBLICATIONS, INC.

The information contained in this book is based upon the research and personal and professional experiences of the author. It is not intended as a substitute for consulting with your physician or other healthcare provider. Any attempt to diagnose and treat an illness should be done under the direction of a healthcare professional.

The publisher does not advocate the use of any particular healthcare protocol but believes the information in this book should be available to the public. The publisher and author are not responsible for any adverse effects or consequences resulting from the use of the suggestions, preparations, or procedures discussed in this book. Should the reader have any questions concerning the appropriateness of any procedures or preparation mentioned, the author and the publisher strongly suggest consulting a professional healthcare advisor.

The author of this book has a financial interest in the product Protective Breast Formula. This does not constitute an endorsement by Basic Health Publications, Inc.

Basic Health Publications, Inc.
28812 Top of the World Drive
Laguna Beach, CA 92651
Phone: 949-715-7327

Library of Congress Cataloging-in-Publication Data

Horner, Christine.
    Waking the warrior goddess : Christine Horner's program to protect against & fight breast cancer / Christine Horner.
        p. cm.
    Includes bibliographical references and index.
    ISBN 1-59120-155-1
    1. Breast—Cancer—Popular works. I. Title.

    RC280.B8H665   2005
    616.99'449—dc22

                                            2004030700

Editor: Jane E. Morrill
Copyeditor: Carol Rosenberg
Typesetting/Book design: Gary A. Rosenberg
Cover design: Mike Stromberg
Illustrator: Skye Gibbins

Printed in the United States of America

10   9   8   7   6   5   4   3

Contents

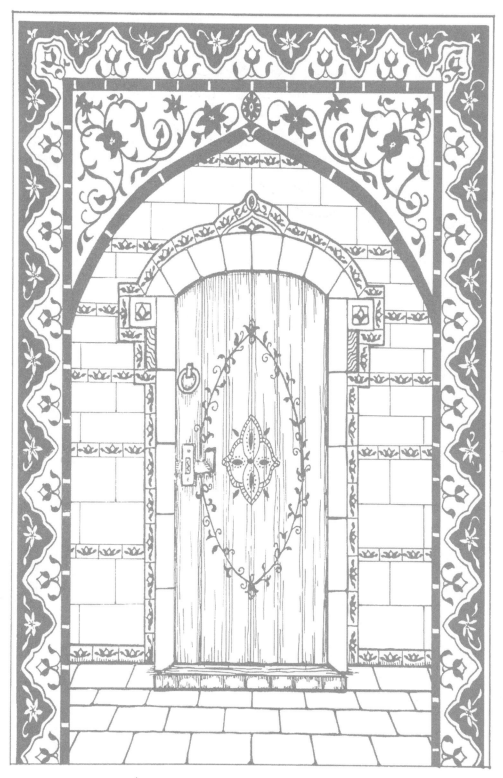

Open the doorway to knowledge . . .

To my mother
and all the women
who have fought battles
with breast cancer

Acknowledgments

The process of writing a book is invariably a personally challenging journey—and one that cannot be done alone. The greatest gift of this process was the reminder that I am blessed to walk this Earth with the support of many friends who are extraordinarily talented, tremendously loving, and generous.

There are many people I would like to thank who contributed their time and intelligence to help birth this book. First and foremost, my thanks go to Paul Schaefer. There are no words that adequately express the gratitude I feel for his enormous contribution to my life and to this book. Paul introduced me to Transcendental Meditation and *Ayurveda*. He then facilitated and supported every step I took to learn more about this extraordinary system of medicine and to teach its ancient truths—the secrets to health—to others. His magnanimous contributions included stimulating intellectual discussions that sparked and shaped many of the concepts in the book, tireless hours of editing, and taking my photograph for the book jacket. His steadfast unconditional support, love, devotion, and encouragement throughout this project were awe-inspiring and served as the wind beneath my wings.

Special thanks also go to my dearest friend, Lucy Morris. Lucy's contributions to my life and this book are profound beyond measure. Her love, feedback, and unwavering commitment to my evolution and the evolution of the world are astounding. I am filled with so much gratitude for her that I sing praises to God *every day* for my good fortune to have her in my life.

There are many kind and remarkable people who gave me valuable feedback and donated their time and talents to editing the proposal for this book: Paula Sellars, Linda Naylor, Antoinette Asimus, Mackey McNeill, Jayn Meinhardt, and Chris Conlan. Heartfelt thanks to Julie Silver, M.D., for believing in me and this book so much that despite her extremely busy schedule as a physician, author, wife, and mother of three young children she made the time to take me under her wing and share her comprehensive wisdom and experience.

I have enormous appreciation for the generosity and expert editing skills of my sister, Carolyn Horner, and her heroic down-to-the-wire effort to help me edit the final version of the manuscript.

Thanks and praise go to my dear friend Janet Greene, M.D., and my niece, Adrienne Horner, who donated their time and expertise during the editing process.

My gratitude goes to Skye Gibbins and her artistic talent in creating the illustrations for this book.

I am also indebted to my dear friend Lisa Curry Gray for her feedback, support, and legal advice.

There are many other people who deserve acknowledgment for a variety of contributions: Cindy Meehan-Patton for sharing her knowledge about nontoxic products for the home; Sandra Ingerman and Chris Kilham for their friendship and generous expert advice as experienced authors; Jade Beutler and Tom Newmark for their support and networking; Vivien and Neil Schapera for helping me with the spiritual work I needed to do before I began the first draft; and Andrew Weil, M.D., Bernie Siegel, M.D., Norman Shealy, M.D., Neal Barnard, M.D., Nancy Lonsdorf, M.D., Jennifer Hawthorne, Marci Shimoff, and Tom Newmark for their endorsements.

Thanks to my agent, Jeanne Fredericks, for "getting" my book and having absolute faith in it and me, and also for her extraordinary professionalism, excellent communication, experienced advice, deep devotion, hard work, and superb negotiating abilities. She deserves additional accolades for her patience and the time that she cheerfully offered to thoroughly answer all my questions. You'll find my name on the *long* list of her author/clients who "can't say enough good things about her."

I have an immense amount of gratitude to all the talented folks at Basic Health Publications, Inc., especially publisher Norman Goldfind for his belief in my book and for allowing me full creative expression; managing editor Carol Rosenberg for her masterful copyediting; editor Jane Morrill for all her hard work; Gary Rosenberg for the book design and typesetting; and Mike Stromberg for the cover design.

Finally, I'd like to thank my mother, Beulah Horner. My mother's courageous battle with breast cancer sparked and fueled my passion and commitment to help stop this epidemic. Her tragic death from this disease was the inspiration for this book. She also was the one who taught me to believe in the message from an old Les Brown tune, "Shoot for the moon. Even if you miss, you'll land among the stars."

Thank you, Mama!

My Journey

hen I heard the news on October 21, 1998, that President Clinton had signed the Woman's Health and Cancer Rights Act into law, I wiped the tears from my eyes and gave my mom in heaven a high-five. "We did it, Mom!" I exulted.

It had been a tough five-year battle to get this legislation passed, but worth every frustration, every heartache, every late night, every dime. The new law meant that if a woman had to have a mastectomy, her insurance company would have to cover reconstructive breast surgery. In the early 1990s many insurance companies, in a misguided effort to save money, had decided to stop paying for this essential restorative operation. Now, coverage would be required, and every patient would have the chance to be made whole again.

This story begins seven years earlier, in the fall of 1991, when I opened my solo plastic surgery practice in the greater Cincinnati, Ohio area. At age thirty-three, I had finally completed twenty-seven years of intense training and education to realize my childhood dream of becoming a surgeon. It was extremely fulfilling to finally be able to help people with my surgical skills.

As I developed my practice over the next two years, I felt a special passion for serving a particular group of patients. They struck a deep personal chord within me because my mother was one of them. These were women with breast cancer.

One day in 1993, a young woman in her thirties sat anxiously in my office as she told me that the treatment of her breast cancer required mastectomies of both of her breasts. She wanted me to reconstruct them. Following her consultation, as required, I sent a letter to her insurer, Indiana Medicaid, requesting authorization to perform the reconstructive surgery. I thought the letter was a mere formality because insurance companies had always routinely paid for breast reconstruction after a mastectomy. But several weeks later, I received a reply saying that the surgery was "not medically indicated." Those words are insurance jargon that usually means, "There's no real reason to deny this surgery, but to cut costs so that we can protect corporate profits and our CEO's huge salary, we're not paying for it."

I thought their decision was an administrative error and wrote to them again. It was not an error. The Medicaid insurance executive was unrelenting. This businessman declared again that the surgery was "not medically necessary."

Outraged, I decided that, no matter what it took, I would fight this horrendous ruling that prohibited my patient from being able to have a normal female form. The appeals process required that I first write several letters and participate in a series of telephone conference calls with various insurance company bureaucrats. The calls continued until I had worked up the entire ranks of Medicaid officials. At each step, their decision was always the same: "No."

Finally, I reached the top rung on the appeals process ladder. The only option I had left was to present the case before a judge at a state Medicaid hearing—the "supreme court" of the state-run Medicaid program. As I was driving to the hearing in a small rural town in Indiana about an hour and a half away from my office, it struck me that the appeals process was intentionally designed to be difficult, time-consuming, and financially costly, so that few, if any, doctors would follow it this far. But I didn't let that stop me. I wouldn't abandon my patient. I could relate too well to what she was going through.

Just imagine being told you have breast cancer. That news alone is horrific enough. But then, you're told you must have one or both of your breasts surgically removed. You're also told you'll be treated with poisonous chemicals that will make you very sick, cause all your hair to fall out, and possibly damage your vital organs. Your mind begins to race with questions that strike terror in your heart. Will this disease kill you? Will the side effects of the treatments make you wish you were dead? Will the postoperative pain be agonizing? Will your significant other still love you and find you sexually attractive? The only comforting news you hear is that you can be restored to physical wholeness with reconstructive breast surgery. A little patch of blue in the stormy sky. But shortly after this, you find out that your insurance company refuses to pay for this surgery. Your world caves in. Imagine.

That much bad news, in my experience as a physician, is too much for most women to bear. That insurance companies could deny a woman the opportunity to be made physically whole again after mutilating and defeminizing surgery strikes me as so incredibly heartless—it seems criminally inhumane. The thought of this injustice lit a fire in me and fueled my ability to persevere through any challenge.

Armed with stacks of published research, I pleaded my case to the judge. I presented studies documenting the enormously beneficial effects of breast reconstruction. They all showed that when women undergo breast reconstruction in the same operation as the mastectomy, they suffer far less emotional trauma. The judge—a woman—agreed, and I won my case.

During the appeals process, I'd realized that denying insurance coverage for breast reconstruction was an appalling symptom of a much larger problem: the widespread insurance-coverage discrimination against women. For example, in one of my appeal letters, I'd asked a simple pointed question: "Does Indiana Medicaid pay for penile reconstruction?" If they do, I'd argued, this was clearly a case of sexual discrimination. The written reply was, "Young lady, you are completely out of line!" That defensive and predictable response confirmed my suspicions.

As I was leaving the hearing, one of Medicaid's representatives, a woman, stopped me in the hall and said, "I'm so glad you won. You were right. Medicaid pays for penile reconstruction. They also pay for penile implants for sexual dysfunction. In fact, Medicaid pays more money every year for that procedure than for any other!"

Winning this case, however, wasn't the end of my battle for breast cancer patients—far from it. A short time later, I was shocked to discover that this case did not set a precedent and had no bearing on any future cases. Every Medicaid case is evaluated separately. That meant I would have to go through the same draining, time-consuming, costly, administrative slugfest for every single Medicaid patient who needed breast reconstruction!

Worse still, Medicaid suddenly wasn't the only insurance company denying breast reconstruction. Private insurers started jumping on the bandwagon. If Medicaid could save money this way and get away with it, they thought they could too. Then one day, a letter from Blue Cross and Blue Shield of Kentucky arrived that proclaimed that breast reconstruction for my thirty-three-year-old patient was unnecessary because there was no medical need to reconstruct "an organ with *no function*."

My eyes fixated on those five words: *an organ with no function.* "An organ with *no function?*" I yelled. "What kind of callous, cold-hearted idiot could say such a thing?" Waving the offensive letter in my hand, I stormed down my office hall, seething, "You just said that to the wrong person. You will pay, and every insurer will pay!"

At the time, by no cosmic coincidence or accident, I was taking a series of courses designed to teach people how to live life more powerfully. I was in the third of a series of three courses called the "Curriculum for Living" sponsored by Landmark Education Corporation. The course was called "Self Expression and Leadership." Our assignment was to use all the skills we had learned to create and lead a project that would benefit others.

Instantly, I knew the goal for my project: Insurance coverage for reconstructive breast surgery for every woman who must have a mastectomy.

I knew this was no simple task because laws would have to be passed. To make matters even more challenging, I was working eighty hours a week in my surgical practice and I knew absolutely nothing about the political process. Worse yet, even with a doctorate, I had always been a little hesitant to speak up because I was afraid of sounding stupid. But I knew that if I kept following my heart, somehow I could make this happen.

And so the adventure began. And what an adventure it was—awe-inspiring, magical, and profoundly spiritual. On the other hand, it was also filled with extraordinarily difficult, frustrating, sometimes shocking experiences that required enormous perseverance, growth, and strength. But the miracles outweighed the obstacles. It seemed like everything and everyone I needed for the project magically fell into my lap. For example, deep into the project, I realized that Senator Ted Kennedy was the best person to sponsor the federal bill because of his success at getting health bills through Congress. I hadn't taken any action or spoken to anyone about this idea. A week later, out of the blue, a visiting plastic surgeon from Boston walked up to me at a state medical meeting and said, "I'm meeting with Ted Kennedy next week. Do you want me to ask him to sponsor your bill?"

From the moment I started this project, seemingly random offers of help and perfectly timed meetings and events like this happened so routinely, I came to expect it. It seemed like I had a direct line to God. "Ask and ye shall receive"— no kidding!

But there were also many challenges—some seemingly insurmountable. When I launched the project, it made sense to focus on passing one federal law, rather than attempting to pass fifty separate state laws. Unfortunately, my legislative initiative came on the heels of the Clintons' failed National Healthcare Plan. The word in Washington was that *no* federal healthcare bills would even be considered. The news was a nightmare. Now, I *had* to pass fifty individual state laws. So, I took a deep breath and began planning, organizing, calling, and writing. Within a year, I had enrolled the help of plastic surgeons, breast cancer survivors, and numerous organizations in every state. And one by one, state laws began to pass.

Then, one morning in 1994, I got the darkest news yet. I learned that our successes in the states basically meant nothing, thanks to a loophole. A law called ERISA—the Employee Retirement Income Securities Act—contains language that excludes most people from the protection of state healthcare laws. To fulfill my commitment, I realized that a federal law would have to be passed, after all.

The challenge and chances of success seemed as intimidating as climbing Mt. Everest shoeless. But something personal and tragic happened in 1994 that cemented my resolve. My mother, the vibrant extraordinary woman who taught me to reach for the stars, was diagnosed with metastatic breast cancer in her bones. She had been treated for "early stage" breast cancer five years earlier. Everyone—her doctors, my dad, my brothers and sister, and I—thought that she was going to be fine. But she wasn't. Nine months later in the hospice, I held her hand and felt her spirit go free as she took her last breath.

She was seventy-five. She shouldn't have died that young. She was a Mac-Dougall—a Scottish clan known for their extraordinary strength, good health, and longevity. Virtually everyone in the family who preceded her had lived to be at least 100. My mom was in perfect health—that is, until she got cancer. She had done all the right things—yearly mammograms and breast self-exams (BSEs). Like me, she believed in Western medicine's advice and reassurance that if we do these "right" things, we can catch breast cancer "early" enough to save our lives. This isn't true for everyone—certainly not my mom. In some cases, it's only wishful thinking. The truth is, with this approach, there's absolutely no guarantee that we can catch breast cancer early enough to stop this killer and save lives.

I didn't want my mother's death from breast cancer to be another meaning-less statistic, a faceless number in the loss column. This abhorrent disease had stripped her of her dignity and cut her life short. I wanted her life, suffering, and untimely death to mean something for the world. Generally, I like to believe that everything happens for a reason. So, I decided my mother died of breast cancer to be a beacon of change for the world—through me. I pledged to myself that her untimely death would be a pivotal event in the worldwide fight against this disease. In addition, it fueled my commitment to get breast-reconstruction leg-islation passed. I decided no matter what it took, or how long it took, I would never give up. I would do it for her. I dedicated the project, now called the Breast Reconstruction Advocacy Project (BRA Project), to her memory.

By the time I faced the monumental task of achieving a federal bill, I had grown more politically savvy. I decided to go straight to the top, instead of work-ing up from the bottom. That meant I had to meet the President of the United States, Bill Clinton. I'd heard it said that we are only three people away from meeting anyone, so everywhere I went I started asking everyone, "Do you know how I can meet President Clinton?" Within two weeks, a friend introduced me to David, a member of the Federal Trade Commission. A few days later, I met David for lunch and told him about my plans. He told me he went to Washington to meet with the President four times a year, and the next time he went, I could go with him.

Two days later, he called me and announced, "We're going on Tuesday."

"What?" I said, looking at my packed calendar with about forty patients scheduled for the office that day.

"Your patients will understand," he explained, "You're meeting *the President*. Oh, and by the way," he added, "there's one other thing. It will cost you $10,000. It's a fundraiser for the 1996 election and that's the minimum contribution."

Incredulous shock paralyzed me for a moment. "There's no way!" I yelped. "I can't do that."

"Look," he reasoned, "you don't understand. This is a once-in-a-lifetime opportunity. You can fundraise from your friends. It's for a good cause."

Suddenly, I had a strong feeling in my gut that said, "Do it." Because my gut rarely fails me, I listened. And so, a few days later, I was in Washington to meet the President.

A vague memory of a picture of Jacqueline Kennedy Onassis in *Life* magazine decades before completely shaped my decision to wear a perfect, black, strapless evening gown and elbow-length, black velvet gloves. I felt like a million bucks as I left my room at the Mayflower Hotel. After waltzing through the metal detector, I gave one final check and adjustment to my gown and gloves and entered the room—where everyone was wearing a business suit!

When I stopped to get my seat assignment, I was told that the President's table was short one woman and that I'd been moved there. The attendant wanted to know if that was okay. Without a moment's hesitation, I responded, "Absolutely!"

As I headed for my table, my embarrassment intensified as heads swiveled in my direction.

"Thanks for dressing for us," one of David's friends quipped as I walked by.

"Oh, you're welcome," I said with a genuine smile, my embarrassment fading. "It was really no trouble at all." I realized I might as well make the best of my faux pas and enjoy myself.

An hour later, the President arrived. He was taller than I had imagined, with a ruddy complexion and gray hair—and yes, he is as charming and charismatic as legend says.

I waited patiently on the receiving line to meet him. When I finally made it to the front, I reached out to shake his hand. "I'm Dr. Christine Horner," I said.

"Yes, I know who you are," he replied, grasping my hand with a firm shake. "You live across the river from Cincinnati and you're working on legislation about breast cancer. And I believe you are sitting at my table tonight, aren't you?"

"Why, yes, I am," I answered, trying to hide my astonishment. He really was amazing! I had been asked to send information about myself before the event because the President liked to be briefed about everyone he would be meeting. I had heard that he never forgot a name or a face, but still, I was impressed.

"I'll see you later at the table," he said as the next person in line moved up to shake his hand.

My place at the large round table was directly across from the President's. The twelve feet between us made it too difficult to have a conversation. Endless streams of people came up to speak to him throughout the meal. As the evening passed and the time for him to give his speech rapidly approached, I was struck with the thought that I had just spent $10,000 to talk to the President, and I might not get to do it. In a mild panic, I leaned as far across the table as I could, caught his eye, and shouted, "I want to talk to you!" He jumped a little and called back across the expanse, "Okay. I'll come and get you after my speech and we can talk."

After giving his twenty-minute speech, he left the podium and, as promised, came by the table and signaled to me to follow him. I rose from my chair and walked behind him. He shook hands, smiled, and bid good-bye to everyone with sweet, laid-back Southern charm. I followed him into the hallway, and the doors closed behind us.

Swarms of Secret Service descended upon him. He began snapping his fingers at his assistants. "Give it to me now," the President demanded. Papers were thrust at him from all directions, and he began signing them with rapid-fire dedication. At the same time, streams of young men updated him on the latest happenings in quick sound bites. Tension was high, and he was working at lightning speed. I looked on in amazement.

Suddenly, he turned to me. "Now, what is it you want to say?" he asked in a relaxed tone that contradicted the chaos.

I was still reeling from the urgency and pressure of moments ago, and my knees felt weak. I felt like Dorothy trembling before the Wizard of Oz. One minute of presidential time seemed equivalent to an hour, so I quickly regained my composure and started speaking as fast as I could. I told him about the problems with insurance companies denying coverage for breast reconstruction and our efforts to get a bill to Congress. He jotted down a few notes and seemed genuinely interested. Then he told me he would look into it and see what he could do. Moments later, he and his entourage left the building.

Three days later, I received a call from a member of the Democratic National Committee. "We like your spunk," he said. "Normally a $10,000 contribution is the cost for two people to attend a fundraising event. Since you came by yourself, we'd like to invite you to meet with the President again when he comes to Cincinnati in two days."

Wearing just the right business suit this time, I listened intently as the President gave his speech at the private luncheon. When he turned to leave, I sprang from my chair. I leaped in front of him, blocking his path up the stairs to the men's room. Dorothy was gone, and Xena the Warrior Princess had taken her place! With less than a half a foot between us, I met his eyes directly and said, "My mother died of breast cancer, and so did yours. We can make a tribute to our mothers' lives by passing breast-reconstruction legislation!"

He snapped his fingers at an assistant and asked for his business card—the one with his private address at the Oval Office printed on it. Handing it to me, he said, "Send me a packet of information at this address."

I did. A few weeks later, I received a letter on White House stationery, personally signed by the President, thanking me for the information and promising he would look into the matter.

That meeting led to more meetings, including several with First Lady Hillary Clinton and her staff in the West Wing of the White House. Suddenly doors began to open. Media coverage for the project exploded. Several major women's magazines called for interviews, including *Glamour, Allure, Elle,* and *Ms.* There were dozens of television, radio, and newspaper interviews. It seemed like everyone across the country wanted to get on board.

I was buoyed with optimism when the bill was introduced to Congress in 1997. Then, it stalled. It was promptly put into legislative committee—"a black hole," as it's also known—where it sat for two years, seemingly dead. I knew that bills rarely, if ever, pass on their own merit; they only make it through by being tagged on to a larger, "moving" bill. But even that wasn't working. The reconstruction legislation was tagged on to every moving bill, but none passed. With only a day left of the 1998 Congressional session, it looked as if the situation were hopeless. Sure enough, I received a phone call that day from a staff liaison for the National Plastic Surgery Society. His words cut through me like a knife. "Bad news, Christine; it's all over. There aren't any other bills to tag it on to."

My heart sank. I couldn't believe that all those years of hard work with such clear divine support could end like this. We had come so close!

The next day, my secretary knocked on the door while I was examining a patient. She rarely interrupted me, and I thought something must be terribly wrong.

"You have an urgent phone call you must take now," she said. My heart raced as I picked up the phone. Then I heard the voice of the same staffer, but his tone was entirely different. He sounded elated.

"It passed!" he said.

"What?" I said. "What did you say?"

"It got tagged on to the budget bill at the last minute and it passed!" he exclaimed.

In a daze I thanked him and hung up the phone. Then I burst into tears, and gave my mom a high-five. My heart spoke the words, "We did it, Mom!" and her spirit filled the room. My mother's great sacrifice *had* made a difference. Her life and death would help millions of women. At least now they could be spared the trauma of not being able to have reconstructive surgery.

During this campaign I met with many powerful, creative, and amazing people: the President, senators, congressmen, and governors. To every one of the elected officials who supported the legislation I give my undying gratitude: President Clinton, First Lady Hillary Clinton, Senator Ted Kennedy, Senator Alfonse D'Amato, Congresswoman Anna Eshoo, Congresswoman Sue Kelly, Kentucky Governor Patton and his wife, Judy Patton, and a whole host of other dignitaries. I also had the pleasure of working with fifty wonderful plastic surgeons who took on leadership roles to pass the legislation in their own states. There was an enormous number of remarkable people who helped along the way. Without every one of them, the legislative project would never have succeeded the way that it did.

But deep within, at the moment of this great victory, something troubled me. One problem was solved, but another, much greater problem remained and clouded the celebration—the growing *epidemic* of breast cancer. In the United States, breast cancer strikes an appalling, ever-increasing number of women. Why was it still growing? How could we stop it? I knew there had to be answers. So began a new and far more important mission: to trace the tracks of this killer back to its root causes and help protect women from developing breast cancer in the first place.

My search began with the collection of all the published medical research, and what I found inspired me, gave me hope, and then outraged me. I found *many* research-proven "natural" ways women can significantly lower their risk of breast cancer. Not only can these foods, herbs, spices, supplements, and lifestyle choices lower the risk, but good solid research published in peer-reviewed journals shows that they can also help women already diagnosed with breast cancer by slowing down tumor growth, preventing metastasis, and even shrinking the size of their tumors. Many of these natural techniques have been found to increase the effectiveness of Western medical treatments (chemotherapy and radiation) and protect against their harmful side effects.

But most doctors, as well as most women, are completely unaware of this lifesaving information. One explanation could be that these techniques—most having roots in ancient traditional systems of medicine—are nonpharmaceutical and nonsurgical. In other words, these techniques are not generally included in Western medicine and won't create any significant financial rewards. So, tragically, our economically driven system of medicine has no incentive to get this information out.

I, however, do.

In 1999, I teamed up with award-winning television news anchor Paul Schaefer to create the first syndicated television news segment devoted to teaching people how to prevent common diseases and stay healthy using the research-proven techniques of complementary and alternative medicine. This segment aired in Cincinnati on the ABC and NBC affiliates and was then syndicated to the Wisdom Television Network.

In 2002, my passion for teaching natural preventative medicine led me to jump off another professional cliff. I retired from my plastic surgery practice to dedicate my life full-time to writing and teaching. First on my agenda was to write this book.

Waking the Warrior Goddess: Dr. Christine Horner's Program to Protect Against & Fight Breast Cancer reveals all the best, research-proven, natural approaches scientists have found that substantially lower the risk of breast cancer. When used in conjunction with standard medical treatments for women with breast cancer, these same techniques can help to improve their chances of survival.

From my work on the legislative project, I learned that powerful and magical things happen when you envision a better life for the future and enroll other people into that vision. With this book I declare the following vision for the world: All women experience perfect health because they recognize and use their powerful inner ability to heal themselves.

How to Use
This Book

*Y*ou have the power and ability to influence your state of health more than you ever imagined. Your choices every day significantly influence your chances of staying healthy or developing a terrible disease such as breast cancer. Genetics and luck have very little to do with your risk of developing most chronic disorders, including breast cancer. This book will teach you how to protect your breasts and your overall health. It includes more than forty different research-proven ways to lower your risk of breast cancer, and if you have breast cancer, these same techniques—when done in conjunction with Western medical treatments—improve your chances of survival. Chapter 28 puts all of the risk-lowering techniques together in an easy thirty-step program.

If you are eager to do everything you can to protect yourself quickly, you can complete the program in thirty days. But don't pressure yourself to adopt all the new habits in thirty days if it's not comfortable. The program can be completed in thirty weeks or thirty months if that works better for you. Each day, week, or month you start doing something new will make a substantial difference in lowering your risk. By the end of the month or year, you'll be doing everything science knows how to do to lower your risk of breast cancer. When added up, the amount of risk reduction you'll enjoy won't simply be the sum of all the parts—it will increase exponentially.

In preparing to write this book, I conducted an exhaustive study of the medical literature on breast cancer. I pulled out all the articles on anything and everything that showed a statistically significant benefit in lowering your risk of this disease. To my knowledge, virtually everything we know to date about lowering the risk of breast cancer is covered in this book. Keep in mind, research shows that almost everything that can help lower your risk of breast cancer can *also* improve your chance of survival if you already have the disease. These techniques and recommendations should not be used as a replacement for Western medicine, but rather as support for the treatments. We will undoubtedly know much more in the near future. For example, scientists have found that nearly all vegetables and fruits have a variety of cancer-fighting properties. As researchers begin to analyze individual plants—vegetables, fruits, herbs, and spices—I'm sure many of them will prove helpful in preventing and fighting breast cancer.

Reading a research-based book can sometimes be a little dry and boring. For that reason, I wrote this book from a slightly different angle. First, I use principles of *Ayurveda,* the oldest and most complete system of prevention-oriented holistic health still practiced today, as a basis for many of the recommendations for natural approaches that protect against breast cancer. Second, I use a metaphor—the Warrior Goddess—for the body's internal healing intelligence.

Ayurveda originated in the *Vedic* culture—an advanced culture that thrived more than 5,000 years ago in the area of the world that is now India. Today, various fragmented forms of *Ayurveda* are practiced in India, Sri Lanka, and southern Asia. About one-sixth of the world's population uses *Ayurveda* as its primary form of medical care.

Although *Ayurveda* treats diseases, in its purest original form it is a comprehensive system of *preventative* medicine. It masterfully teaches people how to become and stay healthy. I think of *Ayurveda* as the cosmic download of all the timeless laws of Nature that help guide us to keep our mind/body strong. It describes thousands of laws governing the intricacies of our complex, sophisticated, and infinitely amazing physiology.

You can use these laws of Nature expressed in the principles of *Ayurveda* to help you make intelligent choices that beneficially impact your health. This knowledge can help guide you to choose only those things that are health-supporting and avoid those things that are not. The *Ayurvedic* principles will also give you a context in which to understand each item presented in this book. They give you a broader and deeper understanding of why each item benefits your health and protects you from developing diseases, especially breast cancer.

At the heart of *Ayurveda* is the recognition of a divine, natural healing intelligence that exists in each of us. According to *Ayurveda,* diseases arise from imbalances that occur when this intelligence is subverted by poor choices, such as certain foods and lifestyles. These imbalances block the full expression of this healing intelligence, eventually weakening it to where it can no longer keep you well. In time, the body begins to break down and diseases begin to manifest. Health is only regained and maintained by enhancing the healing intelligence, keeping it lively and flowing.

In *Waking the Warrior Goddess,* this healing intelligence is personified as a Warrior Goddess. This is not just a creative archetype. When considering the human body and all its extraordinary complex functions, the image that emerges that best represents the managing intelligence is one of a multitasking Warrior Goddess. She is supernatural in strength and power and vastly discriminating in her intellect. Yet, she is delicate and very particular. This metaphor accurately reflects both the mastery and the magnificence of the intelligence that manages the trillions of biochemical reactions simultaneously occurring in our bodies at any given moment. It also provides a new perspective for appreciating the importance of providing attentive care and nurturance for this extraordinary body that each of us has been given. Like a Goddess, this managing intelligence's majesty and splendor depends on respecting its very precise and specific demands. *Waking the Warrior Goddess* teaches a woman about her Warrior Goddess—what weakens her, and what makes her strong and invincible. The symbol of the Warrior Goddess also helps to transform the abstract—but nonetheless phenomenal—physics, chemistry, and biology of the body into an intimate, personal, and powerful friend.

Because every woman's risk of breast cancer is real, I encourage you to begin the thirty-step program immediately. Make it fun. Make it an adventure. Find a girlfriend to join you. Or organize a group of friends, and meet once a week to encourage and support one another and share experiences. Research shows meeting with a group of supportive friends regularly is strong preventive medicine, too. Adopting even some of these simple, but powerful techniques will improve how you feel and lower your risk of breast cancer. Depending on your current state of health, the improvement could be quite dramatic.

My greatest wish, hope, and dream is this: that this knowledge becomes common knowledge; that people use this information and adopt these health-preserving habits; that the incidence of breast cancer radically drops; and that the world is filled with people experiencing perfect health and enlightenment.

Though no one can go back and make a brand new start,
anyone can start from now and make a brand new ending.

—AUTHOR UNKNOWN

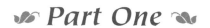
Modern Beast and Ancient Slayer

The Basics of Breast Cancer and *Ayurveda*

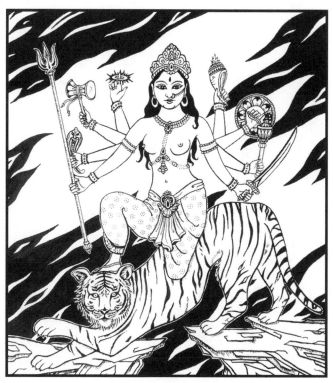

Durga, the Warrior Goddess

Chapter 1

Breast Cancer Epidemic
The Numbers, the Fears,
and the Possibility of Prevention

*When solving problems, dig at the roots
instead of just hacking at the leaves.*

—ANTHONY J. D'ANGELO, *THE COLLEGE BLUE BOOK*

*B*reast cancer is a killer beast with a voracious appetite. Every year it attacks more and more women. It isn't attracted to children, but once a woman reaches her mid-twenties, she will catch its attention and it will start to stalk her. Generally, like most hunters, breast cancer prefers a slower easier target, so it particularly likes older women—in fact, the older the better. And the more meat on their bones—actually, the more extra fat—the better. This savage killer finds women particularly delectable if they have just been brought to their knees by a major emotional trauma. It doesn't care about race, religious beliefs, finances, or marital status.

Breast cancer is a womanizer. It finds most women equally desirable, but there are a few things that make a woman absolutely irresistible. If breast cancer were to place an ad for the female of its dreams, it would go something like this:

> SEARCHING FOR AN OVERWEIGHT, older, American or Western European woman to take on a short, extremely emotional ride; someone who loves to stay up all night drinking alcohol and eating red meat, junk food, and sugary desserts—that is, on the nights she's not working the graveyard shift; a woman who thinks organically raised fruit, vegetables, and whole grains aren't foods; a person who loves to burn the candle at both ends, thrives on stress, isn't into exercising, has been a smoker since she was a teenager, and who puts everyone else's needs before her own.

Not the normal type of ad you'd see in a singles column, but for breast cancer, this type of woman is perfect.

Although breast cancer loves all women in general, the good news is, it has preferences. By being aware of them, you can make yourself much less desirable. This book will teach you how to make yourself as *unattractive* to this monster as possible.

First, let's take a look at the breast cancer battlefield. You need to know a few things about the enemy's current position and force: where it is, how far it has advanced, who is on the front lines and at greater risk, and the current casualty and death toll. Then, you'll learn about its strengths and weaknesses, and together, we'll plan a strategy to slay this beast. What you'll learn in this book will cut the enemy's supply lines and raise a wall of protection. Breast cancer can be conquered. Knowledge is power. Together, we can end this epidemic.

YOUR RISK

Breast cancer is the most common cancer among American women and the second-leading cause of cancer deaths. The older a woman is, the higher her risk. At age twenty-five, her risk is 1 in 19,608. At age forty, her risk climbs to 1 in 217. If she lives to be more than eighty-five, her risk is 1 in 8. The American Cancer Society estimates that in 2004, more than 270,000 women will be diagnosed with breast cancer, and more than 40,000 will die because of it. At any given time in the United States, 2 to 3 million women have been diagnosed, treated, and cured of breast cancer or are currently living with it. From 1999–2003, the incidence of breast cancer rose 21 percent.

The result of these alarming statistics is that most women are terrified of getting breast cancer. One of every three women who are diagnosed with it will die from it. If that isn't bad enough, the treatment of this disease, although it may be effective for many women, is horrendous: mutilating surgery, damaging radiation, and injections of severely toxic chemical poisons. As Dr. Susan Love, author of *Dr. Susan Love's Breast Book* and *Dr. Susan Love's Hormone Book,* says, the treatment of breast cancer is "slash, burn, and poison." No wonder women are terrified.

Examination Isn't Prevention

Doctors aren't taught much about prevention because Western medicine does not make prevention a priority. The priority is to treat a disease you already have, not prevent you from getting it in the first place.

When I was trained as a surgeon and as a spokesperson for the American Cancer Society, I was taught that there was no known cause and no known cure for breast cancer. The belief was, the only thing you can do is to try to catch the disease "early" using mammograms and breast exams. But catching a cancer in a "treatable stage" isn't what you really want, either. Anyone who has been diagnosed with breast cancer (or is close to someone who has) knows that the diagnosis of breast cancer is devastating—no matter when it is detected. Who wants to be slashed, burned, and poisoned? And, after going through all these treatments, there's no guarantee that your cancer is gone. These treatments don't always work, even for cancers that are caught "early." For instance, my mother never missed an annual mammogram and regularly examined her own breasts. Her cancer was caught "early" by Western standards. The tumor was less than 1 cm in diameter and had not spread to her lymph nodes. Statistically, she shouldn't have died from breast cancer—but she did, five years later in 1994.

Although the Western medical community's intentions are good, this approach to mammograms and breast exams is *not* prevention. It only exposes the disease once you have it. Given these facts, it wouldn't be surprising if you believed that there isn't much you can do to decrease your chances of getting breast cancer. You may believe it's all due to bad luck or bad genes.

If you believe that, you're mistaken.

Whoever thought up the word "Mammogram"?
Every time I hear it, I think I'm supposed to put my
breast in an envelope and send it to someone.

—Jan King

Mammograms and Other Technologies

There's no question that mammograms are a useful screening tool. They have helped us find cancers at earlier, more treatable stages and have helped save lives. However, mammograms aren't perfect. This test uses potentially dangerous radiation, can be painful, can't see through "dense" breast tissue (found typically in most women younger than forty), and doesn't work well for women with breast implants. At its best, a mammogram can only "see" breast cancers that produce calcium or significant masses—about 70 to 80 percent of all breast cancers. Regardless of their size, 20 to 30 percent of breast cancers won't show up on a mammogram. So, women with these "invisible" tumors feel falsely reassured by normal mammograms, and diagnosis of their cancers may be dangerously delayed. In addition, *80 percent* of the findings on a mammogram that are "suspicious" enough to lead to a breast biopsy are *not* cancers. In other words, mammograms wrongly suspect the presence of breast cancer *80 percent of the time!* The financial and emotional costs of the "false positive" readings from mammography are enormous. More than 1 million breast biopsies are performed in the United States every year. So, approximately 800,000 women undergo expensive, physically traumatizing, and emotionally devastating surgical breast biopsies *unnecessarily* every year.

Because of the well-recognized shortcomings of mammography, additional tests, such as ultrasounds and magnetic resonance imaging (MRI) scans, are frequently employed. An ultrasound uses sound waves to show images of the tissues in the body. It is safe, noninvasive, and painless. But it doesn't give enough information to be valuable as a screening or diagnostic tool for breast cancer. An ultrasound can only be used to determine whether a breast mass is cystic or solid (solid masses are of more concern). MRI scans use a magnetic field instead of radiation to generate images of the interior structures of the body. These scans are safe for most people, painless, and noninvasive. They are very good at revealing the minute structural changes associated with breast tumors, including those that mammograms might miss. But like mammograms, MRI scans aren't very specific; they frequently show areas that are "suspicious" for breast cancer, but that are actually benign. So MRI scans also lead to excessive numbers of unnecessary biopsies. Another downside of MRI scans is that they are *very* expensive. The average cost for a breast MRI in 2004 was about $2,000—a price too high to make it practical as a primary screening tool.

We need a highly accurate, inexpensive, noninvasive, painless safe test that can show abnormalities at very early stages. Recent research shows that there is a reemerging technology with all these qualities that shows tremendous potential as a screening tool for breast cancer. It's called "thermography."

Thermography uses infrared technology to detect heat. It was first developed by the military in the early 1950s as a way to see enemy forces at night— by sensing their heat and movement. In the early 1960s, thermography was introduced in a very rudimentary form for medical use. It was approved by the FDA in 1982, but unfortunately, this promising technology fell out of favor when it was prematurely, hastily, and haphazardly included in the Breast Cancer Detection Demonstration Project, a large national study of mammography. Poor training, quality controls, and equipment led to misinterpretations and the false conclusion that thermography wasn't a valuable screening tool for breast cancer. But a few individuals, believing in its potential, persevered.

In the last few years, thermography equipment has vastly improved. The digital cameras and computer-software systems that are now available are so sophisticated that their high-resolution images and precise heat-variation calculations generate extremely valuable information. Recent research shows that, unlike mammograms, when thermography suspects something is wrong, it usually is. A study published in the *American Journal of Radiology* in January 2003 concluded that this technology could help prevent most unnecessary breast biopsies: "Infrared imaging (thermography) offers a safe noninvasive procedure that would be valuable as an adjunct to mammography in determining whether a lesion is benign or malignant."

A breast thermogram is a digital infrared picture that reveals the heat and vascular patterns of the breast tissue. These patterns change when a breast tumor starts to grow. Breast cancer cells require new blood vessels to feed them nutrients and oxygen. These new blood vessels don't grow like normal blood vessels. Instead, they grow in characteristically *abnormal* patterns, and they generate increased heat that is detectable by thermography.

Thermography can detect breast cancers much earlier than any other available technology. Because blood vessels ordinarily start to grow *before* any other significant changes and tumor growth, a thermogram can "see" these abnormal physiological processes as early as five to ten years *before* a cancer can be seen by a mammogram, MRI, or ultrasound or felt by a physical exam. What is most exciting is that when these abnormal processes are caught this early, they are *reversible*. The warning patterns seen by thermography have been found to resolve and return to normal after only a few short months of the healthy diet and lifestyle changes presented in this book. Thus, thermography is the first tool we have that shows promise at being able to pick up breast cancers so early— at a stage that involves only precancerous physiological changes—that women can reverse these changes and avoid getting breast cancer by making a few simple diet and lifestyle modifications.

The potential of this technology is electrifying. In the near future, thermography may play a dominant role in the screening and prevention of breast cancer. But before that can happen, many well-designed studies must be conducted to understand what the full potential of thermography really is: its precise capabilities and limitations, how it can best be used, where it fits in with other technologies, and how to properly evaluate and interpret the information it generates.

How to Lower Your Risk

Research shows that there are many natural, nonpharmaceutical, nonsurgical approaches that can substantially lower your risk of developing breast cancer. The medical literature is full of studies that have found strong anticancer effects in many foods, spices, herbs, and dietary supplements. There are also techniques that fit under the umbrella of complementary and alternative medicine that have been shown to be effective. For example, simple regular aerobic exercise can lower your risk of breast cancer by as much as 30 to 50 percent.

The amount of risk reduction associated with each of these items is not small. Many of them lower your risk by as much as 50 percent or more. And their protective effects multiply when you do more than one. For instance, later in this book, you'll learn that the spice turmeric greatly enhances the breast cancer–blocking qualities of soy. And when turmeric is consumed in the same meal with green tea, each makes the other's anticancer properties more powerful: Turmeric makes green tea eight times more effective, and green tea, in turn, makes turmeric three times more effective.

If you have breast cancer, this information can help you, too. Studies show that many of the items that lower your risk also help to improve your outcome and chances of survival if you have the disease. For example, many spices, herbs, supplements, or techniques can help prevent metastasis (the spread of the tumor), decrease the risk of the tumor's coming back, and stop new tumors from growing. Best of all, everything that lowers your risk of breast cancer also decreases your risk of developing a multitude of other diseases. This collection of risk-reducing habits not only lowers your chances of developing breast cancer, but also helps you to achieve an excellent robust state of health.

You're Not to Blame

Don't use the information in this book to beat yourself up. It's not designed for that. It's designed to empower you. It's not your fault that you didn't know these things before. No good comes from blaming yourself or feeling guilty. The most powerful and productive thing you can do is to start taking action now. Accept whatever situation you find yourself in today as simply "what is" with no judgment. It's called the power of living in the "now." You have no power over the past. Your real power exists in the present moment. This belief has been taught by wisdom traditions throughout the centuries. For a clear picture of this empowering way of living, I recommend reading *The Power of Now*, an excellent book by Eckhart Tolle. Then, start the "thirty-step" program (see Chapter 28) and celebrate every step you take.

> *The secret of health for both mind and body is not to mourn*
> *for the past, worry about the future, or anticipate troubles,*
> *but to live in the present moment wisely and earnestly.*
>
> —BUDDHA

Your Doctor's Not to Blame

Don't blame your doctor for not telling you all the facts on breast cancer prevention. Most doctors don't know them; they know only the basics of prevention: don't smoke; don't drink too much alcohol; exercise; and eat more fruits and vegetables instead of hamburgers, french fries, and doughnuts. That's about it. Although it's good advice, this list barely touches upon what you need to know to stay healthy. Medical education concentrates on the surgical and pharmaceutical treatment of diseases—*after* you have them. Most doctors know very little about prevention because it's not taught in medical school. Topics on natural prevention are rarely, if ever, included in traditional continuing-medical-education conferences, either. One reason for this is that most of the money for research comes from the pharmaceutical industry. Doctors would have to attend "holistic" medical conferences, usually sponsored outside their traditional medical society, to learn about natural prevention. The only other option doctors have is to research the medical literature, as I have done. And that takes a lot of time—time most doctors don't have.

It's the system of medicine that's broken. Our current approach to "health-care" is actually one of "disease care." Except for acute care, such as trauma, this system doesn't work very well. If you have a broken bone or a gunshot wound, there's none better, but Western medicine doesn't know much about the prevention or treatment of chronic disorders. The "root causes" of a disease are not part of its vocabulary. The best that you can hope for, for most chronic disorders, is to suppress the symptoms without creating side effects that are worse than the disease itself.

A Quantum Leap

The paradigm of Western medicine and how it views the human body needs a radical shift. In the first half of the twentieth century, physicists discovered that the structure of our universe and how it operates are fundamentally very different from what we had previously thought. The concepts and laws of Newtonian physics were replaced with those of the radically different quantum physics. But surprisingly, Western medicine hasn't caught up with this scientific revolution. It still treats the body as if it were a machine of unrelated parts. It doesn't see the unified field of intelligence described by quantum physics that underlies and coordinates body, mind, and consciousness. It doesn't understand that everything affects the complex balance of your physiology in one way or another for good or ill: everything you eat, everything you do, every thought you think, the company you keep, the music you listen to—everything. Western medicine doesn't understand that all diseases come from imbalances or that correcting those imbalances causes most chronic illnesses to improve and, sometimes, to be cured. It doesn't understand that imbalances caught and corrected early will prevent chronic disorders from manifesting. Worse, it has no technology or diagnostic technique to catch a disease "early." Rather, its tests can only detect diseases at late stages, once they have caused structural changes in the body.

What if I were to tell you that there's a system of medicine that contains very detailed and sophisticated knowledge about how to stay healthy and prevent diseases, such as breast cancer, arthritis, asthma, and heart disease? Even better, what if I were to tell you that this system's in-depth understanding of human health, physiology, and consciousness is so profound that if you follow its advice, you can achieve a state of extraordinary and vibrant health beyond what you thought possible—a state of perfect health? Would you believe me? And what if I told you that this system of medicine has been around for a very long time, that the human race has held the secrets to extraordinary health for thousands of years—in fact, 5,000 years? You'd probably find it very hard to believe, but it's true!

This astounding ancient system of holistic medicine is called *Ayurveda*. The next chapter will tell you about a few basic principles and techniques of this wonderful and profound system of medicine.

Chapter 2

Rediscovering Ancient Healing

Ayurveda: A Comprehensive Holistic Preventative System of Health

*W*hen I went to medical school in the early 1980s, I was taught how to try to fix existing medical problems, but I wasn't taught how to prevent disease or how to achieve and maintain health. Having recently spoken to the medical students at the University of Cincinnati, I can tell you that not much has changed in the last twenty years or so. Almost nothing is taught in medical school about prevention, or about attaining and preserving good health, because Western medicine doesn't know much about these subjects. But *Ayurveda* does.

When I was first introduced to *Ayurveda* and began to study it in 1996, I'm embarrassed to say that I had previously never heard of it, even though 1 billion people—one-sixth of the world's population—use it as their primary form of healthcare. During the past eight years, I have dedicated myself, in large part, to the study of this miraculous system of healthcare, and I have never lost my awe at its power to create perfect health. In fact, my awe simply increases with each passing year.

Ayur means life, and *veda* means knowledge, so *Ayurveda* literally means "the knowledge of life." I'm sure you can get the sense just from its name that the approach of this system of health and its reservoir of knowledge are very different from those of Western medicine.

Ayurveda teaches how to live life to its fullest potential. It's the science of how to live a long, perfectly healthy life by achieving and maintaining a fine state of balance in your physiology. All the techniques and recommendations of *Ayurveda* are designed to bring you into balance and keep you there. *Ayurveda* underscores this core truth: *Perfect balance is the foundation and key to perfect health.*

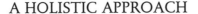

A HOLISTIC APPROACH

Ayurveda is a holistic system of health. It holds that there is no separation between mind, body, spirit, and consciousness or anything seemingly outside you in the universe. Quantum physics has shown that this is true. Everything inside you and everything outside you, at the most finite level, is intimately connected. So, everything affects everything. In other words, any technique—be it mental, physical, or spiritual—has profound effects on your entire physiology. Naturally, it follows that everything in your environment affects your health, as well.

Ayurveda emphasizes the experience of higher states of consciousness, which are characterized by an expanded awareness that brings profound balance to the mind/body. Research shows that people who practice techniques that enliven higher, more expanded states of consciousness regularly enjoy so much balance that they are dramatically healthier than the average American. Studies show that these individuals use the healthcare system, overall, 50 percent less often and have 87 percent fewer hospital admissions for cardiovascular diseases!

But the ultimate intention of *Ayurveda* goes far beyond preventing disease. Its goal is to produce robust perfect health for the mind/body and the consciousness. This level of health is of paramount importance because it helps us to achieve higher states of consciousness—and ultimately, enlightenment. Enlightenment is the highest state of human awareness; it is the ability to see and know the reality of all things and to enjoy mastery over the physical state of being.

Clearly, the goals and objectives of *Ayurveda* are very different from the Western model of healthcare. I like to put it this way: Western medicine is about suppressing the symptoms of disease; *Ayurveda* is about creating profound health. Because we have grown up with a "disease-care" system of medicine (as opposed to "healthcare" system), most Americans have no idea how to create extraordinary health—or even that it's possible. Fortunately, *Ayurveda* can teach us that.

The History of *Ayurveda*

Ayurveda dates back at least 5,000 years and is thought to be the oldest system of medicine still practiced. The *Vedic* culture, a visionary society that lived in an area of the world that is now India, is credited with being the original source of this knowledge. Initially, all the wisdom held in *Ayurveda* was passed down through oral tradition. Then about 2,500 years ago, it was written down in two texts: the *Charaka Samhita* and the *Sushruta Samhita*. Both of these astoundingly comprehensive repositories of ancient knowledge are still used by students of *Ayurveda* today.

Although *Ayurveda* is thousands of years old, it is an extremely sophisticated system of medicine that has many specialty divisions—branches of medicine—that have lasted through time. In fact, they make up the fundamental structure of our medical system today: internal medicine, ENT (ear, nose, and throat), ophthalmology, obstetrics and gynecology, pediatrics, and surgery. As a plastic surgeon, I was fascinated to learn that the preferred surgical technique for reconstructing the nose after trauma or cancer that was taught to me during residency was first described in *Ayurvedic* texts thousands of years ago.

Ayurveda went through some rocky times when the British invaded India. All the *Ayurvedic* medical schools were closed, and practicing *Ayurveda* was declared illegal. After India gained its independence in 1947, attempts were made to reestablish *Ayurveda*. Not surprisingly, much of the ancient knowledge had become fragmented and some of it had been lost. The practice of *Ayurveda* had degenerated essentially into an herbalized form of Western medicine. Prevention and techniques of consciousness were no longer at the forefront of the medical field.

Then, in the early 1980s, Maharishi Mahesh Yogi, the person who brought Transcendental Meditation (TM) to the West, recognized that the world was in desperate need of *Ayurveda*—the original comprehensive *Ayurveda*. He brought the top *Ayurvedic* doctors (called *vaidyas*) together to reconstruct the lost knowledge. They were given the task to carefully read the original *Ayurvedic* texts and then select the most effective techniques that would best suit our culture now. This form of *Ayurveda* is distinguished by being called Maharishi *Ayurveda* or Maharishi *Vedic* Approach to Health (MVAH).

Navigating Alternative Medicine

If you've ever looked into using complementary and alternative medicine (CAM), I'd be surprised if you didn't become confused and overwhelmed. On the surface, it appears to be a smorgasbord of hundreds of different health practices with no apparent link. Without expert guidance, the average person can't select the right combination of techniques or approaches to most effectively meet his or her individual needs.

Most of the techniques used in CAM today have their roots in *Ayurveda,* including such diverse treatments as yoga, massage, meditation, music therapy, sound therapy, aromatherapy, herbs, breathing techniques, special diets, and detoxification, to name just a few. *Ayurveda* also teaches a group of simple but profound principles that provide a broad, yet fundamental understanding of all the different techniques included in CAM. Its basic principles form a framework for understanding these techniques and how they fit together into a comprehensive model of healthcare.

These timeless truths are actually laws of Nature that govern health. They reveal how and why certain techniques work to improve health. Throughout *Waking the Warrior Goddess, Ayurvedic* principles are presented to help give you the "big picture"—a deeper and clearer understanding of each element of the program. If all the methods to lower your risk of breast cancer were presented without teaching you about their underlying *Ayurvedic* principles, they would seem like a long list of unrelated items that you could easily forget. But when you understand them in relationship to the fundamental laws of Nature, you understand them on a much deeper level. They make sense, and they stay with you.

To give you an idea of what I'm talking about, let's look at an example. One *Ayurvedic* principle is: *Food is medicine.* We don't usually think of food as medicine in our culture. For the most part, we are unfamiliar with the medicinal qualities of foods, because Western doctors don't prescribe foods; they prescribe pharmaceutical medications. That's why we're all very familiar with how to approach common, uncomplicated health problems using medications, such as aspirin or Pepto-Bismol. But very few of us know the names of the spices, herbs, and foods that may be just as effective.

Ayurvedic physicians, on the other hand, prescribe food as one of the first lines of treatment. Instead of reaching for aspirin for a painful swollen joint, their patients would most likely seek relief by turning to the cooking spices turmeric and ginger, and the vegetables asparagus and spinach. For acid indigestion, instead of a couple of tablespoons of a bright-pink liquid, they would eat rice, *mung dal* (lentil soup), pumpkin, squash, pomegranate, fennel, cumin, coriander, or turmeric.

Thousands of years ago, the intelligence contained in food was well recognized for its ability to induce balance and increase the healing intelligence of our bodies. Modern science is now confirming what ancient physicians knew: The right food is *powerful medicine.* Part Two of this book reveals the medicinal foods that modern research shows can substantially lower your risk of breast cancer. But protecting against breast cancer isn't the only thing they do. They also lower your risk of most chronic disorders and can dramatically improve your overall health.

Sickness is the vengeance of nature
for violation of her laws.

—Charles Simmons

Two Underlying Principles of *Ayurveda*

All the techniques and principles in *Ayurveda* boil down to two grand underlying principles. The first and foremost one is this:

Perfect balance brings perfect health.

Ayurveda emphasizes that everything you do or eat—every day—either brings you into balance or throws you out of balance. The trick is to know the difference. If you choose only those foods and activities that bring balance, you can create perfect health.

The second most important principle is:

Perfect health is achieved through enlivening your inner healing intelligence.

In other words, all health-promoting foods, activities, herbs, and so on work by making your body *stronger* and *smarter* at repairing itself and resisting disease. At their most fundamental level, all the seemingly unrelated techniques presented in this book lower your risk of breast cancer by enlivening your body's inner healing intelligence and inducing balance.

It's equally important to recognize not only what brings you into balance, but also what throws you out of balance—what to avoid. These are the activities you do or the foods that you eat that weaken you because they violate the natural laws governing your mind/body. Knowing these laws of Nature in advance helps to keep you from making the mistakes or creating the habits that obstruct your inner healing intelligence.

The principles of *Ayurveda* are the keys to understanding all the rules that govern your health. When you know the rules and follow them, you thrive abundantly, avoid catastrophes, and pave the path to the immense pleasure of extraordinary balance and health.

Without a doubt, the medicine of the future will reincorporate these ancient truths. It's already happening. An integrated system of medicine—one that combines the best technologies of Western medicine with those of ancient holistic systems of medicine—will serve us best. Imagine a system of medicine that uses all of the best knowledge and techniques of health from every culture in the world, where rapidly advancing sophisticated technology is built on a base that includes everything we have learned about our bodies and health over thousands of years since the beginning of recorded time.

Chapter 3

The Birth
of the Beast
How Breast Cancer Grows

*I*nside the human body, there is a fascinating universe of spectacular intelligence. In a healthy body, every structure and every cell work together in perfect coordination and harmony. It's important to understand a few basic facts about the anatomy and physiology of the human body because it will enhance your grasp of each subject presented in this book. This fundamental knowledge will help you to comprehend more fully how and why each one influences your risk of breast cancer.

The human body is composed of cells, each of which functions like its own city. The boundary of every cell is defined by a cell membrane—like a protective bubble surrounding the city. Within each cell city, there are many different structures, all with special functions. There are power plants that make energy, construction crews that build new structures and repair damaged ones, and demolition crews that tear things down so that new things can be built in their place.

In the center of every cell (except red blood cells) is a very important structure called the nucleus. It contains the DNA. A simple way to understand DNA is to think of it as the source code for every structure and function in the body. In other words, it supplies the information that tells every cell and every molecule in the body what to do, when to do it, and how to do it. It's like a set of blueprints. DNA comes in strands that form a double helix. Defined sequences of DNA make up a gene. A chromosome is made up of 50,000 to 100,000 genes combined together. Forty-six chromosomes are found in every cell.

New cells are constantly being created to replace old, damaged, or worn-out cells through a process called cell division. When your cells divide to form new cells, the DNA in the cell must make an exact copy of itself. Sometimes, DNA becomes damaged due to environmental toxins, pesticides, radiation, viruses, inflammation, or any of a variety of other factors. When a cell containing damaged DNA divides, a copy of the DNA with damaged genetic information is passed on to the new cell, so some part of the information passed on to the new cell will be wrong.

Depending on where the mistake occurs, it might be the spark that ignites a deadly disease, or it might not create any problems. For instance, let's assume that the part of your DNA that contains the instructions telling the construction workers when to *stop* building becomes damaged. They will start to erect a structure and finish it, but because they receive no instruction telling them to stop, they continue building—*forever.* That's exactly how cancer can form. In a healthy balanced body, DNA controls cell division. However, if the gene that governs cell division becomes damaged, cells may start to divide wildly, initiating the growth of a cancer. Cell division out of control *is* cancer.

ESTROGEN'S ROLE

Estrogen is the hormone that causes female characteristics to develop. It influences the shape of the body, hair distribution, voice, emotions, skin texture, and a myriad of other effects. It also makes breast tissue grow by increasing the rate at which breast cells divide. Too much estrogen causes breast cells to divide too rapidly and to keep on dividing. With every cell division, there's a chance for a mistake to occur that could lead to cancer. So, the faster breast cells divide, the higher the risk of breast cancer.

Scientists have found that it's not uncommon for cancer cells to form as a result of damaged DNA. This is largely because DNA must replicate itself each time a cell divides. This is a complicated process with a high probability of error. Mathematically speaking, the chances of a mistake occurring during DNA replication are extremely high. Consider this: You have 50,000 to 100,000 genes in each chromosome and 46 chromosomes in the nucleus of every cell. That means that between 2.3 and 4.6 million separate pieces of information must be copied each time a cell divides. In other words, there are 2.3 to 4.6 *million* opportunities for a mistake to occur in each cell in your body *every* time a cell divides. And you have *trillions* of cells that are continuously dividing.

With those odds, it should come as no surprise that your body constantly produces cancer cells. Fortunately, you were created with this fact in mind. The extraordinary internal healing intelligence inside you organizes many layers of protection against this normal, but potentially disastrous occurrence. Using the construction analogy again, you have quality-control teams that detect damaged DNA and send in repair crews. If the repair crews are overwhelmed with work, they can't keep up with all the mistakes, and cancer cells may start to grow. Fortunately, there are other workers who back up these repair crews. They flag the newly formed cancer cells and instantly call in another crew to come and destroy it. A tumor only forms when mistakes happen so rapidly and cancer cells form so quickly that the detection and repair crews can't keep up.

The Risk with Estrogen

Breast cancer is considered a hormonal disease because a hormone initiates and fuels it by causing cells to grow and divide. In breast cancer, that hormone is estrogen. The more estrogen you're exposed to, the higher your risk of breast cancer is.

Contrary to a common misconception, the term "estrogen" includes many different types of molecular compounds, not just one. There are three major types of estrogen naturally made by the body: estradiol, estrone, and estriol. Estradiol is the most abundant and the most potent of the three. It's the type of estrogen that contributes the most to increasing your risk of breast cancer. The more estradiol your body makes in your lifetime, the higher your risk of cancer.

When you have a menstrual period, your body produces more estradiol. So the more periods you have during your life, the higher your risk of breast cancer. That's why your risk goes up if you start menstruating at an early age or go through menopause at a later age. For instance, if you were younger than age fourteen when you started having periods, your risk of breast cancer is 30 percent higher than if you started when you were sixteen. If you were ten when your periods started, your risk of breast cancer is 50 percent greater than if you had started at age sixteen. If you go through menopause late—at age fifty-five—your risk is 50 percent higher than it would be if you went through it at age forty-five.

The shorter your menstrual cycles are, the more of them you will have in your lifetime, and the higher your risk of breast cancer will be. You might think that the length of your menstrual cycle is completely controlled by genetics, the phases of the moon, or some other factor beyond your control, but it's not. There are certain foods you can eat to naturally lengthen your menstrual cycles and lower your risk; these foods will be discussed in Part Two.

Pregnancy also influences your risk of breast cancer. If you never had a child or had your first child after age thirty, your risk is higher than if you had a child before you were thirty. The reason, again, has to do with estrogen. When you're pregnant, you don't have menstrual periods, so you don't make much of the strong kind of estrogen (estradiol) that increases your risk of breast cancer.

But, you say, this doesn't sound right. You may remember from high school biology that your body produces high amounts of estrogen when you are pregnant. So, why does pregnancy cause your risk to go down? When you are pregnant, estradiol doesn't go up; a different kind of estrogen—estriol—does. Estriol is the weakest of the three natural estrogens. It is only $\frac{1}{1000}$ the strength of estradiol. That means that for every 1,000 cells that divide in response to estradiol, estriol will cause only one cell to divide. When there's more estriol and less estradiol, breast-cell division is thousands of times slower. The slower breast cells divide, the lower your risk of breast cancer. That's why high estriol levels during pregnancy can significantly lower your risk of breast cancer.

The protective effect of estriol can be substantial. Research shows that when compared to women who have given birth, women who have never had a child have a 20 to 70 percent increased risk of breast cancer by the time they are forty-five. You can lower your risk even more by breastfeeding your baby. Most women don't ovulate or have menstrual cycles during the first few months of breastfeeding.

Your risk of breast cancer goes up as you age. The older you are, the greater the amount of estrogen your body has made. At age twenty, your risk is about 1 in 20,000; at age forty, it is estimated to be 1 in 200. By the time you are eighty, your risk is about 1 in 9. If you live to be eighty-five, it goes up to 1 in 8.

The Estrogen Pathway

Understanding how estrogen is produced, used, broken down, and eliminated from your body—the estrogen pathway—is important. It adds to your understanding of how and why the factors discussed in this book have an impact on your risk of breast cancer. It's a complicated process. Estrogen is produced primarily by your ovaries before you go through menopause. Other tissues make estrogen too. After menopause, estrogen is primarily made by fat cells and by the adrenal glands, which sit on top of the kidneys. A tiny amount is also made by your muscles.

To understand the estrogen pathway better, let's use the analogy of a car ride. Your trip begins in the ovaries where estrogen is made and then is released into the blood. The blood vessels are like highways, and estrogen flows through these blood-vessel highways to get to its target destinations. When estrogen travels in the blood, it either travels alone or is attached to a substance called a "protein binder"—the difference between driving alone in your car and carpooling. When you carpool in certain cities, you can use a special high-speed lane, usually on the far left. In this lane, you can't exit from the highway. If you're driving alone, you can't use these high-speed lanes. You must travel in lanes that have access to the exit lanes. Like the person driving alone, only the estrogen that travels alone—without a protein binder—can exit from the blood-vessel highway. In this case, we are concerned about the off-ramp for only one destination: the breast tissue.

When estrogen reaches the breast, it looks for a place to "park." Parking spaces represent the "estrogen receptors," which estrogen binds to on the breast-cell membranes. There are estrogen receptors all over your body, but the highest concentrations are found in the uterus and breast. Men also have a high concentration of estrogen receptors in their prostate gland. Because of the relatively large number of estrogen receptors in these tissues, they respond more to estrogen than the other tissues in the body do.

When estrogen binds to an estrogen receptor, it "turns it on." A turned-on receptor causes cells to start dividing. Estrogen receptors don't turn on like a simple on/off switch. Instead, they turn on like a rheostat, a light switch with a dimmer.

The rate at which cells divide in response to estrogen is affected by many factors. First, the rate depends on the strength of the estrogen. There are strong and weak estrogens. Strong estrogens speed up cell division and, therefore, increase the risk of cancer. Weak estrogens slow down cell division, decreasing the risk of cancer. You can think of it like this: The driver of the estrogen car, say, estriol or estradiol, starts blowing bubbles, which represent the new cells formed by cell division in response to estrogen. If the driver is strong (estradiol), he or she can blow a lot of bubbles very quickly, creating a big soapy mess in the car (aka cancer). If the driver is very weak (estriol), he or she can hardly blow any bubbles. One or two bubbles doesn't cause any harm.

Parking at an estrogen receptor causes a lot of wear and tear on the estrogen. After a while, it needs to go in for service. So, the estrogen leaves the estrogen receptor and heads for the liver (service station). The liver is the great detoxifier of the body. It breaks down toxins and other natural substances to prepare them for elimination.

Estrogen is broken down in the liver, and is influenced by the presence of certain chemicals. It is either broken down into a "good" kind of estrogen or a "bad" kind of estrogen. For instance, substances in cruciferous vegetables and flax create more of the good kind while environmental toxins create more of the bad. The difference between good and bad estrogen is that good estrogen causes breast cells to divide very slowly, whereas bad estrogen causes them to divide rapidly. Bad estrogen can also cause mutations or mistakes in how the cells grow that increase your risk of cancer even more.

The good estrogen causes no damage and drives immediately to the colon or to the bladder where it leaves the body. The bad estrogen backfires, gets stuck in reverse, and speeds back to the breast where it wreaks havoc (see Figure 3.1 on page 36). If this bad estrogen finds a parking spot on a breast cell, it will rapidly speed up cell division. If you have a lot of bad estrogen in your body, your risk of breast cancer goes up significantly.

In the colon, estrogen is either eliminated or absorbed back into the blood. If it is absorbed back into the blood, it adds to the total amount of estrogen in your body, and therefore, adds to your risk. There's a simple solution: Eat more fiber. Fiber binds to estrogen in your colon and eliminates it. (See Chapter 7 for more on fiber.)

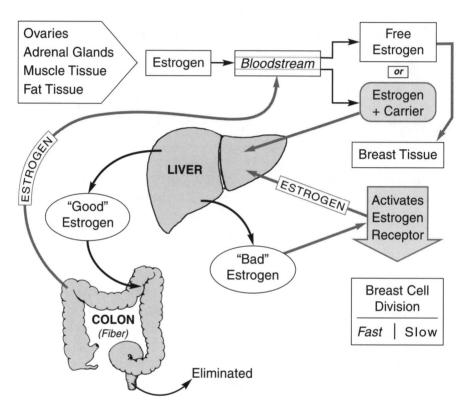

Figure 3.1. The Estrogen Pathway

Now that you understand the fundamental process that links estrogen to breast cancer, we are ready to move on to learning about all the natural ways that you can protect against and fight breast cancer.

Part Two

A Banquet Fit for a Goddess

Foods That Heal

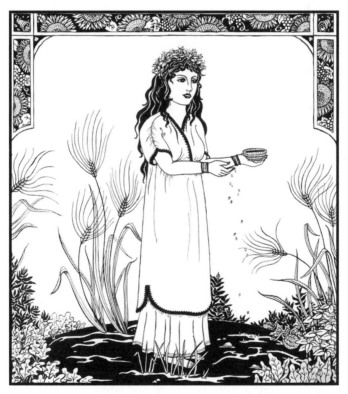

Goddess of Harvest and Fields

Chapter 4

Let Food Be
Your Medicine

Rediscovering a Forgotten
Ayurvedic Pillar of Health

*A*t the heart of *Ayurveda* is your relationship to your inner healing intelligence. It teaches that you can achieve a perfect state of health by enlivening that intelligence with specific foods and behavioral choices. If you make poor choices that sabotage your inherent capacity to heal, imbalances arise that further block the full expression of your healing intelligence. Eventually, poor choices will weaken it to where it can no longer keep you well. In time, your body will begin to break down, and diseases will start to manifest. Health is only regained and maintained by enhancing this healing intelligence and keeping it lively and flowing.

The divine, natural healing intelligence inside you manages trillions of biochemical reactions simultaneously at every moment of your life. The image that emerges for me when I think of this intelligence is one of an extraordinary multitasking Warrior Goddess—supernatural in strength and power and vastly discriminating in her intellect. Yet, she is delicate and very particular.

Like a Goddess, the magnificence of this managing intelligence depends on respecting her very precise and specific demands. When you think of the phenomenal biology, physics, and chemistry that keep you alive and well, embrace them as your Warrior Goddess: an intimate, personal, profoundly intelligent, and powerful friend.

Having the knowledge of what empowers your Warrior Goddess and what drains her strength endows you with the power of choice—the choice about how you treat her and, thus, the direction of your health. But, if you aren't aware of her likes and dislikes, you're like a ship lost at sea, unable to find the course that leads to achieving and maintaining good health. You won't be able to choose the best direction to excellent health—no matter how much you want to— because you lack the skills and equipment for the task. Chances are, sooner or later, you'll crash on the rocks, get stuck on a sandbar, or suddenly find your-self in a hostile foreign land filled with life-threatening diseases. However, if you choose to honor and empower your Warrior Goddess, she will steer you to a land of perfect health—an enchanting place filled with the treasures of clarity, abundance, fulfillment, peace, wisdom, and beauty.

Never does Nature say one thing and wisdom another.

—JUVENAL, *SATIRES*

FOOD FOR A GODDESS

All ancient systems of medicine recognize that one of the most important deter-minants of your health is what you choose to put in your mouth. The right foods bring balance and greatly increase the healing intelligence of your body. The wrong foods can act as poisons—junk foods, for example. They contain health-damaging chemical additives and preservatives, and most of their nutrients have been destroyed during processing. Canned foods, frozen foods, and leftover food all have lower nutritional values. They have qualities that aren't good for your mind/body, and should be avoided.

Your stomach shouldn't be your wastebasket.

—AUTHOR UNKNOWN

Some foods are filled with so many health-promoting and anticancer prop-erties that they can be thought of as medicines. As mentioned earlier, this is an important *Ayurvedic* principle: [*The right*] *food is medicine.* Most medicinal foods come from the plant world. Physicians trained in *Ayurveda* possess an extreme-ly sophisticated knowledge of the medicinal qualities of plants. Because of this, they prescribe fruits, vegetables, grains, seeds, spices, and herbs as the initial approach for the prevention or treatment of any health condition. Not only do they know the medicines contained within each plant, but they also know the ideal harvesting, processing, and mixing procedures to maximize the plant's healing potential.

The most health-promoting foods you can eat are fresh, organically grown fruits, vegetables, and whole grains—especially if they are locally grown. Research shows that eating these foods can have a dramatic effect on lowering your risk of breast cancer. Since these foods also enhance your inner healing intelligence, try to favor them. Think of it this way: Make every meal a banquet fit for a Goddess. When you feed your Goddess what she needs, you arm her with powerful weapons. Her ability to keep you well is amazing. When you give her the right raw materials, she can create a multitude of masterful protective devices. This is why *Ayurveda* places great importance on diet and digestion. In fact, there may be nothing that has more influence on your health.

Together, diet and digestion comprise one of the three pillars of *Ayurvedic* health. The other two are proper lifestyle and rest. According to *Ayurveda,* about 80 percent of all illnesses arise from improper diet and digestion.

What you eat is important, *Ayurveda* says, but *how* you eat is just as important. If you don't digest your food properly, it doesn't matter if you have the best diet in the world; it won't do you any good. You have to digest your food well in order to absorb the nutrients. It's the only way you can be nourished by the food you eat.

The Top 12 Aids to Digestion

Ayurveda recommends twelve ways to help you digest your food properly.

1. Eat your main meal at noon.
2. Don't eat again until your previous meal has been digested (about three hours).
3. Keep regular mealtimes.
4. Don't overeat. Eat to fill three-quarters of your stomach's capacity.
5. Eat in a settled atmosphere.
6. Don't eat when you are upset.
7. Always sit down to eat.
8. Don't talk while chewing.
9. Favor lightly cooked foods over raw foods.
10. Avoid cold drinks.
11. Favor fresh wholesome foods, such as organic fruits, vegetables, and whole grains.
12. Put your full attention on your food.

Most of these recommendations are self-explanatory, but a few of them need further clarification. *Ayurveda* recommends that you *eat your main meal at noon* because your "digestive fires" are at their peak from 10:00 A.M. to 2:00 P.M. In other words, your body's metabolism is revved up during these hours, and you can digest your food better than you can early in the morning or later at night. If you eat a big meal late at night, it won't digest well, and your sleep will be disturbed. I'm sure you've had this unpleasant experience at least once or twice. However, the times you've *eaten light in the evening and gone to bed early,* you more than likely woke up feeling great. Most of the principles and recommendations of *Ayurveda* are as simple as this one, but don't let their simplicity fool you. Their effects can be *very* profound.

Cold drinks should be avoided, especially during a meal, because according to *Ayurveda,* a cool drink cools down and dilutes the digestive fires. In Western scientific terms, cool drinks slow down the action of your stomach's digestive enzymes, which work best at body temperature or a little above. At the temperature of an iced drink, the effectiveness of your digestive enzymes is cut almost in half. If you want to drink something with your meals, *Ayurveda* recommends that you have sips of hot water only. Don't drink too much water with your meal, either, because water will dilute the enzymes in the stomach, making them less effective.

The *Ayurvedic* recommendation to *favor fresh wholesome foods* is a key principle of diet, and it plays a big role in lowering the risk of breast cancer. The 2,500-year-old text of *Ayurveda,* called the *Charaka Samhita,* proclaims the importance of a wholesome diet: "The distinction between health and disease arises as the result of the difference between wholesome and unwholesome diet." Wholesome foods are considered to be primarily fresh organic fruits, vegetables, and whole grains.

According to *Ayurveda,* when foods are lightly cooked they are easier to digest and, therefore, more nutrients are absorbed. Overcooking foods or cooking foods at high temperatures should be avoided because it destroys nutrients and creates harmful substances.

Finally, when you eat a meal, it is ideal to *put your full attention on your food.* Don't watch TV or read the newspaper. When your full attention is on your meal, you're more likely to chew your food well, eat smaller portions, and digest your food better.

If you eat highly nutritious foods and follow these simple recommendations, you can provide your body with the best materials and the most competent and proficient team of builders to design, construct, and maintain the foundation of your health. If you choose poor materials and unskilled workers, your foundation will be weak, and no matter what else you do to support your health, it will crumble. With a strong foundation, you can build a structure so solid that it becomes impenetrable against even the most aggressive and ruthless enemy—breast cancer.

Chapter 5

An Organic Pharmacy

"Chemotherapy" from Organic
Fruits and Vegetables

ruits and vegetables are virtual anticancer pharmacies. Thousands of studies have shown that a diet high in fresh fruits and vegetables is associated with a lower risk of many different types of cancers and chronic diseases. Scientists have found that these plants contain a wide variety of natural chemicals that are extremely powerful at protecting against cancer and help to fight it once it has formed.

The remarkable natural "chemotherapy" found in fresh fruits and vegetables is safe and free of side effects, and it expresses an intelligence of such brilliance that pharmaceutical companies are studying these plants to learn how to create effective, and far less toxic, chemotherapy. *Ayurveda* explains that the reason these plants are so protective is that they contain high amounts of "intelligence." They transfer this intelligence to your body, increasing its natural healing intelligence, its ability to keep you healthy, and its power to ward off disease. Animal-based products, especially those high in saturated fat, tend to have the opposite effect. In other words, they decrease or block the healing intelligence of your body. The result is an increased risk of cancer and other chronic disorders.

Scientists have studied many of these plants to determine what causes them to be so protective. Most fruits and vegetables have several common beneficial properties that are associated with a lower risk of cancer. These beneficial properties are:

1. They are low in fat and high in fiber. (See Chapters 7 and 8.)

2. They are high in antioxidants and vitamins. (See Chapters 12 and 13.)

3. They have fewer calories than animal foods, high-fat foods, and simple carbohydrates, so the people who eat a lot of them on a regular basis generally have less body fat than those who don't.

THE INTELLIGENCE OF PLANTS

Plants contain specific cancer-fighting and disease-battling substances called "phytochemicals," or plant chemicals. Each plant contains anywhere from dozens to hundreds of different plant chemicals. Scientists think that plants developed these phytochemicals to protect themselves against predators, such as insects, bacteria, and fungi. Phytochemicals aren't nutrients and don't provide calories. Rather, they function as medicines—natural medicines with an extraordinary array of healing benefits.

Research has shown that phytochemicals can protect you from cancer in several different ways. Many of them are powerful antioxidants that protect your cells and DNA from damage caused by oxygen free radicals—damage that can lead to cancer. Some plant chemicals inactivate carcinogens and other substances that can damage your DNA and lead to cancer. Others can block one or more of the steps required for a cancer to grow.

Carotenoids

One of the most powerful cancer-fighting groups of phytochemicals is carotenoids. All carotenoids are potent antioxidants, but they each have unique healing properties. For instance, one class of carotenoids might significantly reduce one type of cancer by blocking steps in its growth, but it might have little effect on another kind of cancer. For example, the carotenoid lycopene is very protective against breast and prostate cancer, but it doesn't do much to protect against leukemia.

Carotenoids give a plant its color and contribute to its flavor. For instance, lycopene gives tomatoes their red color, and beta-carotene gives carrots their orange color. But you can't always tell which carotenoids are present by the color of the plant. Sometimes, you can't see the color of a carotenoid, even though it's present in large amounts, because another color is covering it up. For example, lutein has a yellow color and some very important health-promoting qualities; it is found in high quantities in leafy green vegetables, such as kale. You don't normally see the yellow color of lutein in kale, however, because it is camouflaged by the green chlorophyll. When kale starts to age, it loses some of its green chlorophyll, and then you can see the yellow of the lutein. This is exactly what happens to the leaves of deciduous trees in the fall. Tree leaves change their color when they lose enough green chlorophyll to expose the color beneath it.

Carotenoids also help to protect against many other disorders besides breast cancer. For instance, lutein helps to prevent macular degeneration, the most common cause of adult blindness.

Flavonoids

Also called bioflavonoids, these phytochemicals also contribute to the color and flavor of a plant. Flavonoids have powerful anticancer properties, too.

In a study published in 2003 in the *British Journal of Cancer*, one group of flavonoids in particular, flavones (commonly found in leafy green vegetables and herbs), was found to dramatically lower the risk of breast cancer. Just 0.5 milligram (mg) a day of flavones, about what one-eighth of a green pepper contains, decreased the risk of breast cancer by 15 percent. For every additional 0.5 mg of flavones that a woman ate each day, her risk dropped another 15 percent.

Indole-3 Carbinol

Another group of plant chemicals that's particularly helpful in reducing the risk of breast cancer is known as indole-3 carbinol, which is found in all "cruciferous" vegetables. The cruciferous family includes the following:

- Bitter cress
- Bok choy
- Broccoli
- Brussels sprouts
- Cabbage
- Cauliflower
- Collards
- Horseradish
- Kale
- Mustard seeds
- Radishes
- Rutabaga
- Savoy cabbage
- Turnip
- Watercress

Researchers have found that indole-3 carbinol attacks breast cancer with a diversity of weapons. It's like a superhero's Swiss army knife, fighting the deadly disease in many different ways. Here are some of them:

1. Indole-3 carbinol stops breast cancer cells from growing by shutting off a key enzyme necessary for the cells to grow.

2. It interferes in the relationship between estrogen and the estrogen receptors in breast cells. Normally, their interaction ignites the rapid reproduction of cells. Indole-3 carbinol dampens that flame to a mere flicker. In other words, when estrogen binds to the estrogen receptor with indole-3 carbinol present, breast cells don't divide as fast as they usually do.

3. It forces estrogen to break down into a "good" (protective, non-cancer-promoting) type of estrogen. As you saw in Figure 3.1 on page 36, indole-3 carbinol is involved in breaking down estrogen in the liver. The liver converts estrogen into either "good" estrogen or "bad" estrogen. Indole-3 carbinol ensures that more estrogen is transformed into the "good" type.

4. It beneficially influences DNA and the instructions that DNA passes on. For example, it activates a "tumor-suppression" gene, which contains the commands for several internal tactics that stop tumor growth. Not all your genetic material is read or turned on at any one time. Only part of the information in your genes is expressed. Certain substances—indole-3 carbinol, for one—can turn genes on, meaning they give the command for a specific gene's information to be read and the instructions carried out. Certain other agents, such as enzymes, proteins, or other chemical substances, can also turn genes on and off.

Indole-3 carbinol turns on the gene that contains the DNA message to slow down tumor growth. In addition, this tumor-suppression gene sends messages that prevent tumor cells from invading bodily tissues, spreading to other areas of the body, and from adhering together. (Adhesion, which is the ability of cells to stick to one another and other tissues, is necessary for a tumor to grow and spread successfully.)

Of all of these effects, scientists think that indole-3 carbinol's ability to influence the liver to make more of the "good" kind of estrogen and less of the "bad" may play the biggest role in lowering the risk of breast cancer. Researchers have found that "bad" estrogen plays a significant role in causing breast cancer. In one study, the amounts of "good" estrogen and "bad" estrogen were measured in two different groups of women. One group was composed of healthy women and the other group was composed of women who had breast cancer. Those with breast cancer had almost twice as much "bad" estrogen as the healthy women.

If you have breast cancer, indole-3 carbinol's influence on a tumor-suppression gene may be extraordinarily beneficial in improving your chances of survival.

When indole-3 carbinol is ingested, it is converted by stomach acid to a substance called "diindolylmethane" (DIM). DIM is simply two molecules of indole-3 carbinol joined together, and it is the substance that is actually used by the body.

Sulforaphane

Another anticancer phytochemical in cruciferous vegetables, particularly broccoli, is worth noting. It's called sulforaphane, and it helps to stop cancer before it even begins. Sulforaphane increases the activity of the liver enzyme responsible for deactivating or destroying carcinogens and getting them out of your body. It also impedes the spread of a tumor.

D-Glucaric Acid

Cruciferous vegetables, as well as fruits (such as oranges, apples, and grapefruit) also have a high concentration of another phytochemical that's effective in protecting against cancer, especially breast cancer—D-glucaric acid.

The liver manufactures a substance called *glucuronic acid,* which binds to toxins (including the "bad" estrogen) in the liver and deactivates them. But the enzyme beta-glucuronidase can interfere with this effort. It splits the toxins off glucuronic acid and reactivates them (see Figure 5.1 below). Researchers have found that people with a high amount of beta-glucuronidase in the blood have an increased risk of various cancers, particularly the hormone-dependent ones, such as breast, prostate, and colon cancers.

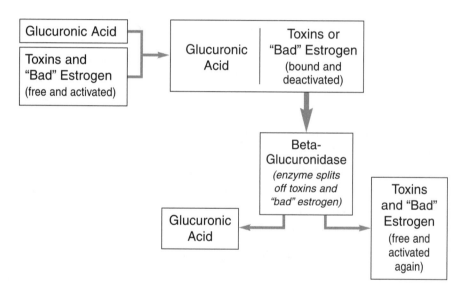

Figure 5.1. Liver Enzyme Action

Here is where the phytochemical D-glucaric acid comes to the rescue: It stops the activity of beta-glucuronidase, keeping the harmful estrogens and other toxins bound to glucuronic acid (see Figure 5.2 on page 48) and deactivated. Simply put, D-glucaric acid strengthens the body's natural defenses against toxins. The liver makes a small amount of D-glucaric acid, but not enough for you to reap the greatest benefits. You can significantly increase the

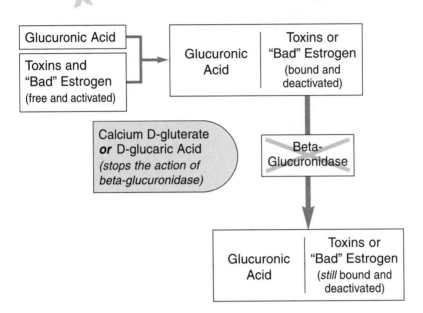

Figure 5.2. D-Glucaric Acid Action

level of this protective substance in your body by eating plenty of cruciferous vegetables and certain fruits or by taking a supplement that comes in the form of a calcium salt called calcium D-gluterate or calcium D-glucarate. Research shows that this supplement is just as effective as natural D-glucaric acid. Taking supplemental calcium D-gluterate may give some added protection against breast cancer, but long-term studies still need to be done.

Eat Your Broccoli!

The results of consuming all the cancer-fighting phytochemicals in cruciferous vegetables are impressive. Researchers have found that women who eat the most cruciferous vegetables have as much as a 40 percent lower risk of breast cancer than women who eat few, if any, of these vegetables.

Chapter 6

Mother Nature
Knows Best

Growing Foods to Enhance
Their Healing Intelligence

If you're going to America, bring your own food.

—FRAN LEBOWITZ, JOURNALIST

he *way* your food is grown can have a powerful influence on the quality of its healing intelligence and, therefore, a significant impact on your risk of breast cancer. Think of it this way: When you eat plants that have been grown with techniques that maximize their quality and vitality, they supply your Warrior Goddess with the highest level of healing intelligence and the most sophisticated weaponry possible to defend against disease.

Conventionally grown foods may look and smell wholesome, but lurking on and under the surface is often a toxic mix of poisons that includes the residues of chemical fertilizers, pesticides, herbicides, hormones, and toxic additives. Organically grown foods, on the other hand, are carefully cultivated to avoid these chemicals. The reasons you don't want your foods grown with synthetic chemicals are simple: They are usually damaging to your health and the environment. Some of these chemicals have been found to increase your risk of breast cancer—and other cancers, as well. Many agricultural and additive chemicals can also disrupt your immune, nervous, endocrine, and reproductive systems.

There is another important health issue concerning conventionally grown food: Some seed producers change the characteristics of a plant by modifying its DNA. This process is known as "genetic modification." The intent is to increase crop production or commercial viability by adding so-called "beneficial" traits to a plant's DNA. For instance, companies add genes to plants to make them grow bigger, to be more resistant to pests, or to increase their shelf life. The problem is that scientists don't know what the long-term effects of eating these types of foods will be on human health—or on the environment. No human studies were done to evaluate their safety before they were put on the market. In other words, you and your family are Guinea pigs in one of the largest non-consensual human experiments in history! This "experiment" *will* find out what happens to humans when they eat these foods over a long period of time—and *we* are the ones who will most likely suffer for it—we and our children and future generations!

Problems are already showing up in several short-term studies of genetically modified organisms (GMOs). In a study conducted at the University of Cincinnati by I. L. Bernstein and published in 1999 in *Environmental Health Perspectives,* allergic reactions were found among farm workers using *Bacillus thuringiensis,* a pesticide that's genetically spliced into corn. There have been many case reports of allergic reactions ranging from mild to severe. Even more alarming, a researcher in England found significant organ damage in rats that were fed genetically engineered potatoes.

The only way to reduce your health risk from GMOs is to buy only organically grown foods. Unfortunately, you can only decrease your risk of consuming GMOs because accidents happen. Genetically altered foods have accidentally been mixed with biologically normal foods. For instance, in 2000, genetically altered corn called StarLink, which had not been approved for human consumption, was found in Kraft taco shells. The problem was traced to a silo in Iowa where StarLink corn had accidentally been mixed with non-GMO corn.

A front-page story in *The New York Times* on June 10, 2001, reported that genetically altered DNA had been found in organic foods. Reporter David Barboza said that the reason was, "More than 100 million acres of the world's most fertile farmland were planted with genetically modified crops last year ([in] 2000) . . . Wind-blown pollen, commingled seeds, and black-market plantings have . . . extended these products of biotechnology into the far corners of the global food supply—perhaps irreversibly." In other words, organically grown plants can become contaminated with genetic modifications. For the most part, however, certified organic foods are free from GMOs and are the only way to reduce your risk of consuming genetically altered foods.

High-tech tomatoes! Mysterious milk! Supersquash!
Are we supposed to eat this stuff? Or is it going to eat us?

—ANNITA MANNING

WEED KILLER COULD KILL YOU

Conventionally grown foods are sprayed with chemical pesticides, herbicides, fungicides, and fertilizers. These chemicals are popular because they are effective, but most of them are also highly toxic. They can damage your health in a variety of ways, causing everything from cancer to nervous, endocrine, and reproductive system damage. Chemicals that damage your nervous system are classified as neurotoxins. They impair IQ, memory, coordination, and the ability to concentrate. Other chemicals, known as endocrine disrupters, disturb the delicate balance of the hormones that regulate your body's functions, including reproductive functions. Most samples of conventionally grown fruits and vegetables contain the residues of several of these dangerous chemicals.

Let's take a close look at one chemical, the pesticide dichlorodiphenyl-trichloroethane (DDT). First developed in 1873, DDT wasn't recognized as a pesticide until 1939 when a Swiss citizen, Paul Meuller, discovered this functional use and was awarded the Nobel Prize in 1948 for his discovery. Initially, DDT was thought to be safe and the answer to the world's pest problems. But then wildlife, especially birds, began to die by the thousands. Certain populations of birds, such as the American bald eagle, dropped almost to extinction. The reason why this happened is because DDT softens the birds' eggshells so much that they can't support a developing embryo.

DDT was sprayed on fruits and vegetables grown in the United States from the early 1950s to the late 1960s. It was found to be harmful to humans by increasing their risk of certain cancers. Because of the serious environmental damage and human-health issues linked to this pesticide, it was banned in the United States in 1972. Unfortunately, DDT is persistent. It doesn't break down quickly and lasts for decades in our soil, water, and bodies. Animals pick up DDT from the environment through the plants, water, and animals they consume. When an animal or a fish ingests DDT from another creature or from the environment, this pesticide concentrates and stores in its fat, and stays there. The level of DDT in an animal's fat is about 700 times greater than the level in its blood.

Each time a bigger animal or fish eats a smaller one, it eats all the stored and concentrated DDT in that animal. So, huge amounts of DDT can accumulate in larger animals after a lifetime of eating smaller ones. This process is called "bio-concentration." Ultimately, when you eat an animal or fish, you ingest all the DDT (not to mention many other concentrated toxins) from all the smaller animals and fish that *that* creature ever ate. That is why the biggest sources of pesticides in your diet are fish, poultry, pork, beef, and other animal products.

You might think that DDT doesn't pose much of a health threat anymore because it was banned so long ago. Unfortunately, that's not true. Despite the ban on using it in the United States, American companies still manufacture DDT and sell it to other countries, such as Mexico, where it's legal. Mexican farmers spray DDT on their fruits and vegetables, and then—you guessed it—they export that produce right back to us. Our government checks only about 1 percent of imported produce, so fruits and vegetables sprayed with DDT, as well as other banned pesticides, come into the United States essentially without restriction. This toxic chemical–boomerang effect is called the "circle of poison." Recent research has found that the levels of many banned pesticides, including DDT, are rising in Americans.

One of the reasons DDT poses such a big threat to breast health is that it mimics estrogen. It acts just like the human estrogen molecule in your body, but with one big difference: This man-made chemical is much more powerful than natural estrogen. DDT significantly increases the rate at which cells divide in the breast—so much so that it dramatically increases your risk of breast cancer.

DDT breaks down in the body into dichlorodiphenyldichloroethylene (DDE). Some studies show that women with the highest DDE levels have a 400 percent higher risk of breast cancer, but other studies don't show any increase at all. Some of the studies that showed no effect, however, were sponsored by the very chemical companies that make DDT. Because of their vested interest, companies have been known to skew the data or design of a study to make their chemicals look safe when they really aren't.

A recent study of more than 400 women in Denmark found that those with breast cancer had significantly higher levels of DDE than those who were healthy. Those with the highest levels of DDE were found to have a 300 percent higher risk of breast cancer. Hundreds of other pesticides have been manufactured, and many currently in use are far more toxic than DDT. For instance, benzene hexachloride (BHC) is nineteen times more powerful as a carcinogen than DDT. To play it safe, avoid chemical estrogens by eating only organically grown fruits, vegetables, and other foods.

The Poison Cocktail

We humans aren't exposed to just one pesticide or harmful chemical at a time. We're exposed to a "soup" of toxins every day. These toxins come from our food, the air we breathe, and the chemicals that outgas in our homes, in the buildings where we work and shop, and in our cars. They also come from dry-cleaned clothes, home-cleaning supplies, and beauty and personal-care products. In addition, some toxins stay in our bodies for decades, creating an ever more complex, chemical cocktail.

The big question is: What happens when these chemicals mix together? Do they interact in some way and become even more toxic? Because most of these chemicals haven't been studied, we don't know; however, the few studies that have been done suggest that this may be *exactly* what happens. A study conducted at Tulane and Xavier Universities in New Orleans found that when two pesticides, endosulfan and dieldrin, were combined together, the estrogenic effect of endosulfan increased 160 times and that of dieldrin increased 1,600 times. When the researchers combined endosulfan with chlordane (a pesticide banned in the United States but still used in third-world countries and sold back to us on the food we import), the endosulfan's estrogenic activity increased 100 times.

ORGANIC: IT'S WORTH IT

Concern over harmful chemicals is probably the biggest reason why organically grown crops and organic products are the fastest growing sector of the agriculture economy, averaging 20 percent growth per year for more than a decade. Another reason may be that organic foods taste better. That's why many chefs at finer restaurants prefer to use them. In addition, most studies comparing the nutritional quality and content of organic foods to conventionally grown foods have found that organic foods fare much better. For instance, a study conducted at the University of California, Davis, found that corn grown without pesticides had 58 percent more antioxidants when compared to conventionally grown corn. Researchers also found that organically grown Marion berries (a type of blackberry) had 50 percent more antioxidants and organically grown strawberries had 19 percent more antioxidants than the same fruits grown conventionally.

There have been about thirty studies comparing the nutritional qualities of conventional (chemically grown) foods to organically grown foods. Drawing accurate conclusions from comparisons can sometimes be difficult, because in any crop—organic or nonorganic—nutrient content can vary. Sunlight, temperature, soil quality, and rainfall all affect the nutrient content of a plant. In addition, fruits and vegetables that are vine-ripened have more nutrients than those picked before they are ripe and held in storage for weeks. Despite these variations, researchers were able to calculate statistically significant differences between organic and conventionally grown crops using more than 300 different comparisons. Organically grown crops were found to have a higher nutritional value 40 percent of the time, whereas conventionally grown crops had a higher nutritional value only 15 percent of the time. Organic crops had an equal or higher nutrient content than conventionally grown foods 85 percent of the time. Three nutrients stood out as being consistently better in organic crops: On average, they have about 20 percent more vitamin C, better protein quality, and about 20 percent fewer carcinogenic nitrates than conventional crops.

Nutrients don't tell the whole story of a plant, however. The best test is to observe what happens to human beings and animals when they eat organically grown crops compared to what happens when they eat chemically grown crops. Are there any differences in their health? Animal experiments have been done with the intent to find the answer to that question. A review of these studies was published in the journal *Alternative Therapies* in 1998. Most of the studies included in the review found a significant difference. The animals that were fed organic foods were healthier. The biggest differences were seen in animals that were sick or very young: The organically fed animals tended to have a higher reproductive capacity, better survival of the young, less illness, and better recovery from illness. Across generations, there was a decline in reproductive ability in the animals fed chemically grown foods: Sperm motility decreased, and ovum production went down.

Organically grown foods are somewhat more expensive than conventional crops, but their superior power as natural medicines makes them well worth the difference. Think of it as a commitment to your health. It's a small price to pay for food that delivers the most nutritional value, tastes better, is free of (or has *very* low amounts of) dangerous carcinogenic chemicals, and is grown in a way that doesn't damage the environment. Remember, too: Buying organic foods saves you money in the long run because cancer, or any chronic disease, costs you time and drains you physically, emotionally, and financially.

Organic Isn't Just About Food

Foods aren't the only products grown with chemicals. Farmers put huge amounts of pesticides on cotton plants grown for fabric. In fact, more pesticides are used on cotton than on any other plant. Every year, one-fourth to one-third of all the pesticides used in the world is used on cotton. Pesticides contaminate the cotton plant and the environment, get into the food chain, and then set up residence in *you* (more on this in Chapter 21). Other dangerous chemicals are used, or created, in the processing of the cotton, too. For instance, when cotton is bleached white, dioxins are created as byproducts of the bleach, and dioxins are the most powerful carcinogen known. Buying organic cotton clothes, towels, and linens will help to stop this unhealthy practice.

New Organic Standards

The United States government approved strict, nationwide organic standards in 2002. The purpose was to guarantee to consumers that all foods labeled as "certified organic" were grown according to uniform standards. Prior to this date, several state agencies, each with different guidelines, certified organic

foods. Because it was difficult for most consumers to know exactly what "certified organic" meant, the federal government stepped in.

All certified-organic foods are now grown according
to the same standards (see the website for the Environmental Protection Agency [EPA] at http://www.epa.gov).
You can identify certified-organic foods by a simple green
and white "USDA organic" label stamped on the front
(see the figure at right).

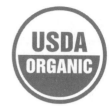

VEDIC ORGANIC AGRICULTURE

"Why do we eat in the first place? We eat to gain a blissful state of life, maximum coherence, health, and vitality." This simple statement by the monk
Maharishi Mahesh Yogi expresses why *Ayurveda* considers high-quality food so
important to your health. Your body and mind are literally created from the food
you eat. Your food *becomes* you. On the horizon is the revival and reestablish-
ment of an ancient agricultural technology that takes certified-organic foods to
the next level, creating maximum quality and vitality in food. It's called Maharishi *Vedic* Organic Agriculture (MVOA).

Ayurveda is based on the quantum laws of the Universe, which modern
physics has only recently begun to explore. For instance, *Ayurveda* acknowl-
edges that everything in life is intimately connected, expertly managed, and
based on the laws of the Universe. So, that which is fundamentally good for
human health is also good for all forms of life, including animals and plants.

MVOA uses the same *Ayurvedic* principles and techniques that govern
human health to help plants grow to their highest potential. For example,
Ayurveda teaches that following the natural rhythms of Nature will enhance
your health and ignoring them will damage it. If you sleep at the proper times
at night, you are working with the rhythms of Nature and your physiology
responds by gaining balance and strength. On the other hand, if you work
against the rhythms of Nature by sleeping during the day and staying awake
all night, your physiology becomes unbalanced, weak, and prone to disease.
Similarly, the health of a plant depends on how well the farmer works with the
rhythms of Nature.

Jyotish and the Rhythms of Nature

Farmers are extremely aware of the rhythms and cycles of Nature. To produce
successful crops, they must work within these laws. For instance, crops are
planted in the spring and harvested in the fall. Crops planted in the fall in
Northern climates are doomed to failure. Everyone knows this because the

cycles of the seasons are so obvious. However, there are cycles and rhythms to Nature that are far more subtle and specific that can also have a significant impact on the growth and quality of plants. MVOA uses a special, ancient mathematical system, called *Jyotish,* to map out these more subtle cycles.

The *Jyotish* calculations help the farmer to determine when to begin certain activities, such as planting and harvesting, with much more precision. Having a deeper knowledge of the more subtle cycles creates a higher probability of success for the crops. For instance, a farmer may know from experience that a crop should ideally be planted by the second week in May. *Jyotish* calculations are much more specific. They can tell the farmer the exact day and the precise time on that day—down to the minute—to begin planting.

The importance of identifying the best day and time to plant and harvest crops is not a strange or foreign concept. One of early America's most influential figures, Benjamin Franklin, recognized the importance of working with the rhythms of Nature to produce the best crops. To help farmers do just that, he published *Poor Richard's Almanack* [sic].

Jyotish calculations go deeper, however. They are based on the influence and movements of the planets and stars. Because all things in the Universe are connected on the quantum level, *everything influences everything.* That's why the planets have a significant effect on us. The influences of the sun and moon are very familiar. The daily cycles of the sun establish the rhythm for every life form on this planet. The moon creates daily and monthly influences. It causes tides to rise, regulates a woman's monthly menstrual cycle, affects moods, and influences the incidence of crime. Some people have a harder time believing that the more distant planets affect us, too, but quantum physics tells us that they do.

Ayurveda uses *Jyotish* to predict the planetary impact on the present and the future. The constantly changing configurations of the planets are mathematically measured, and detailed information can be determined about every aspect of your life, from the probability and timing of potential health problems or accidents, to the best time to begin a new project, such as constructing a new house or getting married. If you know about potential problems *before* they happen, you can do something to try to prevent them and protect yourself. *Jyotish* is said to help you "avert the dangers not yet come." For example, if you know you have a day when the probability of accidents is extremely high, you might choose to not drive on that day. If the *Jyotish* calculations say that there's a strong probability of your developing a particular illness, you might pay closer attention to your diet, rest, and take preventative herbs. In short, *Jyotish* helps you to work with precision with the rhythms of Nature, instead of leaving things up to chance.

Musical Medicine

MVOA uses music and sounds to enhance the growth of plants. Decades of research have determined that certain *sounds and music can induce balance and promote health*—not just in humans, but also in plants. This fundamental principle of health was recognized in *Ayurveda* thousands of years ago, and not surprisingly, this system of medicine contains detailed, sophisticated knowledge about using sounds for health.

The fact that music can affect the growth of plants should come as no surprise. More than thirty years ago, modern scientists rediscovered the powerful effects of music on plants. In the 1970s, classical music was observed to cause plants to grow faster and stronger, whereas hard rock-and-roll caused them to droop and wilt.

Instead of classical music, *Ayurveda* prescribes specific sounds, called primordial sounds, and music, called *Gandharva Veda*. There are many types of *Gandharva Veda* music, and each one is designed to be used during different hours of the day. Precise types of music are also prescribed for various health conditions. MVOA uses these same primordial sounds and music for the benefit of crops. Research has shown that playing primordial sounds, called *Sama Veda,* and the music, *Gandharva Veda,* at prescribed times helps to bring balance and coherence to plants and causes them to grow to their full potential.

In addition to *Sama Veda* and *Gandharva Veda,* there is a wide variety of *Ayurvedic* tools that can be used to help prevent disease, promote growth, and enhance the healing qualities of plants. They include techniques of consciousness, medicinal smoke pots, aromatherapy, herbal medicines, and specially timed and prescribed performances of traditional ancient vibrational chants, called *yagyas*.

The Farmer's Consciousness

Vedic agriculture recognizes that the consciousness of the farmer and those who work on the farm also has a significant influence on the health and nutritive value of a plant. Science shows that people create "field effects," that is, they generate measurable influences on the environment. People are influenced by other people's states of consciousness, too. For instance, if you are in an extreme state of bliss or if you are in a horrible rage, you create a field around you that influences the people and the environment around you.

Research also shows that when people collectively experience higher states of consciousness—particularly during group meditation—the field effect of each individual merges with the others, intensifies, and creates specific and measurable benefits. For instance, when groups of individuals practice a form of meditation called Transcendental Meditation (TM) and an advanced meditation technique called the TM *Sidhi* program, the surrounding geographical area is beneficially affected by a calming influence. In a study published in 1988 in the *Journal of Conflict Resolution,* groups of meditators during the Lebanon war were found to produce an influence that resulted in a significant reduction in war deaths and casualties, when compared to those that occurred on days when no meditators were present. In the summer of 1985, an assembly of thousands of meditators convened in Washington, D.C. During their stay, crime rates went down and the incidence of violence and accidents dropped by 25 percent.

How does the field effect of consciousness work? It works at the quantum level (see Quantum Physics and Consciousness on page 215). Quantum physics says that everything in the universe, when reduced to its finest level—the quantum level—is interconnected and composed of the same material. In other words, if you look beyond the atom, beyond the subatomic parts, you find a nonchanging field of quantum forces/particles that physicists have called the "unified field." This field holds all the laws of Nature. Scientists say that what lies beyond this physical unified field is a unified field of consciousness. The practice of TM strengthens your connection to this unified field of consciousness. When the unified field is directly experienced during the practice of TM, it is enlivened. Because this field holds the laws of Nature, enlivening this field enlivens natural law. The result is that the health of your mind/body is automatically supported and nourished.

Since everything is connected on the quantum level, it's easy to understand how the farmer's consciousness can create a nourishing field of influence on his or her crops. Experiencing the unified field through the regular practice of TM enlivens the laws of Nature, creating a powerful beneficial influence on the plants. You can think of *Vedic* agriculture as quantum-mechanical farming.

Sthapatya Veda Architecture

Because *Vedic* agriculture as a quantum-mechanical science recognizes that all things are interconnected and influence one another, it gives serious thought to the influence caused by the characteristics of the land, its slope, orientation, and other special features, as well as all the buildings on the farm. To optimize a nourishing influence on the growth of the plants, the fields and buildings should be designed according to an ancient form of architecture called *Sthapatya Veda.* Its structures are known to have an extraordinary influence on plant growth. For example, a tree next to a temple in India that was built according to this design blooms twelve months out of the year.

You may be familiar with a similar, but different, form of Chinese architectural design called *feng shui*. Historians believe *feng shui* may have developed from *Sthapatya Veda*. Both systems of architecture are based on the recognition that the structures you live and work in, as well as the characteristics of the land, have powerful effects on your mind/body. The direction in which a building faces, the dimensions and layout of its rooms, the thickness of its walls, the materials used for its construction—all have a predictable influence. *Sthapatya Veda* buildings are designed to create optimal harmony between the individual and all things in Nature, enhancing human physiology and everything in the surrounding area.

On the Vine

A final important step in *Vedic* agriculture is to allow fruits and vegetables to ripen on the vine before picking them. The maximum nutritional benefits of a plant can be achieved only by allowing its produce to vine-ripen. Those of you who have a garden know that there are no words to adequately describe what happens when you bite into freshly picked, vine-ripened food. The explosion of flavor is so incredible compared to "store-bought" foods, it's startling. That's because the taste of vine-ripened food reflects its nutritional qualities.

All the techniques of *Vedic* agriculture are designed to create foods with the highest possible potential for medicines and life-giving nutrients, which then thoroughly metabolize and integrate into your body. As Maharishi Mahesh Yogi so eloquently said, "Conventionally grown foods poison you; organically grown foods won't hurt you; and MVOA foods produce a blissful state of life, maximum coherence, health, and vitality." (See Resources under Maharishi *Vedic* Organic Agriculture.)

Chapter 7

Fields of Gold

How Whole Grains
and Fiber Protect You

*P*icture rolling hills covered with amber fields of whole grains dancing in the wind. Their majestic beauty hints at their special power.
The rustling sound they make as they gently brush against one
another whispers the suggestion that Nature has bestowed upon us another
plant food that contains powerful medicine. These fields of gold are teeming
with plant medicines—medicines so potent and varied that they protect against
breast cancer and other diseases in a multitude of ways. For your Warrior Goddess, they are mighty shafts of intense potential—fundamental instruments of
focused plant intelligence that can fortify you against even the fiercest of foes.

Whole grains have been a primary food staple in the diet of many cultures
for thousands of years, and for good reasons. They are rich in antioxidants, vitamins, trace minerals, fiber, and lignans, all of which promote health and protect
against diseases, especially cancer, cardiovascular disease, diabetes, and obesity.
Not surprisingly, researchers have found that people who consume diets high in
fresh organic fruits, vegetables, and whole grains have the lowest risk of chronic disorders. For example, women who regularly eat these foods cut their risk
of breast cancer by more than 50 percent.

A FEAST OF FIBER

Most plant foods are rich in fiber, particularly whole grains. Fiber is much more
than an effective laxative. It has many medicinal qualities that make it extremely adept at preventing and combating breast cancer. Research shows that women
who eat a high-fiber diet have a 54 percent lower risk of breast cancer.

There are two major types of fiber: soluble and insoluble. Each is important
for good health, and each has special anticancer properties.

Soluble fiber is found in fruits, vegetables, and certain grains, such as oats.

This type of fiber is processed by intestinal bacteria and converted into a powerful deactivator of carcinogens in the colon. Think of it like a bomb squad deactivating bombs. This is one of the reasons why high-fiber vegetarian diets are associated with a much lower risk of colon cancer.

Soluble fiber doesn't add much bulk to your stool, but *insoluble* fiber does. It, therefore, assists in regularity. When there's a lot of bulk to your stool, the time it takes to pass through your colon is much shorter. The faster carcinogens in your stool get out of your colon, the less likely they are to cause damage.

Insoluble fiber is found in large amounts in wheat bran and corn bran. This type of fiber also absorbs and retains water like a sponge—an important characteristic when it comes to protecting against cancer. Insoluble fiber absorbs so much water that it dilutes carcinogens, making them less dangerous. But this is no ordinary sponge; it's a special weapon against breast cancer, absorbing and binding all kinds of potential enemies.

Take, for example, the fact that insoluble fiber binds to estrogen in the colon and eliminates it. If you review Figure 3.1 on page 36, you'll see that estrogen is broken down by your liver, and then sent to the colon to be eliminated. If there is insoluble fiber in your colon, it will bind to the estrogen and facilitate its removal from your body. As a result, the total amount of estrogen in your body will be reduced. Experimental animals fed high-fiber diets (containing both soluble and insoluble fiber) were found to excrete twice as much estrogen in their feces as animals fed low-fiber diets.

Fiber has the same beneficial estrogen-lowering effects in humans, too. In a study of women who ate wheat bran, researchers found that the more wheat bran a woman consumed, the lower her estrogen levels were.

There are several other ways that fiber helps to lower the risk of breast cancer as well. Insoluble fiber takes away much of the threat of certain adversaries, such as simple carbohydrates (including refined sugars) and harmful fats, by slowing down their absorption. But its cancer-fighting abilities don't stop there. Insoluble fiber regulates insulin and glucose, two high-threat opponents that can significantly elevate the risk of breast cancer. Glucose is the principal form of sugar that your cells use for energy. High glucose and insulin levels are one of the biggest risk factors for breast cancer (see Chapter 16).

High-fiber diets also lower the risk of obesity by promoting weight loss. Obesity is thought to be responsible for 20 to 30 percent of all breast cancers diagnosed after menopause. In addition, fiber cuts your risk of obesity and breast cancer by decreasing the amount of fat you absorb from your food, thereby lowering blood-fat levels. High amounts of saturated fats and certain other types of unhealthy fats are also associated with a higher risk of breast cancer.

Whole grains and bran are also rich in antioxidants, vitamins, and trace minerals, all of which support the exceptional ability of your internal healing intelligence to keep you healthy and ward off disease. In addition, whole grains are endowed with generous amounts of a substance called "lignans." Lignans are what give stiffness to the structure of a plant. They are extremely medicinal and can have a big impact on lowering your risk of breast cancer. Scientists have mapped out at least a dozen different ways that lignans help to reduce your risk. The cancer-fighting properties of lignans are discussed in detail in Chapter 9.

Chapter 8

Fats: The Good and the Bad

Fats That Poison and Fats That Protect

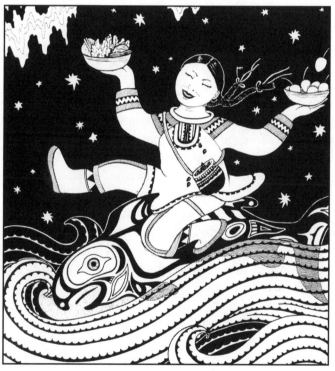

Goddess of Good Oils

Intellectuals solve problems; geniuses prevent them.

—ALBERT EINSTEIN

*F*ats aren't ambivalent when it comes to breast cancer. They're either miraculous in their power to protect or terrible in their power to destroy, accelerating the initiation and growth of breast cancer. Contrary to a common misconception, *not all* fats are bad for you. In fact, certain fats are life-sustaining and absolutely essential to enable your body to function properly. Your Warrior Goddess finds a multitude of uses for these fundamental substances of life. When she is given proper amounts, her energy is boundless, her movements are as agile and lyrical as a dancer's, and her complexion is luxuriant and glows like the full moon. She exudes these qualities because you have provided her with the resources she needs to stay strong and supple. You have also given her the material she needs to craft her many sly and slippery modes of defense against disease. In order to more fully understand how she does this, it is important to first discuss basics about nutrition.

The food you eat each day is composed of nutrients. These nutrients supply your body with fuel for energy production, with building blocks for tissue repair and construction, and with all the substances your body needs to initiate chemical reactions and carry out body functions. The nutrients you consume influence your risk of breast cancer. Depending on what you eat, they can either increase your risk, decrease your risk, or have no effect on it whatsoever.

There are two broad categories of nutrients: macronutrients and micronutrients. Macronutrients are the nutrients that we need in relatively large amounts. They are carbohydrates, fats, and proteins. All packaged-food labels list the amounts of these three macronutrients. Because we also need water in large amounts each day, some nutritionists consider water a macronutrient, too. Micronutrients—vitamins and minerals—are discussed in Chapter 12.

Your body is constantly rebuilding itself, and carbohydrates, fats, and proteins supply the fuel and building materials. Most of the cells in your body have preprogrammed deaths. That means they are designed to live for a certain amount of time and die. New cells then replace these worn-out cells. This process is called "cell turnover."

Cell turnover plays an important part in your risk of cancer. Certain cells in your body turn over at a faster rate than other cells. For example, the lining of the intestines and breast and prostate cells turn over fairly frequently. The faster the cells turn over, the higher the risk is of a cancer developing. That's why cancers of the breast, prostate, and colon are so much more common than cancers in other parts of your body, where cells turn over slowly or, perhaps, not at all, like the heart.

There are different kinds of proteins, carbohydrates, and fats, and each of them has a different effect on your body and on your risk of breast cancer. Later in the book we will look at certain proteins and carbohydrates and how they affect your risk of breast cancer. Meanwhile, let's take a closer look at fat.

FATS AREN'T ALL BAD

Fat has gotten a bad rap. It's a substance that we have been taught to avoid, but the truth is certain fats are vital to life. For instance, every cell in your body has a membrane that is composed primarily of fat. Without proper amounts of fat in your diet, your cells can't function well. All your nerve cells, including those in your brain, are coated with fat. And this fatty sheath is what enables electrical impulses to travel through them. If there's a problem with this fatty sheath, as there is in multiple sclerosis, the ability of nerve impulses to move along these pathways is severely impaired and, as a result, so is your ability to move and think. Fat also serves as your body's main storage unit of fuel. It provides insulation, assists in wound healing, is used to make hormones, and protects you from trauma.

Fats make up the fundamental structure of every cell membrane. You've heard the cliché "You are what you eat." This statement is absolutely true. Your body can only use the materials you supply to rebuild itself. That means the type of fat structuring your cell membranes can *only* be the type of fat you have eaten. The specific type of fat that predominantly makes up your cell membranes determines how well those membranes will function. It also affects how well your whole body functions. If your cell membranes are composed primarily of health-promoting fats, they will be able to carry out their duties with perfect competence and ease. If health-destroying fats have the upper hand, the ability of your cell membranes to perform their tasks will be severely impaired.

Here's a good analogy: Your car needs certain fats—oil—to run properly. If you don't put oil in the engine, you're headed for big trouble. The engine will soon suffer irreversible damage. If you put the wrong kind of oil in the engine, it won't run very well or very efficiently, either. Over time, this misguided choice of oil will clog the engine. However, if you put the ideal high-quality oil in your car, the engine will run extremely well. And if you keep using top-grade oil in the right amounts, your car's engine will continue to run well for a long time.

Balance Is Everything

Although you need fats for your body to run well, too much of a good thing can be bad. This concept is expressed through the *Ayurvedic* principle: *The right things in the right amounts at the right times will bring balance.* Remember, perfect balance means perfect health. If you eat the wrong things in the wrong amounts at the wrong times, you cause imbalances, and all diseases start as imbalances.

Eating excessive amounts of fat, especially certain types of "bad" fats, significantly increases your risk of several types of cancer, including breast cancer, as well as other serious diseases. High-fat diets increase your chances of developing breast cancer because they amplify the production of estrogen in your body. Remember, the more estrogen your body makes, the higher your risk is. Researchers have found that diets high in saturated animal fats may boost your risk of breast cancer by 50 percent or more. If you have breast cancer, eating a diet high in fat may decrease your chances of survival. Out of fourteen studies looking at women with breast cancer and their intake of dietary fat, eight showed that the women who ate a high-fat diet had a higher death rate than those who ate diets that were lower in fat.

The good news is, if you reduce the amount of fat in your diet, you can substantially lower your risk of breast cancer. A study published in the *British Journal of Cancer* confirmed this fact. The women in the study were put on a low-fat diet. Their daily intake of calories from fat normally made up about 30 to 40 percent of their total calories. They were given a diet in which fat supplied only 15 percent of their daily calories. The amount of estradiol (the most common and most potent type of natural estrogen in your body and the one that correlates to your risk of breast cancer) in their blood was measured before they went on the low-fat diet. It was measured again after they had followed the low-fat diet for two years. Researchers found that the level of estradiol in these women dropped by 20 percent over the two years. That means that their risk of breast cancer dropped substantially *more* than 20 percent, because small changes in estradiol translate into big changes in your risk.

Another study investigated the influence of a low-fat diet on total estrogen levels (all three types of natural estrogens—estradiol, estrone, and estriol) after a much shorter period of time. The women in this study had a 20 percent drop in their estrogen levels after an average of only five to six months on a low-fat diet.

BAD FATS

Certain types of fat are very bad for your body. They damage your overall health and significantly increase your risk of breast cancer and other serious diseases. The worst types of fats are saturated fats—especially animal fats—and fats that have been chemically altered, called trans fats or hydrogenated fats.

Saturated Animal Fats

Eating a diet high in saturated animal fats, like those found in red meat and high-fat dairy products, notably increases your risk of breast cancer. A study published in the *Journal of the National Cancer Institute* in 2003 interviewed 90,655 women and found that premenopausal women between the ages of twenty-six and forty-six who consumed the highest amounts of red meat and high-fat dairy had a higher risk of breast cancer than those who ate only a small amount of these fats.

What's interesting, according to the study's principal researcher, Eunyong Cho, is that this study "found that earlier [dietary habits] have a stronger impact on later breast cancer risk. In other words, women had an increased risk if, as young adults, they had a higher intake of animal fat, mainly from meat and dairy fat." But don't think that this means there's nothing you can do now to reverse the damage. You can. Remember, other studies show that decreasing your saturated-fat intake lowers your estrogen levels and significantly reduces your danger of developing breast cancer.

When you eat saturated animal fats, they make the cells throughout your body more insulin resistant and consequently increase the level of insulin in your blood. This seemingly innocent, normal response actually brings on a flood of increased risk; high insulin levels are one of the biggest risk factors and promoters of breast cancer. Women with abnormally elevated insulin levels have a 283 percent higher risk of breast cancer than those with normal insulin levels (see Chapter 16).

Saturated animal fats are a storehouse for concentrated toxic chemicals such as pesticides. Some of these chemicals mimic estrogen and make cell division in the breast speed up rapidly. As you now know, the faster cells divide in your breast, the higher your risk of breast cancer. If the animals and animal products you eat were not organically raised, the level of toxic chemicals in them can be quite high. In addition, these animals are commonly given hormones and growth factors that, when you ingest them, speed up breast-cell division. These hormones are also very dangerous for women with breast cancer, because they cause breast tumors to grow more rapidly.

Organic, but Not Toxin-Free

By law, organically raised animals must be fed only organically grown foods. They cannot be given any antibiotics, hormones, or growth factors. Despite this, organically raised animals aren't always completely toxin-free. Some of them may have small amounts of toxic chemicals concentrated in their fat. Why are there toxins in organic animals? Primarily because, instead up being confined in stalls, they graze in pastures. Although being outdoors is a good thing, our environment is contaminated with hundreds, if not thousands, of toxins. Rainwater may, and often does, contain poisonous chemicals. When it rains, these dangerous compounds fall onto the pasture and into the ponds where organic animals eat and drink.

There's another reason why organically raised animals may contain toxins. Harmful chemicals are generally very persistent in our environment. That means that they don't break down easily. For a farm to become certified organic, no synthetic or potentially unsafe chemicals may have been used on the land for at least three years. But some of these toxins persist in the soil for much longer than three years. In fact, it's not unusual for them to last twenty years or more.

IGF-1: A Top Breast Health Enemy

The body naturally produces insulin-like growth factors (IGFs). In normal concentrations, they play a necessary role in the manufacture of body tissue. However, an elevated level of insulin-like growth factor-1 (IGF-1) is a huge promoter of breast cancer, as well as prostate and colon cancers. In fact, scientists have found that there's nothing we know of that stimulates breast cancer or prostate cancer more than IGF-1! Promoting excessive amounts of this growth factor is like throwing rocket fuel onto the flames of cancer.

You can avoid inundating your body with excessive amounts of IGF-1 by steering clear of conventional dairy products. In the United States, cows are routinely injected with the genetically engineered growth hormone recombinant bovine growth hormone (rBGH). When rBGH is injected into a cow, it causes the natural growth factor IGF-1 to be released into the body of the cow. Cows injected with rBGH have been found to have unusually high levels of IGF-1 in their fat and milk. When you consume IGF-1 in animal products, it normally breaks down in your stomach and causes no harm. But when IGF-1 is consumed in milk, it doesn't break down. The protein in milk, called casein, prevents IGF-1 from breaking down, so it's all absorbed into your body.

A study published in the British journal *The Lancet* in 1998 documented the enormous risk associated with high levels of IGF-1. The risk of breast cancer among premenopausal women younger than fifty-one who had the highest levels of IGF-1 in their blood was found to be 700 percent higher than the average.

The reason that the IGF-1 bite is so venomous is because there are IGF-1 receptors on breast cells, just as there are estrogen receptors. Research has found that IGF-1 and estrogen interact. According to a study from Georgetown University published in 2002, estradiol and IGF-1, through a complex "cross-talk" mechanism, stimulate normal breast cells to start dividing.

In summary, when you eat the nonorganic saturated animal fats found in meat and dairy products, your risk of breast cancer escalates from a triple threat:

1. High insulin levels (as a response to the saturated fats),

2. High IGF-1 levels (from rBGH-injected cows), and

3. Toxic estrogenic hormones and chemicals (either injected into or fed to the cows).

This is why you should avoid nonorganic red meats and dairy as much as possible. If you simply must have dairy products, you can minimize your risk by eating only those that have been organically produced and are low in fat.

Trans Fats: Another Top Enemy of Breast Health

Of all the fats you can eat, trans fats are the most dangerous. Trans fats are man-made. They are natural fats that have been chemically altered by adding extra hydrogen atoms. That's why they are also called "hydrogenated" or "partially hydrogenated" fats. Chemical engineers created these fats in an effort to make processed foods taste better and to increase their shelf life. They were successful. Hydrogenated fats make foods such as potato chips crispier, and they increase the shelf life of processed foods such as crackers, chips, cookies, and baked goods. But what the engineers didn't know was that the fats they created would also promote serious diseases, including heart disease and cancer.

The reason trans fats are so bad for you is because they promote oxygen free radicals—molecules that cause damage to your cells and DNA, damage that can lead to cancer. (For more about oxygen free radicals, see Chapter 13.) Trans fats also encourage inflammation, which, in turn, creates more oxygen free radicals. Chronic inflammation has been identified as a key factor in the initiation and progression of breast cancer.

All these ill effects add up to a high probability of developing breast cancer. Research has found that women with the highest amounts of trans fats in their bodies have a 40 percent increased risk. And if that isn't bad enough, cancer isn't the only disease provoked by chronic inflammation. It's thought to play a large role in many degenerative diseases, including heart disease, the number-one killer of American men and women.

Omega-6 Fatty Acids

Fats are made up of smaller units of molecules called fatty acids. Omega-6 fatty acids are needed by your body to function properly. But if you eat too much of them, they increase your risk of breast cancer. Studies have found that women with the highest amounts of omega-6 fatty acids in their bodies have a 69 percent increased risk of breast cancer. If you have breast cancer, eating large amounts of omega-6 fatty acids can make your prognosis—and your chance of survival—worse. A high intake of these fatty acids increases the likelihood that your cancer will metastasize, spreading to other parts of your body. The following is a partial list of the foods and oils that are high in omega-6 fatty acids.

- Borage oil
- Commercial salad dressings
- Corn oil
- Cottonseed oil

- Grape seed oil
- Margarine
- Mayonnaise
- Peanut oil

- Primrose oil
- Safflower oil
- Sesame oil
- Soybean oil

Omega-6 fatty acids are essential for your body to function properly, so don't eliminate all omega-6 fatty acids from your diet. In the following section "Omega-3 Fatty Acids," there's more information on the best amounts to consume. Also, see the section "Conjugated Linoleic Acids (CLAs)" on page 75 for a discussion of this health-promoting type of omega-6 fatty acid.

GOOD FATS

As the ancient Chinese described, there is a yin (dark) and yang (light) side to all things; fats are no exception. The devastation caused by destructive fats is inversely proportional to the powerful shielding force of protective fats. Certain types of fats have extraordinary healing benefits. These "good" fats help your body to function properly and noticeably reduce your risk of such diseases as heart disease and cancer.

Omega-3 Fatty Acids

The most health-promoting type of fat you can eat is composed of omega-3 fatty acids. They reduce your risk of breast cancer considerably in two major ways. First, omega-3 fatty acids decrease the power of estrogen in the breast, so that cells won't divide as quickly in response to estrogen. Second, they act to subdue inflammation.

Omega-3 fatty acids also help to fight breast cancer if you already have it, and they do so very impressively. Research has found that they cause breast tumors to shrink in size and prevent them from metastasizing. In fact, omega-3 fatty acids are so powerful in subverting the spread of tumors in the body that women with the highest levels of omega-3s in their bodies have only one-fifth the incidence of metastasis that occurs in women with the lowest levels.

The best plant source of omega-3 fatty acids is flaxseeds. Flaxseeds contain considerably more omega-3s than any other known edible plant. When it comes to combating breast cancer, flaxseeds exhibit superhero power. But an abundant supply of omega-3s is only one of the reasons flaxseeds are so beneficial. For more information about flaxseeds, see Chapter 9.

Omega-3 fatty acids can also be found in notable amounts in other foods—for example, walnuts and certain fish, such as salmon and herring. But—and this is a *big but*—*fish is now one of the most toxic foods you can eat* because we've polluted our lakes, rivers, and oceans so badly. In fact, fish contain more concentrated amounts of dangerous chemicals than any other food source.

If you think eating farm-raised fish is safer, think again. An article published in *The New York Times* on July 30, 2003, reported findings by the Environmental Working Group, a nonprofit environmental research and advocacy group, on ten samples of farmed salmon bought at markets on the East and West coasts. (Farmed salmon accounts for 60 percent of all salmon eaten in the United States.) All the fish samples were contaminated with polychlorinated biphenyls (PCBs) at levels far higher than any other protein source, including all other types of seafood. (See Chapter 21 and the inset "What Are PCBs?" on page 74.) For this reason, I don't recommend eating fish to get your omega-3s. (Instead, choose flaxseeds and other good omega-3 sources such as walnuts, pumpkin seeds, hemp seeds, soybeans, some dark green leafy vegetables, winter squash, and ground oregano.)

When it comes to omega-3 and omega-6 fatty acids, it's the ratio that you consume of them that makes all the difference—how much you eat of one compared to the other. The body functions best when you eat a 4:1 ratio of omega-6s to omega-3s. The typical American diet has a dangerous ratio of about 20:1. As you now know, consuming excessive amounts of omega-6 fatty acids is extremely dangerous.

Omega-9 Fatty Acids

Those who follow a Mediterranean-style diet have only half the breast cancer risk of those who follow the standard American diet. Researchers think there are two main reasons for this. First, the Mediterranean diet is high in fruits and vegetables, and second, it includes a lot of olive oil, which is high in omega-9 fatty acids. Omega-9s have a neutral effect in the breast; by themselves, they neither increase nor decrease the effect of estrogen. But researchers have found that women who eat copious amounts of olive oil have a lower risk of breast cancer. So, what's the reason?

All the fats that you eat compete with one another for a place in your body. It's like a game of musical chairs. When you eat more omega-9 fatty acids than bad fats, the bad fats are overwhelmed by the large number of omega-9s vying for a spot in your body. The more omega-9s there are, the fewer the number of

What Are PCBs?

PCBs are a group of 209 different compounds. They were first brought to the market by the Monsanto Corporation in 1929. (Monsanto is also the company principally responsible for creating genetically altered foods.) PCBs were used in electrical transformers, adhesives, fluorescent lighting, flame retardants, and paints. Their primary use, however, was as a dielectric fluid in electrical equipment. Because of their stability and resistance to thermal breakdown, as well as their insulating properties, they were the fluid of choice for transformers and capacitors. As a matter of fact, they were required by some fire codes due to their exceptional fire resistance.

But after a few decades of use, it was discovered that PCBs caused an alarming number of serious health problems, so corporations were forced to stop manufacturing them in the late 1970s and early 1980s. These health problems include suppression of the immune system, headaches, depression, numbness, abnormal heart rhythm, impaired long-term memory, loss of coordination, liver failure, disruption of the endocrine system, and cancer. Pregnant women with high PCB counts are more likely to have children with physical, behavioral, and cognitive problems.

Even though PCBs are no longer made, an estimated two-thirds of all the PCBs manufactured between 1930 and 1970 are still in use or are in waste dumps, slowly leeching into our water supply. PCBs are extremely resistant to degradation. So, scientists say that the remaining one-third are still somewhere in our environment. Disturbingly, experts expect that they will persist for hundreds of years.

PCBs are a huge problem in the Great Lakes. They are thought to have entered the lake water from contaminated landfills, leaking tankers, rainwater, and birds. The levels of PCBs in lake water measure between 5 and 60 parts per thousand (ppt). PCBs, like other toxins, become concentrated in animal flesh, and it is this "bioconcentration" phenomenon that poses significant danger to us. Here's how it works: Medium-sized fish eat hundreds of small fish, each with concentrated toxins stored in their flesh. The toxins from these hundreds of small fish then concentrate into the medium-sized fish's flesh. Then, a bigger fish eats hundreds of these medium-sized fish and concentrates all of their toxins into its flesh, and so on. This is why fish that are large enough for human consumption usually have perilous amounts of toxins. For example, commercial-sized fish from the Great Lakes are found to have PCB levels as high as 17,000,000 ppt. This level is considered extremely dangerous to your health. Women who eat the most fish from the Great Lakes give birth to children with a multitude of problems, especially attention deficit hyperactivity disorder (ADHD), learning disabilities, and reproductive disorders.

bad fats that can successfully grab a position in your breast cells. In addition, olive oil is a rich source of cancer-fighting antioxidants.

When you purchase olive oil, *always* remember to buy certified organic. If your local grocery store doesn't carry it, ask the manager to order it. (See the Resources section under Organic Foods.)

Conjugated Linoleic Acids (CLAs)

Conjugated linoleic acids (CLAs) are a mixture of unique omega-6 fatty acids that have a slightly different molecular structure from the omega-6s associated with an increased risk of breast cancer. CLAs have the opposite effect of normal omega-6 fatty acids; they lower the risk of breast cancer. CLAs occur naturally in certain foods, but not in sufficient quantities. Therefore, to benefit from their anticancer properties, you must take a daily supplement. Research shows that supplemental CLAs help to prevent the initiation of breast cancer by toxic chemicals. If you have breast cancer, CLAs are beneficial for you, too. They encourage cancer cells to stop growing and deter the tumor from spreading to other parts of your body.

One way CLAs appear to work is by reducing the effect of estrogen (in some yet-to-be-identified way). CLAs also cause structural changes in breast tissue that make it more resistant to damage from oxygen free radicals and toxins known to initiate breast cancer. According to a study conducted in Finland, these protective effects are profound: Women with the highest amounts of CLAs in their blood had the lowest incidence of breast cancer.

Another way that CLAs may help to lower the risk of breast cancer is by promoting higher lean-muscle mass and lower body fat. That's why bodybuilders use CLAs as a supplement. Remember, fat cells make estrogen, and the more estrogen your body makes, the higher your risk of breast cancer. So, reducing body fat is one effective way to lower your risk of this terrible disease. (By the way, when figuring your 4:1 ratio of omega-6 to omega-3, you do not need to take your supplemental CLA into account.)

Chapter 9

A Fortress
of Seeds

Flax—The Medicine Within

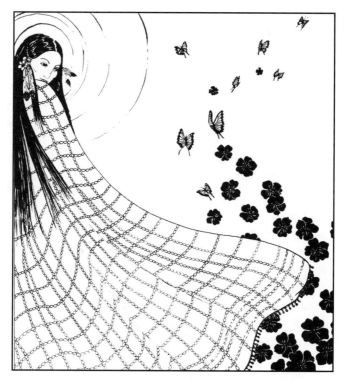

Goddess of Flax

Flowers and fruits are only the beginning.
In the seed lies the life and the future.

—MARION ZIMMER BRADLEY

*H*ippocrates said, "Let food be your medicine and medicine be your food." *Ayurveda* recognized that foods could be a source of medicine thousands of years before Hippocrates and proclaimed, *Food should be the first medicine you take, because without a proper diet, no medicine will work; with a proper diet, no medicine is necessary.* The ancient Chinese agreed, stating, "He who takes medicine and neglects diet wastes the skill of the physician."

If you were given only one choice of a food to take as medicine, your best choice would be the tiny seeds from the flax plant. Flaxseeds have more potent medicinal qualities—especially those that fight breast cancer—than any known edible plant. This small seed provides a fortress of protection against this killer.

1. OMEGA-3 FATTY ACIDS

The intelligence contained in flax is so spectacular that it coordinates a sensational offense against breast cancer. Flax has three notable distinctions. First, it's the richest plant source of omega-3 fatty acids. Research has found that women who eat the highest amounts of omega-3s have the lowest risk of breast cancer.

Omega-3 fatty acids help to lower the risk of breast cancer by quieting inflammation and by decreasing the rate at which breast cells divide in response to estrogen. Inflammation is a key factor in the initiation and progression of a variety of diseases including heart disease, rheumatoid arthritis, skin diseases, and cancers (such as breast cancer). If you have breast cancer, omega-3s have been found to help shrink breast tumors and prevent them from spreading to other parts of the body.

2. LIGNANS

The second exceptional quality of flax has to do with lignans. Lignans are natural plant compounds that help to give plants their stiff structure. They also possess extraordinary anticancer properties, with an astonishing ability to help protect against and fight breast cancer. Lignans are found abundantly in certain fruits, vegetables, beans, seeds, and legumes—including garlic, carrots, broccoli, asparagus, dried apricots, and prunes. But the amount of lignans in these plants is miniscule compared to that in flaxseeds. Flaxseeds contain at least 100 times more lignans than any other known edible plant!

Lignans deter and arrest the growth of breast cancer in a multitude of ways. First, they act as a weak estrogen (similar to how genistein acts in soy; see Chapter 10). Second, lignans change the structure of the breast, making it more resistant to the toxins that induce cancer. Third, if you have breast cancer, lignans can stop the tumor cells from growing and help to prevent the metastasis of your tumor. They do this by decreasing two growth factors that fuel the fires of breast cancer: insulin-like growth factor-1 (IGF-1) and epidermal growth factor. As you may recall, IGF-1 is thought to be one of the most dangerous and potent risk factors for breast and prostate cancer.

There is another cancer-enhancing growth factor that lignans thwart, called "vascular endothelial growth factor" (VEGF). VEGF aids in the growth of cancer cells by stimulating new blood vessels to grow. How can new blood vessels affect the rate of growth of cancer cells? Here's how: In order for a tumor to grow larger, it needs more nutrients—nutrients that can be delivered only by new blood vessels. So, the more blood vessels that grow into a tumor, the more food that is delivered to it, and the faster it will grow. In fact, without new blood vessels, tumors can't grow larger. Cancer specialists recently discovered that this anti-cancer tactic used by lignans—blocking VEGF—is so powerful at stopping tumor growth that they have created a new anticancer drug that works this same way. It is called Avastin (bevacizumab) and was released on the market in 2004. Avastin is currently approved only for the treatment of metastatic colon cancer and must be given in combination with another chemotherapeutic drug called 5-FU.

Lignans have several additional ways that they reduce the risk of breast cancer. They create more of the "good" kind of estrogen (similar to how indole-3 carbinol works), and reduce the production of estrogen by fat cells. According to a 1993 study from the University of Rochester, flaxseeds high in lignans also lengthen the menstrual cycle. For example, if a woman has a menstrual period every twenty-eight days and then starts consuming flaxseeds, her cycles may lengthen to every thirty-two days. The longer your menstrual cycles are, the fewer the number of cycles you will have over your lifetime, and the less estradiol you will produce. Simply put, the longer your menstrual cycles are, the lower your risk of breast cancer is.

All of the very effective schemes that lignans use to combat breast cancer add up to lots of protection. Research shows that women with the highest amounts of lignans in their urine—a reflection of how much they consume in their diet—have the lowest risk of breast cancer.

In the fall of 2003, a new supplement that is made of isolated, purified, and concentrated lignans from flaxseeds, called Brevail, was released on the market. The dose in one daily capsule was strategically designed to create levels of lignans in the body that are in the same range as those found in women with the lowest risk of breast cancer. There are two major benefits to taking supplemental lignans. First, the amount of lignans in flax can vary from crop to crop by as much as 300 percent, whereas those in the supplement are standardized so you always get the optimal amount. Second, studies show that the lignans in Brevail are absorbed eighteen times more effectively than they are from ground flaxseeds. So, taking lignans in this supplemental form guarantees that you get the healthiest dose of lignans every day. Brevail is not recommended for women who are pregnant or currently breastfeeding, not because it isn't safe, but because no studies have been conducted yet on this special group of women to analyze the effects and proper dose.

Taking Brevail with other cancer drugs is also not recommended because this product hasn't been studied in women currently undergoing cancer treatment. However, that may change in the near future. A study published in the journal *Breast Cancer Research and Treatment* in July 2003 found that lignans enhance the effectiveness of the common cancer medication Tamoxifen. Researchers J. Chen and Lillian Thompson found that lignans and Tamoxifen, alone and— better yet—in combination, reduce the ability of estrogen-receptor-negative tumor cells to stick together, invade, and migrate—all important properties in cancer's metastasis. More research is needed to determine the exact role this supplement may play in cancer treatment.

Brevail is standardized to one type of lignan found in flax, "secoisolariciresinol diglycoside" (SDG). Of all the lignans found in flax, SDG is the one found in the highest amounts and is possibly the most potent. If you decide to take Brevail, I think it's a good idea to eat flaxseed, too. In addition to the advantages of lignans, flax has many other anticancer properties that you wouldn't want to miss out on.

I recommend eating at least 3 tablespoons of *ground* flaxseeds a day. The hard seeds can't be digested, so grind them in a coffee grinder until they become a fine nutty powder. Add the ground seeds to just about anything you like: vegetable dishes, salads, smoothies, baked goods such as muffins, and cereal.

3. FIBER

The third property of flax that lowers your risk of breast cancer is its abundant fiber. High-fiber diets are associated with a 54 percent lower risk of breast cancer. Fiber helps to lower the amount of estrogen in your body by binding to it in your intestines and then expelling it from your body.

A MAGNIFICENT CAPE

To put the power of flaxseeds into perspective, consider this: If your Warrior Goddess were to create a majestic cloak of divine protection for herself, she would require a fabric made of the finest natural substance possessing a multitude of miraculous powers. She would search the world until she found the most magnificent fiber she could to create her cape of supernatural strength. Her expedition would end the moment she encountered the flaxseed. Her refined intuition would instantly tell her that this tiny seed was no ordinary seed. Rather, flax is the source of a rare and astonishing intelligence, the perfect material for creating a barrier against breast cancer.

Chapter 10
Asian Defense
Soy Foods

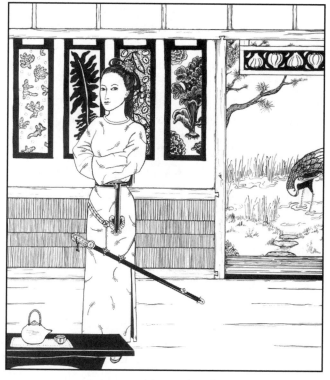

Asian Goddess of Defense

Never be afraid to try something new.
Remember, amateurs built the ark;
professionals built the Titanic.

—AUTHOR UNKNOWN

*T*he East is known for its martial arts: elegant beautiful forms of movement that can be used to induce balance and healing or to deliver deadly blows to ward off formidable foes. Several foods in the traditional Asian diet, especially soy foods, strengthen the physiology, and attack and defend against breast cancer with the skill of a *Ninja* warrior. These foods are some of your Warrior Goddess's favorite weapons against this enemy—eating these foods is like arming her with *samurai* swords, *nunchucks,* and *shurikens* (throwing stars).

Soy—a superstar in your arsenal against breast cancer—has been a food staple in the Asian diet for thousands of years. Asia has far lower rates of cancer than the United States does, and researchers think that eating a lot of soy may be one of the reasons. Japanese men and women eat about ten times more soy than American men and women. According to many studies, if you eat an adequate amount of soy often enough, your risk of breast cancer will drop by 30 to 50 percent. For instance, a study published in the *Journal of the National Cancer Institute* in June 2003 found that women who ate three bowls of miso soup (a soup made with soybean paste) a day had a 40 percent lower risk of breast cancer. Those who ate two bowls of miso soup a day cut their risk by 26 percent.

GENISTEIN—SOY'S MOST IMPORTANT PHYTOCHEMICAL

There are several substances in soy that are active against breast cancer. A particular type of phytochemical called genistein appears to be one of the most important protagonists. Genistein is classified as a phytoestrogen, or plant estrogen, because it has a weak estrogenic effect. Two other major phytoestrogens in soy are daidzein and glycitein. However, genistein is the most abundant and well researched of the three and is usually the only one that is listed on the label of soy products.

Research shows that genistein is extraordinarily effective at reducing the risk of breast cancer. It has been shown to stop tumor growth, prevent metastasis, and shut off new blood vessels in growing tumors. One reason why genistein is able to prevent and fight breast cancer is because it blocks the cancer-promoting estrogens from attaching to the estrogen receptors on breast cells.

Let's review how this beast grows. Breast cancer is a hormonal disease. That means that a hormone causes the cancer to develop by inciting cells to grow and divide. For breast cancer, that hormone is estrogen. The more estrogen you are exposed to, the higher your risk of breast cancer is.

Estrogens come in different strengths and behave differently. Strong estrogens increase your risk of cancer because they tell cells to grow and divide rapidly. Phytoestrogens and other weak estrogens decrease your risk of cancer

Understanding Phytoestrogens

There is currently a lot of confusion and misinformation about phyto-estrogens. It is important to understand that plant estrogens are *not the* same as the estrogens our bodies make or the synthetic estrogens found in hormone replacement therapy (HRT) or birth control pills. They are very different. Most act more like selective estrogen modulators (SERMs), such as the cancer medication Tamoxifen, and as inhibitors of the enzyme aro-matase (which is used in the production of estrogen), like the new anti-cancer drug Arimidex. In other words, phytoestrogens act more like estrogen blockers than like estrogen. They act in so many complex ways that we may never fully understand them all.

because they slow down cell division. Genistein acts like a weak estrogen in the body. It blocks the effects of strong estrogens and slows down cell division. Genistein is very weak—in fact, less than $1/100$ of the strength of estradiol (the most potent type of natural estrogen). So, if genistein attaches to an estrogen receptor, the rate of cell division is only $1/100$ of the speed that it is if estradiol attaches to the receptor. The more genistein there is to compete with estradiol, the slower the rate of cell division and the lower your risk of breast cancer.

This is an extremely simplistic look at a very complicated process. Remember, soy is composed of hundreds of components all interacting together. Genistein doesn't act alone. If it's extracted from whole soy foods and then isolated and consumed without the other soy ingredients, it can actually have detrimental effects (see The Soy Controversy on page 84).

SOY CONSUMPTION IN PREPUBESCENT GIRLS

Many studies show that young girls who eat soy products before they go through puberty have a substantially lower risk of breast cancer later in life. One explanation for this finding is that a woman's breast tissue is considered "immature" before she has had her first baby. Immature breast tissue is more sensitive to environmental toxins and other carcinogens. Soy has been found to help mature the breast tissue, making it more resistant to environmental toxins. According to a study published in *Carcinogenesis* in 2004, exposure to soy prior to puberty triggers another protective action—it "up-regulates" the breast cancer 1 (BRCA1) gene, a tumor-suppression gene. In other words, soy turns on a gene that suppresses tumor growth—and keeps it on.

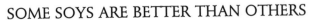

SOME SOYS ARE BETTER THAN OTHERS

There are dozens of different types of soy foods available, but when it comes to nutrients and health-promoting qualities, not all soy products are the same. Some soy foods are far better for you than others. Here are six great ones:

1. **Steamed or boiled soybeans in the pod, also called *edamame*.** Only the beans are eaten; the tough, fibrous pod is discarded.

2. **Dry roasted soybeans.** These make a great snack food. There are several different flavors to choose from, including ranch and, my personal favorite, Cajun.

3. **Tempeh.** This traditional Asian and Indonesian food is growing in popularity, so you can find it in most grocery stores. It's a cultured soy cake that sometimes has other grains or spices added to it. You can cook tempeh a number of ways: sauté it in olive oil, bake it, crumble it into salads or stews, use it as a sandwich filling, or add it to a stir-fry dish.

4. **Tofu.** Made from soymilk curd, tofu looks a little like cheese. Its own flavor is very mild, but it will pick up the flavor of any dish you add it to. You can use it in at least 101 different ways, so I suggest you get a good tofu cookbook and experiment. (For a list of some tofu cookbooks, see the Recommended Reading section.)

5. **Miso.** Miso (fermented soybean paste) is a salty condiment that can be used to flavor a variety of dishes. Added to boiling water, it makes an excellent soup.

6. **Natto.** This form of soy is made from fermented cooked whole soybeans. It comes in a variety of flavors and is commonly used in sushi rolls and with rice in Japanese restaurants. It's less popular than other soy products, so you are more likely to find it in an Asian market than at your local grocery store.

How much soy should you consume each day to lower your risk of breast cancer? Experts say about 4–12 ounces of a quality soy product. However, if you want to eat a little less soy than that but still get the same (or even better) cancer-fighting effects, you can add certain traditional Asian spices to your soy dishes. (See the inset "Add a Little Spice to Your Life" on page 85.)

THE SOY CONTROVERSY

Some physicians warn their patients not to eat soy foods because they fear that soy may increase the risk of breast cancer instead of decreasing it. Their mistaken fear comes primarily from one study from the University of California,

San Francisco, published in October 1996. In this study, women were given 38 grams of genistein a day for one year. It's important to note that these women were not given genistein as it occurs naturally in whole soy foods. Rather, they were given genistein that had been extracted and isolated from soy foods and prepared as a supplement—a supplement composed *only* of genistein with none of the hundreds of other nutrients in soy.

The researchers were surprised to discover that instead of having a protective effect, the genistein supplement appeared to be harmful. After one year on the genistein supplement, the women had elevated the amounts of estradiol in their blood and their breast cells showed signs of stimulation and increased growth. This unexpected result concerned researchers. Could soy actually *increase* the risk of cancer? Hundreds of other studies show that women who eat the most soy have the lowest risk of breast cancer. So, how could a genistein isolate have the opposite effect? Remember the *Ayurvedic* principle: *Favor fresh whole foods.*

The women in the controversial study didn't eat fresh whole soy foods. They were given an isolate of genistein—something that doesn't naturally occur in Nature. When you isolate a substance from the whole, it often behaves differently. Your body was designed to eat, digest, and metabolize fresh *whole* foods, which contain hundreds, even thousands, of substances all interacting with one another. Those interactions can be critically important. One substance may balance the effect of another, make it more or less effective, take away its toxic effects, increase its absorption, or modify how your body uses it in some important way.

Add a Little Spice to Your Life

When you cook soy, you can exponentially enhance its anticancer power by simply adding a pinch of turmeric or cumin. Both of these spices defend against and sabotage the growth of breast cancer in many clever ways (see Chapter 11).

A 1997 study from Tufts University in Boston found that when turmeric and genistein are combined, they have a synergistic effect. In other words, each one makes the other more effective. Researchers used certain highly estrogenic pesticides, endosulfan/chlordane/DDT, to start some breast cancer tumors—estradiol for others—growing in the laboratory. Both genistein and curcumin (an active ingredient in turmeric and cumin) prevented the growth of the tumor cells—but not completely. When they were added together, the effect was so strong, all tumor-cell growth stopped.

Research shows that when genistein is consumed as part of whole soy foods, it's absorbed very differently from how it is in an isolated supplemental form. Genistein in whole soy is activated by intestinal bacteria during digestion, whereas genistein taken as an isolated supplement is absorbed *before* it reaches the bacteria in the intestines. This may be part of the reason that genistein supplements appear to have an effect different from that of whole soy foods. So, until research shows otherwise, stay away from genistein supplements and eat whole soy foods.

The Problem with Isolated Plant Elements

The isolated "active" ingredients of a plant don't express its full intelligence. Products that contain only certain elements of whole plants can miss out on all the other healing qualities of the plant delivered in the way Nature intended. Worse, sometimes isolates can have undesirable health effects because we are consuming substances in a concentration and form not found in Nature.

A whole plant contains hundreds, if not thousands, of different substances all interacting together. When you disrupt the balance in the plant, it's more than likely that you will disrupt the balance in yourself. Good health is all about balance. You don't want to take something for its medicinal qualities if it's going to throw the rest of you out of balance, sparking the development of another disease that may be worse than the one you're treating or trying to avoid. This is a common problem with pharmaceutical medications. They treat one problem, but often create others.

Ayurveda, on the other hand, contains an extremely sophisticated knowledge of the ideal way to administer herbs so that they *don't* create imbalances. *Ayurvedic* herbal medicines are usually mixtures of several different herbs acting synergistically, one enhancing or balancing the effects of another. So, according to the ancient time-tested principle of *Ayurveda,* isolating the "active ingredient" is a step in the wrong direction, away from trying to create an ideal medicine.

This brings up another important *Ayurvedic* principle: *Never sacrifice health for the sake of a cure.* Treatments should not create imbalances or disease. All the herbs and treatments in *Ayurveda* are formulated and designed to enhance balance and increase the body's healing intelligence. If an herb is used to help suppress a symptom, other herbs are also used to balance its effects or enhance the strength of the whole body. That's why eating a

ANOTHER SOY CONTROVERSY

Another controversy regarding soy comes from a preliminary study published in 2000. There's a large ongoing study, called the Honolulu-Asian Aging Study, which is following 3,734 elderly Japanese-American men for thirty years. At this still-early stage, it appears that the men who consumed the most tofu during midlife had up to a 2.4 times *increased* risk of Alzheimer's disease later in life. There also appears to be a link between a higher incidence of brain atrophy (shrinkage) in men who ate two or more servings of tofu a week. Experts stress

wide variety of whole organic foods is important, too. If you eat the same food every day, you'll miss out on important plant synergies and certain nutrients. There's a good chance that you will develop imbalances and eventually get sick.

When you compare certain pharmaceutical drugs to their herbal or natural counterparts, the reasoning behind the principle of favoring whole foods becomes very clear. Herbs are composed of whole plants or whole parts of a plant, such as the leaves and the roots. Pharmaceutical drugs take the active ingredient out of the plant, synthesize it, and then make it into a pill. Usually, the results are an effective substance, but with a catch—unwanted, potentially toxic, side effects. One-third of all patients admitted to the hospital are there due to iatrogenic causes (that is, health problems inadvertently induced by a physician, healthcare providers such as nurses, aides, and therapists, medical treatment, or diagnostic procedure). Each year, an estimated 250,000 people die from iatrogenic causes and, according to Dr. Gary Null and Dr. Carolyn Dean, that number may be much higher. In a paper they coauthored in 2003, "Death by Medicine," the total number of annual iatrogenic deaths they calculated (based on medical peer-review journals) may be closer to 784,000. That means that the "American medical system is the leading cause of deaths and injury in the United States!" Approximately 106,000 of those deaths are due to adverse drug reactions and interactions.

Herbs aren't just weak pharmaceuticals. They're completely different. When taken properly, they work in harmony with the body and create an abundance of side *benefits*. When taken properly, herbs rarely have side effects. If they do, the side effects are usually mild. Similarly, whole foods work in harmony with the body by increasing its healing intelligence in many ways. Isolated elements of foods aren't foods; they're pharmaceutical preparations of a single, concentrated active ingredient.

that the conclusions in this study are preliminary at this point. The link between tofu consumption and brain atrophy is speculative and hasn't been proven.

Some researchers have found substances in soy that may interfere with the absorption of certain minerals and other nutrients. They hypothesize that soy could cause a problem with the brain if it actually does obstruct the absorption of nutrients so much so that their levels become dangerously low. These questionable substances are broken down when soy is fermented. Because of that, some doctors recommend that you should eat only fermented soy products such as miso, tempeh, and natto. If you have healthy intestines, the bacteria in your intestines ferments soy, so nonfermented soy shouldn't interfere with your body's ability to absorb minerals, either.

My personal opinion is that you should eat a wide variety of whole foods, including soy foods. Add spices to your foods to increase the anticancer properties. Don't make your diet all about one food. There are many different foods that fight cancer. Your diet should include as many of them as possible. This concept is expressed in another fundamental *Ayurvedic* principle: *A balanced diet should include a wide variety of fresh wholesome foods.* The greater the diversity of plants that you eat, the broader the spectrum of Nature's healing intelligence that you import into your body.

Chapter 11

Magic Mushrooms and Much More

Specialty Foods with Spectacular Powers

oy isn't the only Asian food that mounts an impressive assault against breast cancer. There is a wonderful array of exotic specialty foods—all with Asian origins—that have their own magical and spectacular powers against this killer beast. These foods include a fungus, a beverage, a spice, an herb, and two types of seaweed!

THE MAITAKE MUSHROOM—TUMOR-CELL ASSASSIN

Mushrooms have been used for thousands of years as medicines in Asian cultures. One type of mushroom that has been used by the Japanese as a medicine for more than 2,000 years is the maitake mushroom. Hidden within this enchanting fungus is a powerful army of therapeutic chemical weapons against cancer.

Maitake mushrooms (*Grifola frondosa*) grow in clusters on hardwood trees and are indigenous to the Northern Hemisphere. In Japanese, "maitake mushrooms" means "dancing mushrooms." As legend has it, the name comes from how the ancients danced for joy when they found these extremely valuable mushrooms.

Research shows that the cancer-fighting chemicals in maitake mushrooms arrest the growth of tumors, cause them to shrink, and prevent them from spreading to other areas of the body. Maitake mushrooms also stimulate and boost the immune system by increasing the number and function of two important cells in the immune system—macrophages and T cells.

Three broad categories of cells make up the immune system: two types of lymphocytes, called B cells and T cells, and a third type of cells called macrophages. T cells make up 70 to 80 percent of all the lymphocytes in the blood. They lead the body's resistance force against bacterial infections, viral diseases, and tumors, and help to regulate the immune system. After an initial frontal attack by the immune system's lymphocytes, macrophages (or scavenger cells) strike from the rear to gobble up unwanted invaders in your body, including bacteria and cancer cells.

Most of the medicinal effects of this mushroom are thought to come from a special polysaccharide (a type of sugar). Found in what scientists call the "D fraction" in the maitake mushroom, the polysaccharide contains a substance called "beta-glucans," which, research shows, stimulates the immune system.

Maitake mushrooms' cancer-fighting effects go far beyond just boosting the immune system. This fungus can also kill tumor cells. In a laboratory study from Japan published in the journal *Molecular Biology* in 2002, liquid extracts of maitake mushrooms killed 95 percent of prostate cancer cells within twenty-four hours. In a human study, patients diagnosed as having stage 2, stage 3, or stage 4 breast cancer were given a combination of whole maitake powder and the "D fraction" of maitake mushrooms. Tumors shrank and symptoms improved in 68.8 percent of the patients. Researchers found that the mushrooms also helped to shrink cancers of the liver and lung.

These amazing mushrooms can also be very beneficial for patients on chemotherapy. Normally, chemotherapeutic drugs dramatically weaken the immune system. But research shows that maitake mushrooms can counteract that effect and keep the immune system strong.

Consuming Maitake

Maitake mushrooms come fresh or dried to be used in cooking. Supplements are also available as powder, capsules, or liquid extracts. The recommended dose of maitake mushrooms is 3–5 grams of the dry powder or capsules each day, or 10–30 drops of the liquid extract three times per day.

OTHER CANCER-FIGHTING MUSHROOMS

Many other mushrooms have nonspecific ways of helping to ward off cancer, such as boosting the immune system. Others, such as the reishi mushroom (*Ganoderma lucidum*), have specific actions against breast cancer. In 2004, researchers at UCLA found that an alcohol extract of reishi mushroom spores stopped the growth of breast cancer cells in a dose-dependent manner. That means that the higher the concentration of the reishi mushroom extract, the more breast cancer cells it can kill.

Reishi mushrooms also appear to have many other anticancer effects. For example, they can shut off new blood-vessel growth to tumors and suppress cell adhesion and migration. These qualities mean that reishi mushrooms may reduce the ability of a tumor to invade both surrounding and distant tissues. Therefore, reishi mushrooms may be a valuable dietary supplement for women who already have breast cancer.

GREEN TEA—THE #1 ANTICANCER BEVERAGE

More than 4,000 years ago, the Chinese began brewing the leaves of a plant and drinking it as a hot beverage. They called the infusion *cha*, their word for "tea." Now, more tea is consumed around the world every day than any other liquid except water. Research shows that drinking tea, especially green tea, is a wise choice because tea has been found to have many potent health benefits.

Research has shown that green tea is very effective in hampering the growth of at least eleven different types of cancer, including cancers of the esophagus, stomach, colon, bladder, prostate, skin, ovaries, and breast. Green tea also reduces the risk of lung cancer in smokers, non-Hodgkin's lymphoma, and leukemia. That's why green tea is considered the number-one anticancer beverage. You might think that the impact of a few cups of tea each day on lowering the risk of these cancers would be small, but it's not. Cancers of the digestive tract are as much as 68 percent lower in tea drinkers.

One of the reasons why green tea is so potent against so many cancers is because it contains an exceptional blend of powerful anti-inflammatories and antioxidants. Green tea also has the remarkable ability to amplify the power of the enzymes in your liver that detoxify your body of poisons and carcinogens. Researchers believe that most of the health benefits of green tea come from substances within it called polyphenols. The three polyphenols considered most important are gallocatechin (GC), epigallocatechin (EGC), and epigallocatechin gallate (EGCG). Of the three, EGCG is the most potent.

Japanese researchers found that among healthy women, those who drank green tea had a lower risk of breast cancer. And those women with breast cancer who drank green tea lived much longer than those who didn't. For instance, women with stage 1 or stage 2 breast cancer, who were green-tea drinkers before they were diagnosed, were found to have a much better prognosis for survival. Also, a 1998 study found that drinking green tea lowered the risk of breast tumors metastasizing and stopped them from recurring after the women had been treated.

Several studies show that EGCG inhibits the growth of breast cancer and decreases the incidence of its metastasizing to the lungs. A Japanese study of rats with mammary tumors found that 93.8 percent of the rats given green tea survived, compared to only 33 percent of the rats that weren't given green tea. The rats given green tea also had smaller tumors than those that weren't given it.

Scientists have mapped out seven different ways in which green tea combats breast cancer. For one, it increases the number of protein binders in the blood, and the more protein binders there are in the blood, the more estrogen it binds and the less estrogen there is available to attach to estrogen receptors in the breast. Green tea also lowers estradiol levels and increases the number of estrogen- and progesterone-sensitive receptors in breast cancers found in postmenopausal women. This is important, because tumors with receptors sensitive to these hormones respond better to treatment and have a better prognosis.

This stellar brew also helps to block the growth of new blood vessels into the tumor—a quality that is technically referred to as antiangiogenic. If you are on chemotherapy, green tea can enhance its effectiveness and at the same time protect against many of its dangerous side effects. Japanese researchers T. Sugiyama and Y. Saduka published several studies between 1998 and 2003 showing that green tea and some of its individual components increase the concentration of chemotherapeutic agents, such as doxorubicin and Adriamycin, in tumors by 2.1 to 2.9 times, and decrease the levels of these drugs in normal tissue.

The results are that when you drink green tea while you're taking these chemotherapeutic drugs, tumors shrink more than they usually do without the green tea. In addition, organs that are commonly damaged by these anticancer drugs, such as the heart and liver, are protected from injury by drinking this potent green brew.

Major Health Benefits

Hundreds of studies show that green tea has many other impressive health benefits, as well. It decreases your risk of heart attacks and strokes by lowering levels of cholesterol and blood pressure, as well as by slowing the development of atherosclerosis ("hardening" of the arteries). Green tea is also superb at killing certain bacteria, especially in the bladder. Its flair for stopping these bladder bugs from propagating is revealed in this statistic: Tea drinkers have a 40 percent lower incidence of urinary tract infections. Green tea also aids digestion by increasing the number of helpful bacteria in your intestines while decreasing the number of harmful ones. In addition, green tea is a thermogenic agent. Thermogenics speed up your metabolism and help you lose weight. And if you're concerned about osteoporosis, drink this healthy brew often. A study published in the *American Journal of Clinical Nutrition* in April 2000 found that women aged sixty-five to seventy-five who drank at least one cup of green tea a day had significantly higher bone densities than those who didn't.

Choosing and Preparing Green Tea

Green tea (*Camellia sinensis*) is processed by steaming the tea leaves at high temperatures. When prepared in this way, the health-promoting polyphenols are preserved. (During the processing of black tea, some of these polyphenols are destroyed, which is probably why green tea has more potent medicinal properties than black tea.)

When you choose a green tea, it's important to buy organically grown tea. A recent analysis of several nonorganic brands found that they contained traces of the banned estrogenic pesticide, DDT. You don't want to drink something to *reduce* your risk of cancer if it also contains something that may *increase* your risk! Be safe and use organically grown green tea.

To create the best-tasting cup of tea with the highest medicinal qualities, steep your tea bag or tea ball in hot water for three to five minutes. For the maximum protection, drink eight to ten cups of green tea a day. Yes, green tea does contain some caffeine, but there are substances in the tea that seem to modify caffeine's side effects to the point that most of the people who drink it aren't adversely affected. Removing the caffeine from green tea actually *weakens* its anticancer power; the caffeine appears to be an important component of the tea's antitumor effects. If you don't think you can drink this much green tea each day, take a green-tea supplement. Two 250-milligram (mg) tablets a day are recommended.

TURMERIC—A MEDICINAL SPICE OF THE HIGHEST ORDER

From the healing powers of green, we move to the medicinal marvels of blazing yellow-orange. The Indian cooking spice turmeric, responsible for the intense color of curry, is even older and wiser than green tea when it comes to promoting and protecting health. This indigenous plant of Asia and India has been a star of *Ayurvedic* and traditional Chinese medicine (TCM) for more than 5,000 years—and for good reason. More than 1,300 studies published in medical journals confirm that this spectacular spice is one of Nature's most intelligent creations. These studies show that of all the known herbs and spices, turmeric possesses more anticancer qualities and healing benefits than any other.

Turmeric (*Curcuma longa*), a plant with beautiful, very large, long lily-like leaves, is indigenous to India and southern Asia. But it's what you don't see—under the ground—that possesses all the magic. The medicinal part of turmeric is its *rhizome* (root); it looks very much like ginger root. That's not surprising because turmeric and ginger are considered cousins. They are members of the same botanical family: *Zingiberaceae*.

The big difference between ginger and turmeric can be seen when you cut open the *rhizome*. Ginger root has a pale, plain white interior, but when you slice into turmeric, what you see is anything but drab. A vibrant, almost irides-cent, bright-orange pigment radiates from its interior. Turmeric's visual hue gives a clue to the power of the medicine it holds.

Scientists have confirmed that the substance responsible for the spellbind-ing color of turmeric—curcumin—has many medicinal benefits. In fact, hun-dreds of studies show that curcumin possesses almost all of turmeric's healing benefits. However, a 1997 study indicates that curcumin may not be the whole story of turmeric. Researchers removed the curcumin from a sample of turmer-ic, and then tested the curcumin-free turmeric for antitumor effects. They found that the anticancer qualities of curcumin-free turmeric were *more potent* than those of whole turmeric with its curcumin intact.

Like green tea, turmeric stands out from all the other plants in its class in its ability to impede cancer. Research shows that turmeric substantially thwarts at least eight different cancers: lung, mouth, colon, liver, kidneys, skin (mela-noma), breast, and blood (leukemia). That's why this amazing spice is consid-ered the number-one anticancer spice.

Turmeric helps to break down toxins in the liver and prevent carcinogens from forming, possesses dramatic anti-inflammatory properties, has potent antioxidants (300 times the power of vitamin E), and stimulates the immune system. Turmeric also emulsifies fat, so it helps to promote weight loss. Keep-ing your weight down is important, because obesity raises the risk of many can-cers including breast cancer. And if you have cancer, turmeric enhances the effectiveness of chemotherapy against your tumor while it protects your organs from the damage that these drugs often cause.

Turmeric works with your liver in an ingenious way to get rid of the toxins in your body. Your liver has two sets of enzymes, called "phase 1" and "phase 2" enzymes. When a toxin or carcinogen, such as *benzopyrene,* which is found in cigarette smoke and charcoal-broiled meats, comes to the liver, phase 1 enzymes activate it. In other words, the toxin isn't a carcinogen until the phase 1 enzymes in your liver turn it into one. Why would your body want to *create* carcinogens? Because they are easier for phase 2 enzymes in your liver to recognize. Phase 2 enzymes attack carcinogens, break them down, and get rid of them. The prob-lem comes when you overwhelm this system. When too many toxins come into the liver, some of them will escape the mechanisms designed to eliminate them.

Your risk of cancer can be reduced by *blocking* the activity of phase 1 enzymes, reducing the number of carcinogens formed or activated, or by *enhanc-ing* the action of phase 2 enzymes, eliminating more carcinogens. One of the reasons that turmeric is so effective against cancer is because it has the ability to *both* block phase 1 and enhance phase 2 enzymes!

If you think the ability of a spice or an herb to protect your body from toxins isn't very strong, think again. Turmeric has *remarkable* abilities. Here's an example of just how amazing it can be. Mutagens (agents that can cause DNA mutations leading to cancer) are in the food you eat, the air you breathe, and in many things you come in contact with every day. They are activated and broken down in your body. The amount of mutagens in your body can be determined indirectly by measuring the concentration of their metabolites (byproducts of metabolism) in your urine.

The average smoker, not surprisingly, has a lot of carcinogenic metabolites in his or her urine. In a study published in the journal *Mutagenesis* in 1992, researchers measured the mutagen metabolites in the urine of sixteen chronic smokers and sixteen nonsmokers. Then, the smokers were given 1.5 grams of turmeric a day for thirty days. The nonsmokers were *not* given turmeric. At the end of thirty days, the urine of the smokers and nonsmokers were tested for mutagen metabolites. What the researchers found was nothing short of astounding: The level of mutagen metabolites was *lower* in the smokers taking turmeric than it was in the nonsmokers!

Turmeric has many general anticancer effects. It also has a number of amazing properties that specifically prevent and fight breast cancer. One way it lowers the risk of breast cancer is by blocking the toxins that are known to cause it. Some pesticides, such as DDT and chlordane, mimic the estrogen molecule in your body and thereby increase your risk of breast cancer. Turmeric can block the pesticides' estrogenic effects. It also impedes breast cancer tumors from forming in response to estrogen and environmental toxins. Genistein in whole soy foods stumps the pesticides, too.

Researchers at Tufts University in Boston found that genistein and turmeric work synergistically, meaning that each one makes the other's ability to block estrogen and environmental toxins more effective. When genistein and turmeric were combined together, their ability to hinder estrogenic environmental toxins was extremely impressive. In one laboratory study, the combination of genistein and turmeric inhibited 95 percent of chemically induced breast cancer cell growth. In another study, they stopped 100 percent of the growth—*no* cancer cells grew despite heavy loads of estrogenic environmental toxins!

Turmeric also "down regulates" the estrogen receptor. That means it decreases the sensitivity of the estrogen receptor, reducing its normal response to estrogen. In other words, turmeric affects the estrogen receptor in such a way that when estrogen attaches to it, the rate at which breast cells divide is much slower than normal.

Another one of turmeric's very beneficial attributes is that it inhibits or blocks an enzyme that plays a key role in the initiation and growth of breast cancer, as well as several other types of cancer. It's called the COX-2 enzyme. (There's a lot more about this harmful substance in Chapter 14.) The number of COX-2 enzymes found in breast cancer tumors is frequently much higher than in normal cells. Scientists call it an "overexpression of the COX-2 enzyme."

The COX-2 enzyme is responsible for a long list of dangerous deeds. It encourages tumor cells to divide, prevents the death of tumor cells, stimulates the growth of new blood vessels, makes tumor cells better at invading the surrounding tissues, blocks the important tumor-suppressing effects of the immune system, increases the risk of metastasis, and speeds up the production of mutagens. That's an impressive list of horrific actions, but turmeric can put an end to all of them. It shuts down the COX-2 enzyme and thwarts *all* its harmful actions.

If you have breast cancer, turmeric's anti-COX-2-enzyme abilities can be tremendously helpful. Turmeric prevents tumors from growing, induces apoptosis (cell death), and inhibits cell proliferation. It also stops the growth of new blood vessels that tumors need in order to grow and halts the production of a substance called IL-6 (by your immune system), which makes cancer cells grow faster. Turmeric has anti-invasive effects, too; it helps to prevent tumors from invading surrounding tissues. And if you're on chemotherapy, turmeric can increase its effectiveness and protect against the organ damage it may cause.

Turmeric and green tea also have a synergistic effect. Green tea causes turmeric's anticancer effects to be three times stronger, and turmeric enhances green tea's anticancer capabilities by a factor of eight.

Turmeric's Other Healing Effects

Turmeric has an impressive array of other health benefits, too. If you have gallstones, it encourages your gallbladder to expel them. Turmeric aids digestion by increasing stomach secretions and decreasing the amount of gas produced in the intestines. It also protects against stomach ulcers. Turmeric lowers your risk of heart disease by decreasing cholesterol and the formation of plaque in your arteries. It promotes wound healing by decreasing inflammation and stimulating the growth of new blood vessels.

One of the more fascinating features of turmeric is that it clearly expresses its own intelligence. Turmeric *blocks* new blood-vessel growth in cancer to stop further growth of a tumor while it *stimulates* new blood-vessel growth in wounds to help speed healing. The key is that turmeric "knows" when to do each one. It can tell the difference between cancerous tissue and normal tissue and respond appropriately. No doubt, researchers will eventually uncover the elegant mechanisms responsible for this behavior.

In addition, turmeric shields your organs from chemical attack. It minimizes the damage to your brain caused by alcohol, as well as chemical damage to your liver. Elevated liver enzymes are an indication of liver injury. The higher the enzyme level, the more extensive the injury is. When turmeric is ingested, liver enzymes drop, indicating that it effectively helps the liver repair itself. Turmeric also strengthens your connective tissue and prevents the formation of adhesions or scar tissue. And it stimulates muscles to regenerate after trauma.

You can apply turmeric topically to your skin for another whole set of benefits. Turmeric can kill bacteria. If it's exposed to sunlight, its talent for exterminating bacteria improves. It is also effective for treating fungal infections, such as athletes' foot, and skin conditions, such as psoriasis.

There's no other known substance that you can eat or put on your skin that will do all that. All those healing effects from just one miraculous plant? It may sound impossible, but more than 1,300 studies in medical literature prove each and every one of them. When it comes to medicinal plants, turmeric is a superstar. This plant beautifully demonstrates an important *Ayurvedic* principle regarding medicinal plants that is worth remembering: *Plants hold intelligence, and they help us to heal by importing their intelligence into us.*

Taking Turmeric

Turmeric is prepared by soaking and then drying the root. After that, the dried root is ground into a fine powder. Turmeric powder can be found in the spice section of most grocery stores. Remember, organic is always best. *Ayurvedic* physicians recommend adding about one-quarter teaspoon to your food near the end of cooking. Turmeric works more in harmony with your body when it is cooked—but not overcooked.

You can also take turmeric as a supplement. Two 500-mg capsules a day is the recommended dose. In addition, it comes in a combination of delicious Indian healing spices called "*churnas.*" *Churnas* are precise recipes of several different spices that can be added to any dish, either during cooking or afterward. *Churnas* usually aren't composed of "hot" spices like chili; rather, they are a delightful mixture of mildly flavorful natural medicines.

GARLIC—A CANCER NEMESIS EXTRAORDINAIRE

For more than 5,000 years, before even the earliest Chinese dynasties, garlic has been used as a medicine in central Asia. Prized for its health-promoting and health-protecting qualities, it was brought further and further West until it reached Egypt about 4,000 years ago. The earliest surviving written records describing garlic as a medicine are found in the Egyptian Ebers Papyrus written around 1500 B.C.E. Garlic was introduced into Europe in the first century A.D.

With this long history of cultivation, garlic is no longer found in the wild; it is strictly a plant grown by people. Today, it's produced and enjoyed for its excellent taste and diverse medicinal qualities by nearly every culture in the world. One of its distinctive traits is its ability to lower the risk of breast cancer.

An Iowa study of 34,388 postmenopausal women found that those who consumed garlic regularly had a noticeably lower incidence of breast cancer. Eating just one clove of garlic a week made a significant statistical difference.

There are several ways that garlic helps to protect against and fight breast cancer. Overall, garlic is a good cancer fighter because it has more antioxidants than any other vegetable ever tested. Antioxidants protect your body from the oxygen free-radical damage that can lead to cancer. Garlic usually has abundant amounts of selenium, and this mineral stimulates the production of glutathione, one of the body's natural antioxidants.

Research has found that garlic also boosts the immune system. Specifically, it enhances the activity of natural killer (NK) cells. These immune-system cells are important because, as their name indicates, they naturally kill things you don't want in your body, such as cancer cells, bacteria, and viruses.

Laboratory studies have revealed some of the precise ways that garlic prevents and fights breast cancer. Garlic decreases the formation of carcinogens in breast tissue by as much as 50 to 70 percent. It helps to avert the initiation of breast tumors by preventing toxins from binding to DNA in breast cells. Garlic has also been shown to inhibit or prevent breast tumor cells from growing and dividing. In addition, research shows that garlic is very effective at lowering the risk of stomach cancer.

Cancer isn't the only disease that garlic helps to prevent. The main problem in AIDS patients is that the HIV virus destroys the immune system. The number and function of NK cells, in particular, drop to very low levels. A 1989 study found that garlic was effective at increasing the activity of NK cells in AIDS patients.

Garlic is especially good for your heart's health. It decreases cholesterol and triglycerides, prevents blood clots, improves circulation, and decreases the risk of atherosclerosis (hardening of the arteries). Garlic also reduces blood pressure. Studies show it can reduce systolic blood pressure (the first or higher number in a blood-pressure reading) by 20–30 millimeters (mm) of mercury (Hg) and diastolic blood pressure (the second or lower number) by 10–20 mm Hg.

Garlic: Nature's Antibiotic

Garlic can kill a whole army of unwanted invaders: bacteria, viruses, fungi, and parasites. In 1858 Louis Pasteur, who developed the "germ theory," discovered that garlic kills bacteria. This was an important revelation, because there were no antibiotics then. For nearly half a century after his discovery, garlic juice was put on wounds to help prevent infections. It was one of the principal antibiotics used during World War I and until the availability of penicillin in 1942.

Many modern-day studies have shown that garlic is effective in killing a wide variety of bacteria including tuberculosis and *Staphylococcus aureus,* a common skin pathogen that frequently causes infections. Studies conducted in the 1980s and 1990s found that garlic is also a good antiviral, antifungal, and antiparasitic medicine.

The Magic Inside

As with any whole plant, it's difficult to describe exactly how garlic works because there are thousands of constituents all interacting together. But a few substances have been identified in garlic that have clear medicinal benefits and specific actions. Something called "allin" holds many of garlic's health-promoting properties. Allin is just one of thirty sulfur compounds found in garlic. When garlic is crushed or broken, the enzyme allinase is released, and it converts allin to allicin—the actual active compound. Allin doesn't have any health-supporting effects until it becomes allicin. So, to gain the full potential of the allicin in garlic, you should crush it and wait at least fifteen minutes before you eat it. Other plentiful health-enhancing compounds found in garlic are selenium and vitamins A, B, C, and E.

Getting Your Garlic

Garlic can be eaten fresh or taken in standardized doses as capsules and tablets. The general recommended daily dose is 600–900 mg, or one or two fresh cloves. Many of the antioxidants in garlic are destroyed if you cook it too much. So, eat it raw, or only lightly sautéed, and add it to foods near the end of cooking. If you are concerned about having "garlic breath," there is an odorless form of garlic available in capsule form.

Side effects have been reported with therapeutic doses of garlic, but they are mild and rare. They include heartburn, flatulence, headaches, muscle soreness, fatigue, dizziness, and allergic reactions. Garlic is *not* recommended if you are on anticoagulants or blood thinners, because it also thins your blood.

SEAWEED—BREAST MEDICINE FROM THE SEA

The last of the Asian secret weapons against breast cancer comes from the sea. A prehistoric plant, seaweed has been gathered from the oceans for centuries and is a prominent vegetable in Japanese cuisine. It is rarely consumed in this country, despite evidence that it is a powerful ally in the fight against breast cancer.

Two types of seaweed—wakame and mekabu—suppress the growth of breast cancer by causing cell death. In other words, these seaweeds kill breast cancer cells—and with quite a bit of might. A study published in 2001 by Japanese researcher H. Funahashi found that mekabu seaweed killed breast cancer cells and stopped the growth of tumors *more effectively* than a common chemotherapeutic drug used for breast cancer. Better yet, this seaweed did not cause normal cells to die as chemotherapeutic drugs often do.

The reason these seaweeds are so potent against breast cancer is because they are high in iodine. Iodine is toxic to breast cancer cells. It is also involved in the production of antioxidants that protect cells from oxidative damage that can lead to cancer. Not surprisingly, low amounts of iodine in the diet are thought to contribute to the risk of breast cancer. Women with thyroid diseases including hyperthyroidism (overactive thyroid), hypothyroidism (underactive thyroid), thyroiditis (inflammation of the thyroid), and nontoxic goiter have a higher incidence of breast cancer. Many of these thyroid conditions are associated with low dietary iodine, but low iodine doesn't fully explain the association between thyroid disease and breast cancer. At this point, we don't have a clear understanding of why women with thyroid cancer or other thyroid conditions have a higher incidence of breast cancer.

Iodine is a trace element that is normally only taken up by the thyroid gland to make thyroid hormones. Embryologically, the breast and thyroid are derived from similar cells. Breast cells have only a temporary ability to uptake and concentrate iodine during pregnancy and lactation—the purpose being to supply the baby with this important substance through the breast milk. Researchers have found that iodine is also taken up by breast cancer cells, but *not* normal breast cells or any other cells in the body. This fact creates an exciting future possibility for treating breast cancer—using radioactive iodine instead of chemotherapy. Radioactive iodine is a substance used to treat thyroid cancers, and it might also prove to be highly effective against breast cancer. Because iodine is not taken up by any other tissues in the body except the thyroid, radioactive iodine—unlike standard chemotherapy—is harmless to the rest of the body. And the damage caused to the thyroid by radioactive iodine is easily treatable with thyroid hormones.

Although no guidelines have been established for breast cancer prevention, the Food and Nutrition Board of the U.S. National Academy of Sciences recommends that normal healthy adults take 150 micrograms (mcg) of iodine a day. Higher amounts are recommended for certain disease states. (Approximately 1½ teaspoons of seaweed has about 225 mcg of iodine.)

MORE NATURAL DEFENSE

Most plants contain substances that protect against and fight cancer. The anticancer properties of some plants, such as soybeans and flaxseeds, have been well recognized for decades. But there are many other plants, especially herbs and spices, with excellent abilities to ward off breast cancer. Isaac Cohen, a doctor of oriental medicine, licensed acupuncturist, and one of the leading authorities in the field of cancer treatment and traditional Chinese medicine (TCM), reported in the book *Breast Cancer: Beyond Convention* that several Chinese herbs, including ginseng, show good anticancer activity against breast cancer. He points out that it is not unusual for plants to be effective against cancer—in fact, more than 60 percent of the chemotherapeutic drugs currently being used are derived from natural substances.

Other researchers concur that many of the herbs used in TCM are effective at stopping the growth of breast cancer cells in the laboratory. For instance, in 2002 researchers at the Cancer Research Laboratory in Indianapolis, Indiana, found that licorice root (*Ganoderma lucidum*)—a shrub native to southern Europe and Asia and one of the Chinese herbs used in the prostate cancer herbal mixture PC-SPES—showed strong activity against highly invasive breast cancer cells. Another study published in 2002 in the journal *Anticancer Research* found that of seventy-one extracts of Chinese medicinal herbs, 21 percent (fifteen) of the extracts demonstrated greater than 50 percent growth inhibition on at least four of the five breast cancer cell lines. In 2000, researchers at Memorial Sloan-Kettering Cancer Center in New York found that Huanglian, a Chinese herbal extract used in the treatment of gastroenteritis, also inhibits the growth of human gastric, colon, and breast cancer cells.

Some common cooking spices have excellent cancer-fighting properties, too. For example, research shows that the spice rosemary protects against the initiation of breast tumors. When rats were fed rosemary before the administration of breast cancer–inducing chemicals, they developed 74 percent fewer tumors than the rats that weren't fed rosemary. Another study published in the *European Journal of Cancer* in 1999 found that rosemary, like green tea, improves the concentration of the chemotherapeutic agents (doxorubicin and vinblastin) in breast cancer tumor cells. That means that this aromatic spice may be helpful as a complementary treatment for women with tumors that are resistant to these drugs.

According to researchers at the New York College of Osteopathic Medicine, extracts of several weak estrogenic herbs including hops, black cohosh, and chaste-tree berry also inhibit the growth of breast cancer cells in the laboratory.

We have just begun our exploration of the vast and wondrous intelligence contained in plants. As more research is completed, the array of anticancer herbs will assuredly continue to grow.

Part Three

Secret Weapons for Your Warrior Goddess

An Arsenal of Nutritional Supplements

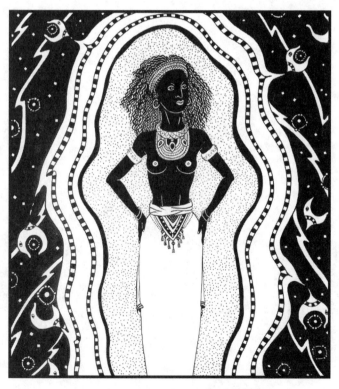

Goddess of Dynamic Defense

Chapter 12

Mighty
Micronutrients

Vitamins That Defend

*J*ust like the old saying, "Some of the best things come in small pack-
ages," some of the best weapons you can give your Warrior Goddess to
help her successfully fend off breast cancer are very tiny. But don't let
their size fool you. Only small amounts of these tiny molecules are needed
because they pack a mighty wallop against breast cancer.

In biology, it's normal for microscopic structures to contain immense potential. For instance, think of a single cell: It's so tiny that it can be seen only with
a powerful microscope. Yet, contained within the nucleus of that cell is your
DNA. Imagine how tiny the double helixes of protein are, and they contain the
potential to manifest a complete human being—trillions of cells, a multitude of
specialized organs and structures, and a mind-boggling number of functions, all
working in perfect coordinated harmony!

If you give your Warrior Goddess a few micrograms of four different
micronutrients, folic acid and vitamins B_{12}, D, and E, every day, she gains
enough power from these "special forces" to provide you with significant protection against breast cancer. By definition, vitamins are organic compounds that
you need only in very small amounts, but they play a big role in keeping you
healthy. Vitamins aren't metabolized for energy—they don't supply any calories—but some of them are important in energy production. The primary function of vitamins is to assist enzymes, which are tiny, vitally important proteins
that drive all the chemical reactions in your body. Because enzymes play such a
critical role, it is vital to take vitamins in the proper daily amounts to maintain
your health.

The word "vitamin" originally meant a nutrient that your body can't make.
This definition isn't always appropriate because your body can make some vitamins, such as vitamin D. The vitamins you can't make—or don't make enough

of—you should get from your food. Most vitamins are absorbed and assimilated more effectively if you consume them in foods, especially fresh, organically grown vegetables, fruits, nuts, and whole grains. But under certain circumstances—for instance, if you don't eat enough of these nutrient-rich foods—taking supplemental vitamins is a good idea. Vitamin supplements derived from whole foods are more readily absorbed and assimilated by the body than those made synthetically. (You may have to call the manufacturer to find out if the supplements you are considering purchasing are derived from whole foods.)

FOLIC ACID

Folic acid (also known as folate) is involved in the process of making proteins. It is a crucial element in constructing and repairing DNA and in normal cell division. Without it, cells can't divide properly and can turn cancerous. Folic acid helps to prevent DNA from making the mistakes that can lead to cancer. Think of it as a built-in proofreader. Certain chance mistakes can turn the messages of DNA traitorous. For example, instead of dispatching communications for health, the DNA may accidentally spawn messages for cancer. Folic acid can prevent this from happening. This may explain why low levels of folic acid in the body are associated with a significantly increased risk of breast cancer.

In a 1992 study from the University of Vermont, researchers found that DNA mistakes or mutations increase with age and cigarette smoking. They also discovered that folate helps to prevent those mutations, including mutations that increase the risk of breast cancer.

Alcohol consumption causes folate levels to drop. (The perils of alcohol with regard to breast cancer are discussed in Chapter 18.) Women who drink alcohol and have low folate levels may be at high risk of developing breast cancer. Harvard University conducted a very large prospective study, called the Nurses' Health Study, which followed 88,818 women from 1980 to 1996. (A prospective study is one that follows the subjects into the future; it is considered one of the best study designs for obtaining significant and reliable information.) The study found that women who had the highest risk of breast cancer drank at least 15 grams (about a half ounce) of alcohol a day and had low folate levels.

Good Sources of Folic Acid

Folic acid is found in eggs, asparagus, whole wheat, dark-green leafy vegetables, and brewers yeast. It's also found in certain meats and fish. But eating large amounts of meat and fish is a double-edged sword, since the toxins in these foods considerably increase the risk of breast cancer. Folic acid is available in supplement form. About 400 micrograms (mcg) a day is all you need. As with all good things, don't take too much folate. *The Physicians Desk Reference for Nutritional Supplements* reports no incidences of folate overdosing in the medical literature, but taking too much folic acid can be a problem for people who have a vitamin B_{12} deficiency. When vitamin B_{12} levels are very low and supplemental folate is taken, the neurological problems and damage associated with low levels of vitamin B_{12} can worsen.

Birth control pills, alcohol, and nonsteroidal anti-inflammatories (such as aspirin and ibuprofen) lower folate levels. So, if you take any of these medications or drink alcohol regularly, make sure you take supplemental folic acid.

VITAMIN B_{12} (COBALAMIN)

Vitamin B_{12} is known as "Nature's most beautiful cofactor," because its crystalline structure is a stunning dark red, like that of a rare ruby. Vitamin B_{12} works *with* folic acid, so it's also a fundamental part of the DNA construction and repair team. Without it, the quality of DNA would never pass inspection. Vitamin B_{12} is vitally important for keeping your DNA messages correct and free from cancer-inducing mistakes. Research shows that women with the lowest B_{12} levels in their bodies have the highest rates of breast cancer.

Vitamin B_{12} may also be very valuable for women who already have breast cancer. In the laboratory, scientists found that when vitamin B_{12} was applied directly to breast cancer cells, it stopped them from growing.

This vitamin is also essential for a healthy nervous system and energy production.

The richest sources of vitamin B_{12} are certain animal organs—especially liver, brain, and kidney. Clams, oysters, sardines, and salmon have significant amounts of this vitamin, too. It is also found in egg yolks and fermented soy products, such as tempeh. Because eating meat and fish *increases* your risk of breast cancer, getting B_{12} from other sources is probably a good idea.

It's not uncommon for those who follow a vegetarian diet to be deficient in vitamin B_{12} since it is found mostly in animal products. Although a vegetarian diet is the most healthful of diets and is associated with the lowest risk of breast cancer, it's important that vegetarians (and others who avoid meat and shellfish) take B_{12} in supplement form. About 3–30 micrograms (mcg) a day—about the weight of one-tenth of a water droplet—is all you need for B_{12} to perform its miracles.

To be absorbed into your body, vitamin B_{12} requires "intrinsic factor," a substance secreted by the cells in your stomach. As you age, you make less intrinsic factor and, therefore, absorb less B_{12}. So, you must consume more B_{12} as you age to absorb amounts similar to what you got when you were younger. For this reason, supplemental B_{12} is a great idea for everyone who is over age sixty. If you have certain conditions, such as the autoimmune disorder pernicious anemia, or if you have had partial or total surgical removal of your stomach, the amount of intrinsic factor you make will be low. Pancreatic insufficiency, disorders of the small bowel, certain drugs, and a variety of other conditions can also interfere with B_{12} absorption. In all these situations, it's very important to take supplemental vitamin B_{12}.

VITAMIN D

Most famous for making bones and teeth strong by helping the body to effectively use calcium and phosphorus, vitamin D has another notable talent. Research shows that this vitamin protects against and fights breast cancer. It helps to make your breast cells more resistant to toxins, decreases the ability of breast cells to divide, stops tumor cells from growing, causes the death of tumor cells, prevents new blood vessels from growing into a tumor, and boosts the immune system, especially the activity of natural killer (NK) cells.

Vitamin D is unique because your body can make its own supply. The secret catalyzing agent is not from this world; it comes from a star—the sun. Sunlight reacts with chemicals in your skin to produce vitamin D. Just fifteen minutes of sunlight a day makes enough vitamin D to reduce your risk of breast cancer by as much as 40 percent. Of course, too much sunlight isn't a good thing, either. Here is another example of the ancient principle of *balance*. Too much of a good thing can cause imbalances and lead to health problems, just as too little can. The ultraviolet radiation in sunlight damages the DNA in skin cells. If you get too much sun, especially if you have lightly pigmented skin, the damage can be severe. Serious ultraviolet-radiation damage to your skin can cause premature aging, leathery skin, deep wrinkles, discolored spots, and potentially deadly skin cancer.

But a little sunlight is important to enable you to make enough health-promoting and health-protecting vitamin D. Fifteen minutes in the early morning or late afternoon—when the sun's rays aren't so intense—is ideal. Combine it with a brisk walk, and you double your benefits. Taking daily walks is an ancient *Ayurvedic* recommendation. It is called your "constitutional" walk. *Ayurveda* recommends *a brisk walk in the morning and another in the evening to maintain good health.*

If you live in a climate that doesn't see much sun, especially during the cold winter months, taking supplemental vitamin D is a must. Fatty fish (for example, salmon and mackerel) are about the only foods with natural vitamin D. Most of the vitamin D in our diet comes from foods that are fortified with it, for example, certain dairy products and breakfast cereals. Most multivitamins contain the recommended daily amount of vitamin D, which is about 200–400 international units (IU).

VITAMIN E

Vitamin E is another vitamin with special abilities to help protect against breast cancer. In the laboratory, scientists have found that vitamin E helps to decrease the risk of breast cancer and improve the chances of survival in at least four ways:

1. Vitamin E is an excellent antioxidant.

2. It slows the speed at which tumor cells grow and divide.

3. It promotes tumor-cell death.

4. It prevents new blood vessels from growing in the tumor.

Each of these wonderful anticancer properties has a significant impact when it comes to preventing breast cancer. Research shows that women who regularly eat foods rich in vitamin E, such as avocados, almonds, sweet potatoes, leafy green vegetables, wheat germ, and salmon, have a lower risk of breast cancer.

You can also take vitamin E as a supplement, but research shows that you don't absorb vitamin E in supplement form as well as you do the vitamin E in your food. This is a perfect example of another *Ayurvedic* principle: *Fresh wholesome foods are the best medicines.* If you do take supplemental vitamin E, make sure it's made with a natural form of vitamin E, rather than a synthetic one. Synthetic vitamins absorb very poorly and probably won't do you much good. The recommended daily dose of vitamin E is 400–800 IU. By the way, researchers have found that other antioxidants, such as vitamin C and CoQ$_{10}$ (see Chapter 13), make the antitumor effects of vitamin E even stronger.

Chapter 13

Defense Shields

Preventing Damage
with Antioxidants

*T*here is a phenomenal class of natural substances that act as the body's antiaircraft and missile-defense system against oxygen free radicals, the enemy's smart bombs. Oxygen free radicals are unstable molecules of oxygen normally created as byproducts of cellular metabolism. You need them to drive all the chemical reactions in your body. But if there are too many of them, they turn into ammunition for the enemy, causing biological devastation. Excess oxygen free radicals seek out and attack their preferred targets: your cell membranes and DNA.

In the aftermath of their deadly assault, the body sends in a repair and reconstruction team. But if the damage is too extensive, the repair teams can't keep up. The DNA wounds that are left unattended can initiate and fuel chronic degenerative diseases, such as atherosclerosis, heart disease, strokes, emphysema, diabetes, arthritis, senility, accelerated aging, and cancer. Pollution, pesticides, tobacco, alcohol, and grilled red meat are just a few of the things that can penetrate your defenses by pouring excess oxygen free radicals into your body and, thus, are good things to avoid.

The only defenses against this unstable oxygen enemy are antioxidants, special weapons favored by your Warrior Goddess. She uses them to create a dynamic defense shield around every cell in your body. Unlike metal shields, which are inert and static, this shield is alive and composed of swarms of molecules, each acting like the protagonist in the old video game Pacman, gobbling up oxygen free radicals as fast as they can.

Your body makes its own antioxidants, but it can't usually create enough to win the battle. It needs a constant supply. Fresh organic fruits and vegetables hold an army of antioxidants. Research shows that a diet rich in antioxidants significantly lowers your risk of breast cancer. Each plant contains specific antioxidants, and each antioxidant has unique abilities to fend off chronic diseases, including cancer. For example, lycopene, the antioxidant responsible for the red color in fruits and vegetables such as tomatoes, is especially effective at lowering the risk of breast and prostate cancer.

Those fruits and vegetables with the most antioxidants ("antioxidant powerhouses") are listed below.

- Beets
- Blackberries
- Blueberries
- Broccoli
- Brussels sprouts
- Cherries
- Garlic
- Kale
- Kiwi
- Oranges
- Plums
- Red grapes
- Red bell pepper
- Spinach
- Strawberries

Although fresh organic fruits and vegetables are excellent sources of antioxidants, in this age of widespread pollution, toxins, and stressful lifestyles that fuel an ever-increasing attack of oxygen free radicals, you need a more powerful supplemental defense—beyond what you can get from even the best food—to keep the enemy at bay.

That's where antioxidant supplements come in. Selenium, vitamin C, vitamin E, CoQ_{10}, and an *Ayurvedic* herbal preparation called *Amrit Kalash* are all potent antioxidants. Research has proven that taking supplemental amounts of these antioxidants better equips you with the ammunition you need to fight the battle against breast cancer.

SELENIUM

Selenium is a mineral and micronutrient that your body needs for a number of very important functions. It plays a big role in preventing several different kinds of cancer, including cancers of the breast, prostate, lung, and colon. Research shows that most women who have breast cancer have much lower selenium levels than those who don't have the disease.

One of the reasons selenium is so effective in lowering the risk of cancer is that it causes your body to make more of its own powerful antioxidant—an enzyme called "glutathione peroxidase." Selenium makes up a fundamental part of the structure of this enzyme and, therefore, affects its function. Without selenium, the enzyme can't work.

Selenium helps to fight cancer in several other ways, as well. Research has shown that it can prevent cancer cells from growing, cause cancer cells to die, foil the formation of new blood vessels needed for cancer to grow, and enhance the immune system, especially natural killer (NK) cells and T-cell function. In addition, selenium has anti-inflammatory effects. When selenium is combined with the iodine found in seaweed (see Chapter 11), it becomes even more effective.

With all these anticancer effects, it's easy to understand why a growing mountain of evidence asserts that taking selenium can be enormously helpful in preventing and treating cancer. In a double-blind, randomized prospective study published in 1996, patients were given 200 micrograms (mcg) of supplemental selenium every day. After six years, the patients taking selenium had only half as many deaths from cancer as the patients who weren't taking it. In other words, in this study the number of people who died of cancer in the group taking selenium was 52 percent lower than the number of people who died in the group that wasn't taking selenium. The subjects who were taking selenium also had 35 percent fewer new cancers diagnosed. So, taking selenium not only lowers the risk of developing cancer, it also appears to lengthen the lives of those who already have it.

Since 1996, numerous other studies have confirmed these same impressive statistics. The conclusion of the vast majority of studies looking at the relationship between selenium and cancer is that taking supplemental selenium or eating a selenium-rich diet reduces your risk of most types of cancer, including breast cancer, by as much as 50 percent and improves your chances of survival if you already have it.

There's a large prospective study currently being conducted in France to determine the long-term health effects of taking supplemental selenium. Of the 12,000 people enrolled in the study, half will take selenium supplements for eight years. Researchers want to determine whether taking more than adequate amounts of selenium every day provides significant health benefits. Specifically, their intent is to definitively answer the question: Can taking supplemental selenium effectively prevent or treat disease, and if so, which diseases?

Taking Selenium

Your main source of selenium is the plants you eat. Selenium is found naturally in soil and is absorbed by plants as they grow. But the amount of selenium in the soil varies considerably from region to region. If there isn't much in the soil, there won't be much in the plants growing there. Research shows that the amount of selenium in the soil and the rate of cancer in that location are inversely proportional. In other words, the areas of the world that have the *highest* selenium levels in the soil have the *lowest* rates of cancer. On the other hand, those with the lowest levels of selenium in the soil have the highest rates of cancer.

The best food source of selenium is Brazil nuts. Just one ounce of Brazil nuts a day gives you 1,200 percent of the recommended daily allowance. Other foods high in selenium include garlic, onions, leafy green vegetables, mushrooms, and whole grains, especially whole wheat. If you choose to take selenium in supplement form, about 200 mcg a day is recommended.

Don't take megadoses of selenium—or of any vitamin or food supplement for that matter. Remember that your body requires a delicate balance. The prudence of choosing just the right amount to achieve balance was introduced to most us of at a very early age by the fairytale "Goldilocks and the Three Bears." (Fairytales often reveal profound archetypal wisdom.) Goldilocks is remembered for one prominent personality trait: She evaluated the size or amount of anything she needed, from a chair to porridge, and always chose whichever was not too big and not too little, but "just right." Goldilocks lived her life according to the most important principle of *Ayurveda:* balance.

Ayurveda teaches that good health is *only* achieved and maintained by making choices that bring balance. In other words, always doing or taking the proper amount of the right things, at and for the ideal time, is the key to good health. In the case of selenium, if you take too much of it, you can develop the syndrome selenosis. Symptoms include hair loss, gastrointestinal upset, white blotchy nails, and mild nerve damage. To prevent these problems, don't take more than 400 mcg of supplemental selenium a day.

VITAMIN E

Vitamin E is another excellent antioxidant that helps to lower your risk of breast cancer. Chapter 12 discussed the details about this vitamin and how it battles this disease.

COENZYME Q_{10} (CoQ_{10})

CoQ_{10}, also known as ubiquinone, is a vitamin-like substance that is found in every cell in your body. It is absolutely essential to the process of cellular energy production. It's also a powerful antioxidant. Research has shown that CoQ_{10} levels are much lower in tumors than they are in normal tissues. When CoQ_{10} has been given to cancer patients, some spectacular results have been seen.

In a study from Denmark published in 1994, thirty-two patients with high-risk breast cancer were treated with antioxidants (vitamins C and E, selenium, and beta-carotene), essential fatty acids (gamma linolenic acid and omega-3 fatty acids), and 90 milligrams (mg) of CoQ_{10}. The breast tumors shrank in six of the thirty-two patients.

The researchers wondered what would happen if they increased the dose of

CoQ_{10}. So, they decided to raise the daily dose of CoQ_{10} to 390 mg in just one of the six patients. They got a big, pleasant surprise. In one month, the tumor in this patient had become so small that it could no longer be felt. In another month, a mammogram showed that the tumor had completely disappeared. With these startling results, the researchers wanted to see if these higher doses of CoQ_{10} would shrink tumors in other breast cancer patients. They selected a woman with breast cancer, gave her 300 mg of CoQ_{10} a day, and waited with great anticipation. In just a few months, her tumor disappeared. In the eighteen months that the patients in this study were treated with CoQ_{10}, none of them died or showed further signs of metastases. The number of women who had been expected to die, as predicted by the stage of their tumors, was four.

Encouraged by these results, the researchers continued their study of CoQ_{10} in breast cancer patients and published a report the following year. They gave all their breast cancer patients 390 mg of CoQ_{10} each day. One patient was a forty-four-year-old woman with numerous metastases of her breast cancer to her liver. After a few months of taking CoQ_{10}, *all the metastatic tumors disappeared!* After six months of taking CoQ_{10}, another breast cancer patient, who had had a metastatic tumor to the lining of her lung before taking the CoQ_{10}, had no signs of the tumor left. More research is needed to determine the effectiveness of CoQ_{10} in stopping the growth of breast cancer, but the results of these studies look very promising.

CoQ_{10} has been shown to help prevent the organ damage caused by chemotherapy, and it may even improve a woman's chance of surviving breast cancer. Chemotherapeutic drugs kill cancer cells, but they also kill normal cells. Certain drugs, such as Adriamycin, are toxic to the heart, and it's not uncommon for them to cause heart damage. The damage Adriamycin causes to this vital organ can be so severe that, if given to elderly patients with hearts already compromised by disease, it can kill them.

The reason Adriamycin damages the heart is directly related to CoQ_{10}. Normally, CoQ_{10} is found in high concentrations in the heart. Adriamycin causes CoQ_{10} levels to drop. Apparently, this drug can only damage the heart if the amount of CoQ_{10} in its muscle cells is low. So, when patients on Adriamycin are given a CoQ_{10} supplement, the levels in the heart muscle remain normal, and heart-muscle cells with normal CoQ_{10} levels aren't damaged by the drug. (For more information on CoQ_{10}, see the inset "The Story of CoQ_{10}" on page 116.)

Taking CoQ_{10}

CoQ_{10} is fat soluble. In other words, it's more easily absorbed when it's in fat. When CoQ_{10} is taken in a soy-oil suspension contained in a soft-shell capsule,

The Story of CoQ$_{10}$

CoQ$_{10}$ (ubiquinone) was discovered by accident in a research lab at the University of Wisconsin in 1957 when a group of postdoctoral students was performing experiments on beef-heart mitochondria. (Mitochondria are the structures in your cells where energy is produced. They are considered the power plants of your cells. CoQ$_{10}$ is used by mitochondria to help drive the chemical reactions that produce energy.)

The students noticed a yellow frothy substance that kept rising to the top of their test tubes. When they looked at it under a microscope, these graduate students were viewing CoQ$_{10}$ for the first time. Incidentally, Peter Mitchell, the scientist who figured out specifically how CoQ$_{10}$ is used by the cells for energy production, received the Nobel Prize in 1978 for this discovery.

Although CoQ$_{10}$ is found in nearly every cell in your body, its highest concentrations are in the cells that make up the organs that need lots of energy, such as the heart, kidneys, liver, and lungs. Your body makes its own CoQ$_{10}$, but you also get additional amounts of it from outside sources—foods such as broccoli, spinach, and fish.

As you age, your levels of CoQ$_{10}$ begin to drop. If the amount of CoQ$_{10}$ in your cells falls too low, you can develop serious health problems. Certain disease conditions, such as congestive heart failure, are commonly associated with CoQ$_{10}$ deficiencies. When patients with congestive heart failure are given supplemental CoQ$_{10}$, their symptoms sometimes improve dramatically.

The Japanese were the first to find a way to make CoQ$_{10}$ in large enough quantities for commercial use. They began to use it extensively to treat hospital patients and soon discovered that the patients with diseases associated with low CoQ$_{10}$ levels, such as congestive heart failure, got a lot better. The Japanese now routinely treat all heart patients with CoQ$_{10}$.

Over the past few decades, there have been hundreds of studies documenting the significant health benefits of supplemental CoQ$_{10}$ for the treatment of many conditions other than heart disease. Some of these disorders are high blood pressure, periodontal (gum) disease, type 2 diabetes, male infertility, chronic fatigue syndrome (CFS), immune-system disorders such as AIDS, sickle-cell anemia, cancer, and neurological disorders including Parkinson's disease.

it is more readily absorbed than if it's taken in a dry tablet or capsule. That means you need a higher dose of the dry form of CoQ_{10} than you do of the oil suspension to attain the same level of it in your body. If your goal is to lower your risk of breast cancer, 30–100 mg of CoQ_{10} a day is recommended. If you already have breast cancer, you'll need to take more.

Case studies from Denmark showed that breast tumors shrank in women given 300–390 mg of CoQ_{10} a day. If you are taking chemotherapeutic drugs that decrease CoQ_{10} levels, such as Adriamycin, you'll definitely want to take higher doses of CoQ_{10} to combat any potential organ damage caused by these drugs. Most CoQ_{10} is synthetically made. But a few companies produce a naturally fermented form of CoQ_{10} made from whole foods that studies show your body absorbs and uses much more efficiently. A study from the University of Scranton found that fermented CoQ_{10} had twenty times more antioxidant activity than the standard synthetic preparations of CoQ_{10} and that only 22 mg of the fermented CoQ_{10} they tested was equivalent to 400 mg of synthetically made CoQ_{10}.

Be sure to tell your doctor that you are planning to take this supplement. Let him or her help you determine how much to take. Also, because supplemental CoQ_{10} improves heart health, a person who takes heart medication may need his or her dosage adjusted while taking this supplement.

High blood pressure medications such as propranolol (Inderal), statin cholesterol-lowering drugs, and red yeast rice (a cholesterol-lowering dietary supplement) bring CoQ_{10} levels down, so you should always take supplemental CoQ_{10} when taking these substances.

AMRIT KALASH

Dr. Yukie Niwa, a Japanese researcher, studied more than 500 different antioxidants over a period of thirty years. He found that the most powerful and effective antioxidant of all those tested is an ancient *Ayurvedic* herbal preparation called *Amrit Kalash*. Research shows that the antioxidant capabilities of *Amrit Kalash* are at least 25,000 times more powerful than those of vitamins C and E. Taking it is like supplying your Warrior Goddess with a *Star Wars* deflector shield. This astounding ambrosia is composed of forty-four different herbs and fruits that seem to work synergistically, enhancing the natural strength of one another's antioxidants. The phenomenon of synergy, where each substance makes the other more effective, is a beautiful example of another marvel of Nature and *Ayurvedic* principle: *The whole is often greater than the sum of the parts.*

Due to its extraordinary antioxidants (and countless other health-protecting and wellness-enhancing nutrients), *Amrit Kalash* defends against cancer in significant ways. Research shows that it prevents tumors from starting, slows down tumor growth, and even shrinks tumors.

Several notable studies have been conducted at Ohio State University showing that *Amrit Kalash* is highly effective against breast cancer. *Amrit Kalash* is actually a two-part formula referred to as MAK-4 and MAK-5. In these studies, the two compounds were studied individually and then together. In one study, animals were fed MAK-5 before they were exposed to chemical carcinogens that often induce breast cancer. After eighteen weeks, 67 percent of the control animals (the animals not given MAK-5) had developed breast cancer. Of the animals that were given MAK-5, only 25 percent developed breast cancer.

The researchers then tested the other part of the *Amrit Kalash* formula, MAK-4, to see if it would have similar anticancer effects. The animals that were given MAK-4 before being exposed to chemicals known to cause breast cancer had 60 percent fewer tumors than the control animals. The tumors that *did* grow in these animals were only about 12 percent of the size of the tumors that grew in the control animals.

In another experiment, animals with fully formed tumors were given both MAK-4 and MAK-5. Researchers found that all the small tumors (less than 1 centimeter in diameter) in the animals shrank in size but that there was no change in the larger tumors. The conclusion of this study was that *Amrit Kalash* seems to be very beneficial in stopping the growth of small tumors.

There are other dramatic and valuable benefits of *Amrit Kalash,* as well. For one, it's an effective anti-aging supplement (see the inset "An Ancient Anti-Aging Formula" on page 119). For another, it alleviates many of the horrendous side effects of chemotherapy. In a 1994 study, breast cancer patients undergoing chemotherapy treatments were also given *Amrit Kalash.* For most of these patients, many of the side effects they were experiencing from the chemotherapy—especially nausea, vomiting, weight loss, dropped blood counts, and fatigue—went away or significantly diminished. These patients also reported that their overall sense of well-being improved when they took this supplement. Most important, *Amrit Kalash* alleviated all these side effects *without* interfering with the effectiveness of the chemotherapy.

THE ANTIOXIDANT/CHEMO CONTROVERSY

There's some controversy surrounding the use of supplemental antioxidants during chemotherapy and radiation. Why? Because certain chemotherapeutic agents (especially alkylating agents such as cyclophosphamide) and radiotherapy are known to generate and use oxygen free radicals to kill cancer cells. Theoretically, taking supplemental antioxidants could interfere with the effectiveness of these

An Ancient Anti-Aging Formula

Thousands of years ago, *Ayurvedic* physicians created the anti-aging formula *Amrit Kalash*. *Ayurveda* considers *Amrit Kalash* to be a *rasayana*—"that which negates old age and disease." Research has shown that *Amrit Kalash* can indeed slow the aging process because it's such a powerful antioxidant. As you've learned, aging is accelerated by oxygen free radicals, and antioxidants neutralize them. It's incredible that science only recently discovered free radicals and antioxidants but these *Ayurvedic* physicians instinctively "knew" how to create this anti-aging formula—a formula with the most potent synergy of antioxidants of any substance ever tested.

Research shows *Amrit Kalash* may actually *reverse* aging. In a double-blind placebo-controlled study published in the *International Journal of Psychosomatics* in 1990, patients who received MAK-5 improved significantly on an age-related alertness task. Performance of this task is known to highly correlate with age. The older you are, the worse you normally do on this test. This study showed that MAK-5 could enhance the capacity for attention and alertness that predictably declines with age.

drugs at killing cancer cells. (Please take note that consuming antioxidants in foods is not at issue here; levels in whole foods are much lower than they are in supplement form.)

An extensive review of hundreds of studies on this subject was published in 1999. In it, researchers Davis Lamson and Matthew Brignall concluded that the vast majority of studies found that taking antioxidants "produces beneficial effects in many cancers with very few exceptions, and human studies show no reduction in the efficacy of chemotherapy or radiation when given with antioxidants." Lamson and Brignall felt that the argument that antioxidants might interfere with chemotherapy was too simplistic and probably untrue. Most studies showed an "increased effectiveness of many cancer chemotherapeutic agents, as well as a decrease in adverse effects, when given concurrently with antioxidants." The exact mechanisms of how these drugs work aren't yet fully understood.

After reviewing several hundred studies, Lamson and Brignall had only three cautions regarding the use of supplemental antioxidants during cancer treatments:

1. Routine use of N-acetylcysteine (NAC) with the chemotherapeutic agents cis-plantinum and doxorubicin should be avoided.

2. The flavonoid tangeretin found in citrus fruits should not be taken with Tamoxifen.

3. Beta-carotene should not be taken with 5-FU (Carac, Efudex) until the nature of their interaction has been clearly determined through research.

A highly quoted study from Finland shows that when beta-carotene was given to smokers, their risk of lung cancer went up. The theoretical explanation is that there are 500 different naturally occurring carotenoids, or plant pigments. If you take high doses of one of them, it doesn't allow you to get enough of the others. In the *Ayurvedic* view, getting your carotenoids from your food—in the proportions and amounts Nature provides—is the ideal way to consume these natural cancer-fighting substances because it brings balance and enhances health.

Certainly, more investigation needs to be done on all the antioxidants to determine exactly what their effects are on every type of cancer and every anti-cancer drug. By the preponderance of evidence, it certainly seems that taking a combination of different antioxidants cautiously and judiciously and eating foods high in antioxidants in conjunction with chemotherapy is very beneficial. In the vast majority of studies, antioxidants have been shown to actually *enhance* the effectiveness of these drugs, to protect against damaging—and sometimes fatal—side effects, such as organ damage, and to lengthen life expectancy. If I ever had to have chemotherapy, I would definitely—and selectively—take antioxidants at the same time.

Chapter 14

Smothering the Flames

The Anticancer Power of Anti-Inflammatories

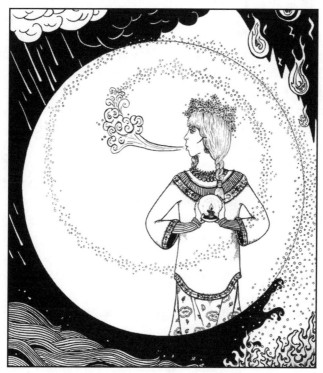

Nordic Goddess That Cools the Fires

*If you have faith in the cause and the means and in God,
the hot sun will be cool for you.*

—MAHATMA GANDHI

*I*nflammation is a normal process created naturally by your body, and it serves an important role. It helps to get rid of unwanted bacteria and other invaders. It also assists your body in cleaning up dead cells from trauma or infection. When inflammation rises to assist your inner healing intelligence in these particular kinds of situations and then quietly wanes when it's no longer needed, no harm is done. But if the inflammation remains beyond its original purpose and becomes chronic (that is, continues as an ongoing process in your body), it turns into a lethal firestorm, breaking down cells and destroying the natural architectural boundaries of the body's tissues, making it easier for tumors to invade and grow.

Your Warrior Goddess can use inflammation as a tool to keep you healthy. It's like having a fireplace in your home where she can build a fire on a cold winter's night to keep you warm. But if you throw too much fuel on the fire, it can quickly grow out of control. Your Warrior Goddess then has to work frantically to keep the fire from burning down your house, destroying everything you own, and killing you in the process. Similarly, if inflammation is not kept under control, it can destroy your health and increase your risk of diseases that can potentially kill you, such as breast cancer.

Researchers have found that chronic inflammation not only plays a key role in the commencement and progression of many types of cancers, it also fuels a wide variety of chronic disorders, including heart disease, arthritis, and Alzheimer's disease.

One major reason why chronic inflammation acts as such a powerful destructive force is because it doesn't act alone. It creates additional destructive ammunition: oxygen free radicals. The cells in your immune system use oxygen free radicals like cosmic ray guns to shoot down bacteria and other offenders. In the presence of inflammation, these cells release showers of oxygen free radicals. And excess oxygen free radicals can cause the kind of DNA damage that can lead to cancer.

Stress and certain foods promote inflammation. Refined carbohydrates, sugar, and certain fats—especially trans fats—are some of the worst offenders. On the other hand, a diet rich in the antioxidants found in fresh, organically grown fruits and vegetables and omega-3 fatty acids reduces inflammation. Taking supplemental antioxidants (see Chapter 13) and practicing stress-reduction techniques (see Chapter 25) are also very beneficial in preventing and reducing inflammation.

THE COX-2 ENZYME

One of the best ways to reduce inflammation is to block the activity of an essential key enzyme in the inflammatory process called "cyclooxygenase-2," (COX-

2). The COX-2 enzyme is stimulated by inflammatory proteins released by cells in the immune system, growth factors, certain types of fat (such as omega-6 fatty acids), and a variety of other substances that encourage tumor growth. When activated, certain genes called "oncogenes" stimulate the growth of cancer. These oncogenes also increase the activity of the COX-2 enzyme.

A relatively new class of pharmaceutical anti-inflammatories targets the COX-2 enzyme and blocks or inhibits it. Celebrex and Vioxx are two examples. But pharmaceutical medications are hard on the body and create imbalances that can result in potentially serious side effects. This is precisely why Vioxx was taken off the market in the fall of 2004. When reaching for COX-2 anti-inflammatories, the wisest choice is to choose those made by Nature. Herbal COX-2 inhibitors not only block the enzyme with as much force as the synthetic pharmaceuticals, but they also import intelligence and balance into the body.

Nature's COX-2-inhibiting pharmacy includes dozens of herbs. The standouts are green tea, turmeric, holy basil, rosemary, ginger, oregano, skullcap (*Scutellaria*), barberry, and the Chinese herbs *hu zhang* and Chinese goldenthread. Researchers at Columbia University are currently studying the effectiveness of the herbal product Zyflamend, which is a mixture of all ten of these potent herbal anti-inflammatories, against prostate cancer. The details of this study are discussed in the inset "Zyflamend and Cancer" on page 125. Leading complementary and alternative physicians, such as Dr. Andrew Weil, prescribe Zyflamend for their patients with inflammatory conditions. It is also used at the Cleveland Clinic Spine Center in Cleveland, Ohio. If you want learn more about the properties of the herbs in Zyflamend, I recommend *Beyond Aspirin: Nature's Challenge to Arthritis, Cancer & Alzheimer's Disease,* an excellent book by Thomas M. Newmark and Paul Schulick.

Cancer and the COX-2 Enzyme

Researchers have found that inflammation isn't the only process that the COX-2 enzyme takes part in. It also plays a key role in the initiation and growth of several different cancers, including colon, prostate, and breast cancer. The COX-2 enzyme stimulates breast cells to start dividing and growing. It also prevents tumor cells from undergoing normal cell death, so more tumor cells remain alive, accelerating the growth of the tumor. The more tumor cells there are, the faster the tumor grows and the bigger it gets. The COX-2 enzyme also encourages new blood vessels to grow into the tumor. New blood vessels are constantly required to deliver enough nutrients and oxygen-laden blood to feed an expanding tumor. The more nutrients and oxygen the tumor gets, the bigger and faster it grows.

Tumor cells can invade normal tissue more aggressively in response to the COX-2 enzyme. This seemingly malicious enzyme also enhances a tumor's ability to metastasize, suppresses the immune system so that it can't fight off cancer cells as effectively, and steps up the production of mutagens (substances that cause mutations in your DNA that can lead to cancer). When you add them all together, these hazardous effects of the COX-2 enzyme powerfully promote tumor growth. It's no wonder studies show that taking anti-inflammatories to block the ill effects of the COX-2 enzyme can reduce your risk of breast cancer by as much as 50 percent.

Some tumors show an "overexpression" of the COX-2 enzyme. This means that these tumor cells have a lot more active COX-2 enzyme in them than normal tissue usually does. The tumors that frequently show this overexpression include cancers of the colon, prostate, and breast. Not all breast cancers overexpress the COX-2 enzyme, but researchers have found that a significant number do—about 50 percent.

According to a study conducted at the University of Innsbruck in Austria and published in the *British Journal of Cancer* in 2003, women with breast tumors that overexpress the COX-2 enzyme are more likely to have their tumors come back a short period of time after treatment. Patients with these types of tumors also have a poorer overall survival rate.

COX-2 ENZYME INHIBITORS

Certain anti-inflammatory pharmaceutical medications, such as Celebrex, are designed to work by blocking or inhibiting the COX-2 enzyme. All the herbs found in Zyflamend inhibit the COX-2 enzyme, too. (The details of a study of this natural COX-2 inhibitor can be found in the inset "Zyflamend and Cancer" on page 125.) Not surprisingly, research has shown that all COX-2 inhibitors have powerful anticancer properties. In experimental animals, they have been found to significantly reduce the formation of breast tumors and the number of tumors that grow in response to a carcinogen. COX-2 inhibitors also slow the growth of tumors once they have formed.

In a study published in 2001, researchers at Ohio State University found a direct inverse relationship between the amount of COX-2 inhibitor that was given and the number of breast tumors that formed in the test animals. The higher the dose of COX-2 inhibitors was, the lower the risk of breast tumors.

ANTI-INFLAMMATORIES AND BREAST CANCER— THE WOMEN'S HEALTH INITIATIVE STUDY

The largest ongoing national study of women's health, called The Women's

Zyflamend and Cancer

Researchers at Columbia University in New York are currently studying the effectiveness of Zyflamend against prostate cancer. This cancer, like breast cancer, can overexpress the COX-2 enzyme. The researchers found in laboratory tests that Zyflamend strongly inhibited the growth of prostate cancer cells by causing the cancer cells to die (a process technically called "apoptosis") and by stopping new blood-vessel growth. The COX-2 inhibiting effects of the ten combined herbs in Zyflamend were found to be greater than those of curcumin, a powerful COX-2 inhibitor and the active ingredient in turmeric.

Encouraged by these laboratory findings, the Columbia researchers are currently conducting more studies on Zyflamend in the laboratory, as well as clinical studies on patients. They have just designed a three-year clinical trial that will follow 100 men. The men will be given Zyflamend and then have biopsies of their prostate gland every six months to see what effect it has. The goal is to determine if Zyflamend effectively prevents prostate cancer. Researchers believe that this herbal COX-2-inhibiting formula will be effective against all cancers that overexpress the COX-2 enzyme, including cancers of the colon and breast. There's also a study just getting underway at Osaka University in Japan to examine the effectiveness of Zyflamend for preventing and treating colon cancer.

All the herbs or isolates of active ingredients in the herbs in Zyflamend have been studied individually to determine their effects in reducing the incidence and growth of cancers. One of the herbs in Zyflamend is turmeric (see Turmeric—A Potent Anti-Inflammatory on page 126). Another is green tea (see Green Tea—The #1 Anticancer Beverage on page 91). In addition, many studies also document the impressive COX-2-inhibiting effects of holy basil, rosemary, ginger, *hu zhang*, Chinese goldenthread, barberry, oregano, and skullcap (*Scutellaria*).

COX-2 inhibitors lower the risk of cancer in two major ways: They reduce inflammation and block the expression of the COX-2 enzyme in tumors. Inflammation creates an abundance of oxygen free radicals, and it destroys natural tissue boundaries making it easier for tumors to grow. The COX-2 enzyme has an unsurpassed talent for promoting the inception and cultivation of tumors because of the impressive array of cancer-promoting techniques that it holds, but COX-2 enzyme inhibitors can block every one of its tumor-fostering processes.

Health Initiative (WHI), recently found that women who had taken aspirin or ibuprofen (a type of nonsteroidal anti-inflammatory drug; NSAID) an average of three times a week for the last ten years had a significantly lower risk of breast cancer. Those who took aspirin had a 28 percent lower risk, and those who took ibuprofen had a 50 percent lower risk.

Since aspirin and ibuprofen have the potential for some serious side effects (107,000 people are hospitalized and more than 16,500 people die in the United States alone each year from bleeding complications related to NSAIDs), many natural-medicine doctors, including Dr. Andrew Weil, and I recommend that you take a safe herbal anti-inflammatory such as Zyflamend instead. Research shows that it works just as well, and rather than causing side effects, it brings a multitude of wonderful side benefits.

TURMERIC—A POTENT ANTI-INFLAMMATORY

Let me say again that the amazing Asian spice turmeric is one of the most brilliant secret weapons against breast cancer that you can give your Warrior Goddess. The broad healing power of this extraordinary rhizome was introduced in Chapter 11, but it has other remarkable attributes, as well. When it comes to natural COX-2 inhibitors, none is as powerful as turmeric. A study published in the *Indian Journal of Medical Research* compared the anti-inflammatory effects of oral curcumin (one of the active ingredients in turmeric and the source of its bright yellow-orange color) against two powerful anti-inflammatory medications: cortisone and phenylbutazone. The study found that curcumin was *just as effective* as these two potent anti-inflammatory medications!

The anti-inflammatory intelligence contained in turmeric enhances your body's anti-inflammatory intelligence in three different ways. First, it stimulates your adrenal glands to release natural, powerful anti-inflammatory substances called corticosteroids. Second, it prevents the breakdown of cortisol, so more of this natural anti-inflammatory stays in your body. Third, it makes your body's cortisol receptors more sensitive. When the receptors are more sensitive, it only takes a small amount of cortisol to produce big anti-inflammatory effects.

Turmeric can also be used as a topical anti-inflammatory and analgesic (pain reliever). When applied over strained muscles, pulled tendons, and arthritic joints, turmeric can help to reduce swelling and pain. It depletes substance P, a chemical produced at nerve endings that causes the sensation of irritation and pain.

Another reason why turmeric is such a powerful anti-inflammatory is because it's also a strong COX-2-enzyme inhibitor—even more grounds for turmeric to be considered the number-one anticancer spice!

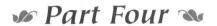

Part Four

Poisoning Your Warrior Goddess

Toxins That Destroy Your Healing Intelligence

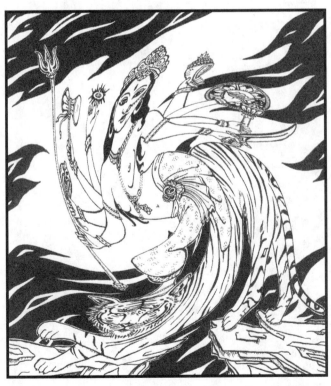

Goddess in Turmoil

Chapter 15

The Four Perils of Red Meat

Your Goddess Is an Herbivore

Nothing will benefit human health and increase chances for survival of life on Earth as much as the evolution to a vegetarian diet.

—ALBERT EINSTEIN

This is the first of seven chapters that put a spotlight on breast cancer's covert allies: the foods and substances that trigger and support its growth. These factors are proven enemies to your breast health. Avoiding them lowers your risk of breast cancer. These "forces of darkness" are the foods, habits, and toxins that destroy your body's inner healing intelligence, help to midwife the cancer monster, and support cancer's rapid growth. These are the things that weaken your Warrior Goddess, strip her of her power, and obstruct her ability to keep you well. They are like Kryptonite to Superman.

Research has shown beyond a scientific doubt that eating red meat is a serious risk factor for breast cancer. You can think of it this way: Breast cancer is a carnivore; your Warrior Goddess is an herbivore. Many studies have shown that women who eat the most red meat have an 88 to 330 percent increased risk of this deadly disease. A German study published in 2002 found that women who consumed the most red meat had an 85 percent greater risk of breast cancer. The numbers were even higher in premenopausal women. A study from Portland, Oregon, published in 2003 in the journal *Cancer Causes and Control,* also found that women who ate red meat regularly had a significantly increased risk of breast cancer.

PERIL #1: ANIMAL PROTEIN

The meat of animals is composed primarily of protein, which is made up of smaller subunits known as "amino acids." It also contains creatine, an important substance that muscle cells use for energy. As you know, protein and amino acids are essential to health, and so is creatine. However, when animal protein is cooked, especially at high heat, structural changes occur in the protein, amino acids, and creatine—changes that create dangerous new carcinogens. A study from Uruguay found that red-meat protein is associated with a *220 to 770 percent* increased risk of breast cancer!

PERIL #2: SATURATED ANIMAL FATS

Saturated animal fats (a type of lipid) from red meat and dairy products are poisonous to your body. These lipids make the cells in your body more resistant to insulin. As a result, your insulin levels go up. High insulin levels are lethal. In fact, they are one of the biggest risk factors for breast cancer. Research shows that women with the highest insulin levels have a 283 percent greater risk of breast cancer.

There are two other ways that saturated animal fat can raise your risk of breast cancer, as well. First, saturated animal fat is converted into a carcinogenic substance by the bacteria in your colon. Second, oxygen free radicals have a tendency to attack and damage these types of fats, changing them into powerful stimulators of inflammation, and inflammation fuels the growth of breast cancer. Worse yet, inflammation and oxygen free radicals engage in a deadly dance with each other, each one increasing the numbers and power of the other. Inflammation produces more oxygen free radicals, and oxygen free radicals, in turn, spark the fires of inflammation.

PERIL #3: CONCENTRATED TOXINS IN RED MEAT

Red meat is a storehouse of concentrated toxins including pesticides, antibiotics, hormones, and growth stimulators. Within this lethal mix is insulin-like growth factor-1 (IGF-1), which, as you've learned, is vile and murderous at higher concentrations. IGF-1 is an extraordinarily potent stimulator of breast cancer. In fact, scientists believe it may be *the most* potent stimulator of breast cancer known.

Eating conventionally raised beef and dairy products is the principal way that excessive amounts of IGF-1 get into your body. In the United States, livestock are regularly fed and injected with growth hormones and stimulators to make them grow bigger and faster and to increase their production of milk. (For more information on IGF-1 and its role in breast cancer, see Chapter 8.)

Environmental toxins, such as pesticides, herbicides, chemical fertilizers, and industrial chemicals, accumulate and are stored in animal fat. Many of these toxins have estrogenic effects. In other words, they act like estrogen in the body and accelerate cell division. Many studies have shown that these pesticides can trigger breast cancer and that those women who have high levels of these pesticides in their bodies have a much higher risk of breast cancer.

PERIL #4: DEATH BY GRILLING

When red meats are cooked at high temperatures, additional carcinogens known as "heterocyclic amines" are formed. These sinister molecules attack DNA, destroying its vital code in a way that seriously increases the risk of cancer. Frying and grilling are the methods of cooking that use the highest temperatures to cook meat, and they are associated with the highest risk of breast cancer. The higher the cooking temperature, the more carcinogenic heterocyclic amines form. How long you cook your meat makes a difference, too. The more well-done your meat is, the more heterocyclic amines it will have, and the more carcinogenic it will be. Research shows that of the women who eat red meat, those who eat both the most grilled and the most well-done red meat have the highest risk of breast cancer.

A study from Vanderbilt University published in 2002 found that women who consumed large amounts of red meat, especially cooked well-done, had a significantly higher risk of breast cancer. If the women were also overweight, their risk was even greater.

Another study, done at the Medical College of Ohio and published in the journal *Carcinogenesis* in 1999, found that an enzyme in breast tissue called "N-acetyltransferase" *activates* the carcinogens in well-done red meat and in cigarette smoke. The study also identified several different subtypes of the N-acetyl-transferase enzyme. The risk of breast cancer in women who had one particular subtype of this enzyme was extremely high. The women who had this dangerous subtype and who also smoked, ate a lot of red meat, or ate well-done red meat were found to have a 400 percent higher risk of breast cancer. In short, eating well-done red meat is always risky, but it is *exceptionally* risky for certain women.

SAFE ALTERNATIVES—MEAT MIMICKERS

If you love the taste and texture of red meat, don't think you have to give it up. The ever-growing and surprisingly delicious vegetable-based meat-substitute cuisine has come a long way. Even committed carnivores will find many of the meat mimickers to be a culinary delight. For instance, my rebellious teenager couldn't tell the difference between a Boca Burger (made with soy protein) and an actual hamburger! Also, some vegetarians (I, for one) think some meat substitutes taste too much like the real thing!

If you *do* like the taste of meat, however, there are delicious substitutes for hamburgers, frankfurters, salami, lunchmeats, chicken, turkey, jerky—you name it. The next time you're at your local health food store, experiment and give one a try. I think you'll be pleasantly surprised. Many chain grocery stores carry them, too.

The list below shows some good substitutes for your old meaty favorites.

- Instead of bacon, try Lightlife Smart Bacon.

- Instead of chicken, try Gardenburger Chik'n Grill or Nate's Chicken Style Nuggets.

- Instead of hamburgers, try Boca Burgers or Morningstar Farms Grillers Prime.

- Instead of hot dogs, try Yves Veggie Cuisine Good Dog

- Instead of turkey, try To-furkey.

Chapter 16

A Dangerous Foe
in a Sweet Disguise

Sugar: Breast Cancer's
Favorite Food

*I*t is estimated that the average American eats almost his or her entire body weight in sugar every year. The average teenage boy eats 34 teaspoons of sugar a day, and the average teenage girl consumes 24 teaspoons. When you add up the amount of sugar in various foods, it's easy to see how this is possible. Sugar is added to virtually all processed foods, especially soda pop. The average can of cola, such as Coke or Pepsi, contains 10–12 teaspoons of sugar! There's a new breakfast cereal with a whopping 18 teaspoons of sugar *per serving;* that's one-third of a cup, or the equivalent of forty-eight Hershey's Kisses.

If you want your Warrior Goddess to stay in top cancer-fighting condition, this sticky substance is one of the worst things you can give her. It's like wrapping her in a spider's web of cotton candy. Caught in this gummy trap, her ability to oppose her mortal enemy, breast cancer, is dramatically hampered.

As Dr. Christiane Northrup says, for some women, chocolate is a food group. I'm one of those women, so it wasn't good news when I heard what I'm about to share with you: the distressing facts about sugar and cancer. But before you become totally dejected, be aware that there are good all-natural sugar alternatives—one, in particular, that tastes great and is good for you.

INSULIN—SUGAR'S ESCORT

Cancer cells love sugar. It's their preferred fuel. The more sugar you eat, the faster cancer cells grow. Your pancreas responds to sugar by releasing insulin, the hormone that escorts sugar into your cells. When you eat refined simple sugars, such as white table sugar, candy, cookies, or other sugar-laden foods, your blood sugar levels rise very quickly. Your pancreas responds by releasing a lot of insulin. That's not good. High insulin levels are one of the biggest risk factors and promoters of breast cancer. Women with high insulin levels have a 283 percent greater risk of breast cancer.

Insulin is capable of extraordinary evil, and the biggest reason is due to the fact that both normal breast cells and cancer cells have insulin receptors on them. When insulin attaches to its receptor, it has the same effect as when estrogen attaches to its receptor; it causes cells to start dividing. The higher your insulin levels are, the faster your breast cells will divide; the faster they divide, the higher your risk of breast cancer is and the faster any existing cancer cells will grow.

There's another wound that insulin can inflict, too. It attacks a portion of the estrogen cycle, making more estrogen available to attach to the estrogen receptors in breast tissue. Insulin regulates how much of the estrogen in your blood is available to attach to estrogen receptors. Look back at Figure 3.1 on page 36. When estrogen travels in the blood, it either travels alone seeking a mate (an estrogen receptor), *or* it travels with a partner (a protein binder, or carrier) that prevents it from attaching to an estrogen receptor. Insulin regulates the number of protein binders in the blood. So, the higher your insulin levels are, the fewer the number of protein binders there will be. Fewer protein binders means that there's more free estrogen available to attach to estrogen receptors.

In other words, when your insulin levels are up, free-estrogen levels are up, too. And both of them speed up cell division. That's why high insulin levels increase your risk of breast cancer so much.

DANGER—SUGAR!

Eating sugar increases your risk of breast cancer in yet another way. It delivers a major blow to your immune system with the force of a prizefighter. Your immune system is your natural defense against such invaders as bacteria, viruses, and cancer cells. Research shows that right after you eat a high-sugar meal, the function of the cells in your immune system drops drastically. In the case of one type of cell in particular—the T lymphocyte (a type of white blood cell)—sugar knocks its defense abilities down by at least 50 percent. This effect lasts for a minimum of five hours! Another researcher found that the function of T lymphocytes dropped by *94 percent* after a high-sugar meal! This means that right after you've eaten a lot of sugar, your body's ability to fight off invaders or destroy cancer cells is tremendously weakened for several hours.

Over a period of time, eating too much sugar can create imbalances that lead to two more deadly diseases: obesity and type 2 diabetes. Both of these diseases dangerously increase your risk of breast cancer, and both have increased alarmingly in the United States in the past two decades. An estimated 60 percent of American adults are overweight, and 5 percent have diabetes. Of those people who have diabetes, 90 percent are also overweight. Not only do these diseases increase your risk of breast cancer, but they also increase your risk of heart disease, high blood pressure, poor circulation, stroke, and infection.

A study conducted by Harvard Medical School and published in 2004 found that women who, as teenagers, ate foods with a high glycemic index (foods that cause blood sugars to soar, such as refined carbohydrates and sugars) had a higher incidence of breast cancer later in life. So, encouraging your teenage daughter to cut back on sugar will help her to lower her risk of breast cancer for the rest of her life.

STEVIA—SWEET RELIEF

Now, the good news: If you have a sweet tooth, you'll be relieved to know that you don't have to suffer. There's a natural sweetener that tastes great, and better yet, research has shown that instead of being dangerous to your health, it actually has several wonderful health-supporting qualities. It's called Stevia, and it comes from the South American plant *Stevia rebaudiana*. What's interesting about this semi shrub, indigenous to Paraguay, is that every part of it tastes intensely sweet. The dried leaves, however, are the only parts that are used for medicinal and commercial purposes. Scientists have found that Stevia's delightfully sweet flavor comes from a group of substances in it called "glycosidal diterpenes."

Compared to sugar, only *very* small amounts of Stevia are needed. That's because Stevia is 300 times sweeter than sucrose, the type of sugar found in table sugar. Stevia hasn't yet been approved by the FDA as a food additive— write your senators and Congressional representatives!—so at this time you won't find it in any processed foods in the United States. In this country Stevia is considered a dietary supplement. Health food stores and national-chain grocery stores that specialize in organic foods, such as Wild Oats and Whole Foods, usually carry Stevia.

Stevia comes in multiple forms: a fine white powder, a green powder, or a liquid. I found that certain brands of Stevia have a bitter taste or leave a strange aftertaste if you use too much. There's one brand, however, that solved this problem by adding some fiber to the Stevia. It is called Stevia Plus by SweetLeaf (see the Resources section). It dissolves well and leaves no bitter aftertaste.

Stevia can also be used in cooking, but it's a little tricky. The amount you should use can vary a lot from brand to brand, so you definitely should use a Stevia cookbook. Many of the companies with Stevia products have their own cookbooks. (See the Resources section for a list of these companies and their websites.)

Stevia has been used for hundreds, if not thousands, of years by the native tribes in Paraguay and Brazil to treat high blood pressure and diabetes. Modern research has shown that it *does* help both conditions. Stevia causes blood vessels to dilate. When the diameter of a blood vessel increases, the blood pressure in it goes down. A double-blind placebo-controlled study was published in the *British Journal of Pharmacology* in 2000 documenting Stevia's ability to lower blood pressure. Researchers found that after only three months, patients with high blood pressure who were given Stevia three times a day had a significant decrease in both their systolic (the upper number) and diastolic (the lower number) blood-pressure numbers.

Stevia is a great sugar substitute for people who really need to avoid sugar, such as diabetics. In addition, Stevia has an added benefit for type 2 diabetics: It seems to have an effect opposite to that of sugar on their bodies; it causes blood sugar to go *down*. Research has also discovered two more Stevia health benefits. First, it can kill certain bacteria and viruses. In a Japanese study published in 2001 by Taka Hashi, et al., in the journal *Antiviral Research,* Stevia was found to have antiviral effects against the rotavirus. This virus can cause severe diarrhea and dehydration, especially in infants. Second, Stevia shows a strong ability to kill a wide range of food-borne bacteria.

Another healthy natural substitute for sugar is also available. It's made from *Luo Han Guo,* the round green fruit of the Chinese plant *Siraita grosvenori. Luo Han Guo* has been used in China as a medicine since the thirteenth century, but it didn't become popular as a remedy for coughs, sore throats, and upper respiratory-tract infections until the twentieth century. In southern China *Luo Han Guo* is also used to enhance longevity. Like Stevia, *Luo Han Guo* is about 300 times sweeter than sugar and is processed into a fine, white crystalline powder. WisdomHerbs makes a sugar substitute using a blend of *Luo Han Guo* and fructose called Sweet & Slender. It can be purchased at most health food stores or on the Internet.

XYLITOL: ANOTHER NATURAL SWEET ALTERNATIVE

Used as a food additive since the 1960s, xylitol is another natural sweetener that appears to be safe and, in addition, sports several health benefits. It is naturally found in fibrous fruits and vegetables, and a variety of hardwoods. The main sources of commercially produced xylitol come from wood scraps and corncobs. Research shows that xylitol is not just an excellent substitute for sugar, it also reduces plaque deposits on teeth, lowers the incidence of dental caries by 80 percent, promotes remineralization of tooth enamel, reduces infections in the mouth and nasopharynx, and decreases bone loss. Xylitol is also good for people with diabetes or who are trying to lose weight. It contains 40 percent fewer calories than sugar and is incompletely absorbed. The portion of xylitol that is absorbed enters the bloodstream very slowly and causes negligible rises in blood sugar and insulin levels. More than 1,500 studies have been published on xylitol confirming its safety. Xylitol was declared to be safe for humans and approved as a food additive by the Federation of American Societies for Experimental Biology (FASEB) in 1986.

ARTIFICIAL SWEETENERS

Artificial sweeteners were created with the good intention of helping you to lower your consumption of sugar. However, most of them are synthetic and not natural to your body. Not surprisingly, a variety of health problems, ranging from the minor to the serious, have been reported by people who have used artificial sweeteners. Saccharine was the only artificial sweetener available on the market through the 1970s. The FDA proposed a ban on this product after a study showed that saccharine caused bladder cancer in male rats. But congress put a moratorium on the ban and, instead, required a warning label on all saccharine-containing products. After several human clinical trials, researchers concluded that with normal usage, the risk posed by saccharine is small. So in 1991, the FDA withdrew their proposal to ban saccharine and President Clinton signed a bill into law in December 2000 removing the required warning label from saccharine products.

More recently, aspartame has become the artificial sweetener of choice. However, it has been reported to cause severe headaches and allergic symptoms and to exacerbate mood disorders such as depression in some people. Aspartame contains aspartic acid, phenylalanine, and methyl alcohol. Methyl alcohol is the chemical that breaks down into formaldehyde and diketopiperazine (DKP), a known carcinogen and neurotoxin. In 1997, eleven-year-old Jennifer Cohen conducted a science experiment in her sixth-grade class that was reported in *The Journal of the American Medical Association* (*JAMA*). Jennifer found that the aspartame present in Diet Coke breaks down into formaldehyde and DKP *at room temperature.*

In 1998, C. Trocho and a team of Spanish researchers found that formaldehyde derived from aspartame binds to DNA and appears to accumulate in tissue proteins and DNA. The problem with formaldehyde interacting with your cells, according to Japanese researchers U. Oyama, et al., in a study published in 2002 in the journal *Cell Biology and Toxicology,* is that it causes cell death and reduces glutathione, one of your body's most powerful natural antioxidants. Lower glutathione levels mean more damage from oxygen free radicals and, consequently, a higher risk of chronic disorders, including cancer. But so far, no clinical studies on humans link any serious health problems to aspartame.

In 1998, the FDA approved the artificial sweetener sucralose (Splenda), which is made by adding chlorine to sucrose. No independent long-term human studies have been done on this product, so we don't know whether it is safe. Before a company can bring an edible product to market, it must conduct "preapproval" research. According to the Sucralose Toxicity Information Center website, preapproval studies on sucralose were found to cause shrunken thymus glands and enlarged liver and kidneys in test animals. Despite this, sucralose is now used in more than fifteen products, including baked goods, chewing gum, salad dressings, processed fruit and fruit juices, tea, and frozen dairy desserts.

From my point of view and that of *Ayurveda,* you should *favor substances made by Nature.* Your body was designed to consume and thrive on the natural plants growing on this planet, not on synthetic chemicals. If you have a choice—and you do—always choose the gifts of the Earth in their most natural form.

Chapter 17

Losing Your
Goddess-Like Figure

Obesity and Breast Cancer

*K*eeping your body fat low reduces your risk of breast cancer as well as your risk of developing many other diseases. You can think of it this way: Your Warrior Goddess likes to keep the figure of an athlete, or at least a Goddess-like figure. It gives her the strength and power to fight off such killer beasts as breast cancer. When she carries too much weight, it slows her down and she can't ward off enemies. For instance, women who are obese (that is, have a BMI over 30) have a much higher risk of postmenopausal breast cancer: 50 to 250 percent higher. About 20 to 30 percent of all postmenopausal breast cancers are thought to be caused primarily by obesity. If you gain weight as an adult, your risk of breast cancer is higher than if you've been overweight all your life. In addition, studies show that obese women with breast cancer are more likely to have advanced breast cancer at the time of their diagnosis and to die from the disease.

There are many other serious reasons why you should avoid gaining too much weight. An estimated 300,000 adults die in the United States each year from obesity-related causes, such as heart disease, high blood pressure, and diabetes, and that number grows every year.

One big reason why obesity is associated with an increased risk of breast cancer is because fat cells produce estrogen. If you look at the estrogen pathway again (Figure 3.1 on page 36), you'll see that estrogen isn't created just by the ovaries. It's also made by fat cells. After menopause, fat becomes the primary site where estrogen is manufactured in your body. So, the more fat you have, the more estrogen your body will produce.

Obesity is also associated with higher levels of insulin and insulin-like growth factor-1 (IGF-1). In Chapter 8, I described the very powerful influences that insulin and IGF-1 have on your risk of breast cancer. They both significantly increase your risk, and if you have the disease, they make your cancer grow faster.

THE OBESITY EPIDEMIC

If you are obese, you're not alone. Recent studies have found the number of obese people in the United States is increasing at an alarming rate. Thirty percent of adults in the United States are obese. Just a decade ago, only 22.9 percent of us were obese. The number of overweight people in the United States increased from 55.9 to 64.5 percent over this same time period, and "extreme obesity"—defined as having a body mass index (BMI) greater than 40—rose from 2.9 percent to 4.7 percent.

Obesity is more common in Blacks and Hispanics. More than half of non-Hispanic Black women over age forty are obese, and 80 percent are overweight. Children are suffering from increased obesity, too. The number of overweight Black and Hispanic children has more than doubled over the past twelve years. For White children, the numbers have increased by 50 percent. In the past, it typically took thirty years for the number of overweight people in the United States to double.

Defining Obesity—Body Mass Index (BMI)

Researchers use very specific measures to define a body as being overweight or obese. The measures include the BMI or body mass index and the percentage of body fat (percent BF). Your BMI is traditionally calculated by dividing your weight in kilograms by your height in meters squared. It can also be calculated by dividing your weight in pounds by your height in inches. Then, that number is divided by your height in inches again, and the result is multiplied by 703. The National Heart, Lung, and Blood Institute has a BMI calculator on its website (http://nhlbisupport.com/bmi/bmicalc.htm), so you don't have to do the math yourself. If you don't know how to convert your weight and height to metric measurements, that's okay; this website can calculate your BMI using standard American measurements.

Ideally, your BMI should be in the range of 18.5 to 24.9. If your BMI is greater than 25, you're overweight. If it's greater than 30, you're considered obese. BMI, however, is not the best measure to determine if you're overweight or obese because it doesn't take body composition into account. Muscle weighs more than fat. For example, bodybuilders may weigh a lot for their height, but their above-normal weight is usually due to their large muscle mass, not excess fat. These toned athletes may have a BMI greater than 30, but they are certainly not obese.

To lengthen your life, shorten your meals.

—Proverb

Percent Body Fat

A better way to determine whether you are overweight, obese, or just "solid" is to measure your percent body fat (percent BF). This measurement is an assessment of your body composition. It evaluates how much of your weight is lean body mass (muscle, bones, and so on) and how much of it is actually fat. There are several different ways to get this measurement. The most accurate way involves completely submerging your body into a tank of water. This fairly expensive test measures the amount of water you displace in the tank and compares it to your height and weight. Fat is lighter than muscle. So pound for pound, fat takes up much more space than muscle. The more water you displace for your height and weight, the higher your percent of body fat.

Body fat can also be calculated by the method known as "bioelectrical impedance." This test is performed by passing a small, low-amp electrical current through your body and measuring the speed at which the current flows through you. Fat doesn't conduct electricity very well, but muscle does. So, the more fat you have, the slower the current travels.

The simplest and least expensive way to measure percent body fat is to use a series of skin-fold measurements. However, calculating body fat using this technique has some limitations and is a lot less accurate than the other methods. The accuracy of this approach very much depends on the skill of the person doing the evaluation. Also, skin-fold measurements are unreliable for estimating the amount of body fat on people who are either extremely thin or very obese.

To calculate percent body fat using this technique, a caliper is used to measure the thickness of skin folds in several very specific areas of the body. The skin and the underlying fat are pinched into the caliper—a device that looks and feels a lot like a vice. Yes, sometimes it hurts a little. The thickness of each skin fold is read from the numbers on the caliper. After all the measurements are taken, they are added up and divided by the person's body weight. That number is then multiplied by a conversion factor to obtain the estimated percent body fat. Certified personal trainers are taught how to take these measurements as part of their certification training. Most gyms and fitness clubs have a personal trainer who can do these measurements for you. You can also make a rough approximation by yourself (see the inset "Calculating a Rough Estimate of Body Fat" on page 142).

Studies have shown that your BMI and percent BF are associated with your

Calculating a Rough Estimate of Body Fat

There's a quick way that you can get a rough estimate of your percent BF without using any fancy or expensive tests, and you can do it by yourself. It's not as accurate as the other techniques, but it will give you a ballpark figure. It involves a lot of simple measurements.

First, weigh yourself (in pounds) in the nude, and then multiply your total weight by 0.732. Take that number, and add 8.987. This number is your weight factor.

(your weight in pounds x 0.732) + 8.987 = weight factor

Then, measure your wrist in inches, and divide it by 3.140.
This number is your wrist factor.

wrist measurement in inches ÷ 3.140 = wrist factor

Next, measure your waist in inches at the navel, and multiply it by 0.157. This number is your waist factor.

waist measurement in inches x 0.157 = waist factor

Now, measure your hips, and multiply that number by 0.249.
This number is your hip factor.

hips measurement in inches x 0.249 = hip factor

Measure the distance around your forearm, and multiply it by 0.434. This is your forearm factor.

forearm measurement in inches x 0.434 = forearm factor

Now, to calculate:
1. Take your weight factor, and add your wrist factor.
2. From that number, subtract your waist factor.
3. Take that number, and subtract your hip factor.
4. To that number, add your forearm factor. This number is your lean body mass.

weight factor + wrist factor − waist factor − hip factor
+ forearm factor = lean body mass

Next, take your total weight and subtract your lean body mass to get your amount of fat in pounds.

weight in pounds − lean body mass = fat in pounds

Now, multiply your fat in pounds by 100, and divide by your total body weight. This number is your percent BF.

(fat in pounds x 100) / weight in pounds = percent BF

Adapted from *Dynamic Nutrition for Maximum Performance* by Daniel Gastelu and Dr. Fred Hatfield (Avery Publishing Group, 1997) with permission.

risk of breast cancer. A study from Sweden published in January 2003 in the *International Journal of Cancer* found that your percent BF has a higher association with your risk of breast cancer than your BMI does. The normal overall range for percent BF in nonathletic women is 16 to 32 percent; the desirable range is 18 to 28 percent.

TOXINS—NOT CALORIES

If you are active and you don't overeat, and yet you are still overweight, a slow metabolism may not be the only reason that weight stays on you. In an article published in the *Journal of Complementary and Alternative Medicine* in 2002, author Paula Baillie-Hamilton presented a new theory about the epidemic of obesity. She said that the amount of obesity that exists in the world today can't be explained by increased calories and sedentary lives alone. She contends that toxins in the environment and in the food you eat may play a significant role in disrupting your body's weight-control mechanisms.

Toxins block the intelligence of your body in many ways. The intelligence that manages weight control seems to be particularly vulnerable to toxins. Growth promoters and hormones are given to animals to fatten them up and increase the amount of milk they produce. When you eat these animals or drink their milk, you also consume the growth promoters. If these substances put weight on animals, you can be sure that they also put weight on humans.

In addition, a variety of synthetic pharmaceutical drugs, including certain antidepressants, anticonvulsants, antihistamines, nonsteroidal anti-inflammatories, antipsychotics, and hormones have been found to cause weight gain. Moreover, studies show that pesticides may cause abnormal weight gain; in fact, animals exposed to pesticides can have *huge* weight gains. In one study, despite no increase in their caloric intake, the body weight of the animals that were given pesticides doubled! Researchers cut the calories in half for other animals that were fed pesticides, and they still gained weight!

At low concentrations, all the chemicals listed below have been shown to powerfully promote weight gain.

- Carbamates (a type of insecticide)

- Heavy metals (such as cadmium and lead)

- Pesticides (organochlorines, DDT, lindane, endrin, and hexachlorobenzene)

- Plastics (phalates and bisphenol A)

- Polybrominated biphenyls (used as a fire retardant)

- Polychlorinated biphenyls (PCBs)

• Solvents (octachorostyrene, decalin, benzene, toluene, 1,1,1-trichloroethane, and trichloroethylene benzene)

Avoiding Chemicals

The best ways to avoid these weight-promoting chemicals are to eat organically grown produce and to use nontoxic products in your home. Common sources of toxins in your home and their nontoxic alternatives are presented in Chapter 22. Eating organic foods and using only nontoxic products in your home are excellent ways to prevent excess quantities of toxins from getting *into* your body, but what about the toxins you already have in your body? Fortunately, there are ways to get most of them out.

The most effective way to cleanse your body of toxins is through *panchakarma*—a series of detoxification procedures unique to *Ayurveda*. The procedures, which are done in a medical spa-like setting, are gentle but powerful. Research shows that just one series of treatments can cut your toxin load in half. If you eat organic foods and go through *panchakarma* twice a year for about five days each time, the levels of toxins in your body will go so low that standard tests won't be able to detect them anymore. Chapter 23 goes into much more detail about this powerfully purifying and rejuvenating technique.

Chapter 18

A Drink
Not to Drink
Alcohol: Thy Name Is Devil

Oh thou invisible spirit of wine,
if thou hast no name to be known by,
let us call thee devil.

—WILLIAM SHAKESPEARE,
OTHELLO, ACT II, SCENE III

*A*s Shakespeare said, alcohol has the potential for such ill effects on your physical, mental, and emotional health that it could appropriately be called a devil. Some doctors and scientists say that drinking a little alcohol is good for you—especially for your heart. But what they don't know, or aren't telling you, is that although a little bit of alcohol may be good for your heart, it's definitely *not* good for protecting yourself against breast cancer.

When it comes to your risk of breast cancer, alcohol truly *is* a devil. It has an alarming aptitude for unleashing this deadly beast. Just a small amount effectively blocks a great deal of your body's healing intelligence. Think of it this way: Alcohol is another substance that, for your Warrior Goddess, is like Kryptonite to Superman—one small drink is enough to strip her of her full power to defend. Numerous studies have found that even one drink a day increases your risk of breast cancer by as much as 11 percent. Two drinks of alcohol a day raise your risk by 22 to 40 percent. Three drinks a day adds to your risk by 33 to 70 percent. The bottom line is this: No alcohol is safe. As far as your heart health goes, a low-fat diet, high in fresh organic fruits and vegetables, regular aerobic exercise, and the daily practice of an effective stress-reducing meditation lowers your risk much more than a glass of wine ever will. And all these suggestions have only healthy side *benefits*.

Researchers have found that alcohol increases the amount of estrogen in your blood. It also causes the release of the hormone prolactin. Like estrogen, prolactin speeds up cell division in the breast. For women who take hormone replacement therapy (HRT), alcohol is particularly dangerous. This hazardous mixture causes estrogen and prolactin levels to skyrocket.

GRAPES INSTEAD OF WINE

Because it contains alcohol, wine sides with the enemy. But research has shown that the sumptuous fruit that wine is made from—grapes—is a powerful ally to breast health. Grape skins contain a wonderful substance called "resveratrol," which prevents the inception of breast cancer cells and inhibits their growth. Scientists have found several reasons why. For one, resveratrol is an anti-inflammatory; it blocks the COX-2 enzyme. (The COX-2 enzyme and breast cancer are covered in Chapter 14.) For another, resveratrol is an antioxidant, and antioxidants prevent free-radical damage to DNA, damage that can lead to cancer.

If you have breast cancer and are being treated with radiation, resveratrol has also been found to assist the radiation in killing more tumor cells. Don't be fooled into thinking that the only way you can get the health benefits of resveratrol is by drinking wine. You can safely consume resveratrol and get all its potent and protective medicine by drinking organic grape juice or a nonalcoholic wine, or by eating a handful of fresh, sweet, organic grapes. (See the Resource section for some nonalcoholic wine alternatives.)

The seeds in grapes also possess many anticancer qualities. One class of phytochemicals in grape seeds, proanthocyanidins, has been found to have powerful antioxidant properties and a broad spectrum of protective benefits. For instance, a study conducted at Creighton University and published in 1999 found that grapeseed proanthocyanidin extract killed breast cancer cells, while enhancing the growth and viability of normal cells. Moreover, in 2003, researchers in California found that grape seeds can decrease the amount of estrogen produced by the body. Therefore, taking grapeseed extract is another way to derive the benefits grapes have to offer.

Chapter 19

Sir Walter Raleigh's Folly

Tobacco: Smoking and Breast Cancer

*N*o one would argue with the fact that smoking is not good for your health. It's an extremely dangerous and costly habit. According to statistics released in 2004 by the American Heart Association, smoking-related illnesses kill an average of 442,398 Americans and cost the nation $157 billion each year. For years we have known that smoking is linked to cancers of the bladder, esophagus, larynx, lung, mouth, and throat; to chronic lung disease, such as bronchitis and emphysema; and to chronic heart disease and cardio-vascular diseases, including strokes, high blood pressure, and poor circulation.

A report released by the Surgeon General in May 2004 revealed that smoking also causes a rash of other diseases: acute myeloid leukemia, abdominal aortic aneurysms, cataracts, periodontitis, pneumonia, and cancers of the cervix, kidney, pancreas, and stomach. There's also evidence that smoking may cause colorectal cancers, liver cancer, prostate cancer, and erectile dysfunction. This report said that smokers die an average of thirteen to fourteen years earlier than nonsmokers. It reports that smoking-related diseases have killed 12 million Americans in the last forty years, continue to kill about 440,000 each year, and cost the nation $75 billion annually to treat these diseases.

For years, it was unclear whether smoking increased the risk of breast cancer or not. Some studies found that it was difficult to separate the risk associated with cigarette smoking from the risk associated with alcohol consumption, because most smokers also drink alcohol, and, as you now know, alcohol is a significant risk factor for breast cancer. But now, researchers have concluded from several well-designed studies that there is a clear and significant association between cigarette smoking and breast cancer.

For all these reasons, your Warrior Goddess despises cigarettes. If you smoke, please do everything you can to successfully stop. Tobacco clouds your

Goddess's awareness, destroys her cosmic intelligence, and strips her of her remarkable ability to outsmart enemy diseases.

YOUNGER START—GREATER RISK

Smoking during the teenage years is particularly dangerous in terms of breast cancer risk. A study from the National Cancer Institute (NCI) found that women who smoked cigarettes during their adolescence had a 50 percent increased risk of breast cancer. This may be because female breast cells generally don't mature until the first pregnancy (immature breast cells are more susceptible to damage from toxins). But smoking can be dangerous at any age. A German study published in 2002 in the journal *Cancer Epidemiology, Biomarkers & Prevention* found that women who smoked had a 50 percent increased risk of breast cancer. The risk for ex-smokers kept going down the longer that they abstained from smoking. But no matter how long it had been since they smoked, their risk was still 20 percent higher than nonsmokers.

These researchers also found that secondhand smoke increased the risk of breast cancer. They documented that women who inhaled passive smoke were 60 percent more likely to develop breast cancer than those who weren't exposed to it. The highest risk was in smokers who also inhaled passive smoke.

Another study published in *The Lancet* in 2002 found that very specific categories of smokers have a particularly high risk. For instance, an unusually high risk of breast cancer was found in women who had been pregnant and who had started smoking as teenagers within five years of starting their period. Women who had never had a baby and who smoked twenty cigarettes a day or more for more than twenty years also had a significantly increased risk.

One of the reasons smoking increases the risk of breast cancer is that cigarette smoke contains carcinogens. A study from Albert Einstein University published in 2002 in the journal *Cancer Epidemiology, Biomarkers & Prevention* identified the specific carcinogens in cigarette smoke: polycyclic hydrocarbons, aromatic amines, and N-nitrosamines. This group of heterocyclic amines is similar to those found in grilled red meat. Certain carcinogens, including these, don't become carcinogens until they are activated by enzymes—predominantly phase 1 liver enzymes—in your body. Breast tissue, like the liver, contains enzymes that can activate the carcinogens found in red meat and cigarette smoke. All these carcinogens can induce mammary tumors, and they have all been found in the breast tissue and breast milk of women who smoke. Researchers have also found the changes in DNA and genetic mutations that are associated with an increased risk of breast cancer in the breast cells of women who smoke.

TO HELP YOU QUIT

If you smoke cigarettes and have tried to quit, you know how hard it can be to break this habit. Of all the addictions you can have, cigarette smoking is one of the hardest to give up. Research shows that the practice of Transcendental Meditation (TM) is extremely successful in breaking the addictive cycle and helping people to quit for good. In fact, of all the programs there are to help you stop smoking, the practice of TM is the most successful. People who practice this simple stress-reducing technique spontaneously quit smoking because they find their desire for cigarettes naturally decreases. Harvard-trained researchers David O'Connell, Ph.D., and Charles Alexander, Ph.D., wrote an excellent book, *Self Recovery: Treating Addictions using Transcendental Meditation and Maharishi Ayurveda,* that reports on all the research showing the impressive success that this mental technique has in overcoming addictions. You'll find out more about TM in Chapter 27.

Chapter 20

Fatally Flawed Pharmaceuticals

Dangerous Medications

*P*harmaceutical drugs are fraught with side effects, some mild and some deadly. The number of reported in-hospital adverse drug reactions to prescribed medications is estimated to be about 2.2 million per year. About 783,000 people die each year in the United States alone from iatrogenic causes (that is, health problems inadvertently induced by healthcare workers, a medical treatment, or a diagnostic procedure). Of those deaths, about 106,000 are from side effects of a drug or combination of drugs.

One horrifying "side effect" of certain pharmaceutical medications is breast cancer. Until recently, little attention was given to the frightening increased risk of breast cancer associated with such medications as birth control pills, hormone replacement therapy (HRT), certain heart medications, various antidepressants, and many other pharmaceuticals. Each of these medications has specific ways that it increases your risk of breast cancer.

Most drugs are metabolized in the liver, and scientists have found that they may interfere with the liver's ability to detoxify carcinogens. When your liver function is impaired, more carcinogens remain in your body, and thereby increase your risk of many different cancers, including breast cancer. That's why your Warrior Goddess prefers that you supply her with foods, herbs, and other natural approaches, rather than pharmaceuticals whenever possible.

"THE PILL"

In a laboratory study published in 1987 in the journal *Cancer,* researchers found that the combination of estrogen and progestin (found in many birth control pills) stimulates breast cells to grow and divide and accelerates the growth of breast cancer. In another study, published more than twenty years ago in the *Journal of Reproductive Medicine,* premenopausal women who used the pill after age forty were found to have a 50 percent increased risk of breast cancer. More recent studies show that women who have a mother or sister with breast cancer and take the pill long term also have a significantly increased risk of breast cancer.

HORMONE REPLACEMENT THERAPY (HRT)

To combat perimenopausal and menopausal symptoms, Western medicine developed synthetic hormones. Drug companies promoted hormone replacement therapy (HRT) as the long-sought-after fountain of youth. HRT, women were told, lowered the risk of heart disease, strokes, Alzheimer's disease, and osteoporosis. But recent studies, including the Women's Health Initiative Study, have found that the opposite is true: Women taking HRT have an increased risk of heart disease, strokes, blood clots, gallbladder disease, and invasive breast cancer. It is true that HRT *does* help to prevent osteoporosis, but not any more so than a little weight-bearing exercise and a diet high in calcium-rich foods.

Pharmaceutical companies, as well as many doctors, still downplay the level of risk associated with these synthetic hormones. But research published in the August 2003 issue of the prestigious journal *The Lancet* found that the risk was considerable. One-quarter of all the women between the ages of fifty and sixty-four in Britain—1 million women—were followed from 1996 until 2002. Those women who took HRT had a 66 percent increased incidence of breast cancer and a 22 percent greater risk of dying from it. Those women who took a combination of estrogen and progestin had a 100 percent higher risk of breast cancer than those women who never took hormones. The women who took estrogen alone had a 30 percent higher risk. And the longer the women took these hormones, the higher their risk became.

Of the women who developed breast cancer, those who had taken hormones had more aggressive tumors than those who had never taken them. Aggressive tumors are very dangerous because they're more likely to spread throughout the body and cause early death. The researchers of this landmark study in England estimated that HRT was responsible for 20,000 cases of breast cancer over the ten-year period from 1992 to 2002.

Several other studies have also found a significant connection between HRT and breast cancer. For instance, the Nurses' Health Study, a large epidemiological study, followed 58,520 women who took HRT from age fifty to sixty. When these women reached the age of seventy, they were found to have a 23 percent higher risk of breast cancer. However, the women who took estrogen plus progestin had a much higher risk of breast cancer—67 percent. Another study published in *JAMA* in 2002 found that long-term users of HRT who took either estrogen alone or estrogen with progestin had a 60 to 85 percent increased incidence of breast cancer.

Researchers have also discovered that HRT causes an unusual type of breast cancer called "invasive lobular carcinoma." The majority of all breast cancers start in the breast ducts. They are called "ductal carcinomas." Lobular carcinoma originates in the terminal lobules or milk glands. A study published in 2003 in *JAMA* found that women who took a combination of estrogen and progestin had a 50 percent higher risk of lobular carcinoma. They also noted that the overall incidence in the United States of this far less common type of breast cancer increased from 9.5 percent in 1987 to 15.6 percent in 1999. HRT is thought to be the primary cause of this alarming escalation.

Taking HRT substantially increases the risk of ovarian cancer, too. Ovarian cancer is a relatively uncommon cancer. The average woman has only a 1.7 percent chance of developing this disease over her lifetime, whereas the risk of breast cancer for the average woman is 13.3 percent. In a 2002 study published by the National Cancer Institute (NCI), women who took HRT for ten to nineteen years had an 80 percent increased risk of ovarian cancer.

Millions of women in the United States have been prescribed HRT. It was one of the top pharmaceuticals sold for many years. In 2002, an estimated 8 million women in the United States were on some form of HRT. With this extensive use, you'd think that this pharmaceutical product would have been thoroughly studied, both before it was put on the market and afterward. But a well-designed study wasn't conducted on HRT until forty years after it was put on the market!

I'm not sure why the long-term health effects of HRT weren't investigated decades earlier. This tragic oversight is estimated to have caused thousands of cases of breast cancer. In other words, thousands of women were brutalized by breast cancer and had their lives cut short by it because they unknowingly took a medication that significantly increased their risk of breast cancer.

Nature's Perfect Design

Prescribing hormones for menopausal symptoms is a perfect example of how the Western paradigm of health care can be so off the mark sometimes, that the consequences can be catastrophic. We seem to forget that Nature designed human beings perfectly. We can't outsmart Nature no matter how hard we try. We shouldn't try to *overpower* it, but rather *work with it*. Menopause, for example, isn't a disease or a condition that needs to be treated or controlled. The hormonal changes that women go through are perfect by design. They are part of the natural progression of life. Symptoms arise from imbalances caused by poor choices in diet and lifestyle. Restoring balance naturally is the solution; suppressing the symptoms of imbalances with supplemental hormones is not.

If you suffer from menopausal symptoms and are looking for relief, or if you want to stop taking hormones, there are many safe and effective natural approaches you can take. Helping you to transition through menopause naturally is beyond the scope of this book, but there are several good books that I recommend. Dr. Nancy Lonsdorf, M.D., wrote an excellent book on the *Ayurvedic* approach to menopause called *A Women's Best Medicine for Menopause.* Two other outstanding books are *The Wisdom of Menopause,* by Christiane Northrup, M.D., and *Dr. Susan Love's Hormone Book,* by Susan Love, M.D.

ANTIDEPRESSANT AND HEART MEDICATIONS

Other types of pharmaceutical medications have been found to increase the risk of breast cancer, too—specifically, two groups of heart medications called "beta blockers" and "calcium-channel blockers" and several psychiatric medications. Each drug may have a number of different physiological interactions that contribute to this calamitous "side effect," but researchers think their influence on melatonin may be one of the biggest factors. Melatonin is an important hormone produced by your body that, research shows, provides powerful protection against breast cancer. People who take these medications have much lower levels of this extraordinary natural cancer-fighting hormone. (For more information on melatonin, see Chapter 24.)

A class of antidepressants called "tricyclic antidepressants"—for example, imipramine (Tofranil) and clomipramine (Anafranil)—provoke the initiation of breast cancer by triggering mutations in your genes. These mutations can lead to breast cancer as long as eleven to fifteen years after taking the drug. According to a Canadian study published in 2002 in the *British Journal of Cancer,* the risk of breast cancer for people who have a long history of taking these genotoxic medications is more than doubled. Even more alarming, another Canadian study published in 2000 in the *American Journal of Epidemiology* found that the risk of breast cancer doubled after only two years on tricyclic medication. The tricyclic antidepressant amitriptyline (Elavil) and the non-tricyclic agent fluoxetine (Prozac) were found by researchers at the University of Manitoba to stimulate the growth of breast cancer by another mechanism—binding to growth receptors.

Natural Approaches to Relieving Depression

Fortunately, there are many alternatives to antidepressant medications that, research shows, may be just as effective. Antidepressants work by altering chem-

Antibiotics and Breast Cancer?

A study published in the February 2004 issue of *The Journal of the American Medical Association* (JAMA) found a possible link between frequent use of antibiotics and an increased risk of breast cancer. However, because of the way the study was designed, it's impossible to determine if antibiotics really were the culprits. Infectious diseases that require treatment with antibiotics can also cause chronic inflammation, increase free-radical production, and depress the immune system—all three of which are known to promote breast cancer. It may be that the true source of the increased risk has everything to do with these well-known cancer-encouraging conditions and nothing to do with the antibiotics. Although this issue obviously requires further study, designing clinical human trials with antibiotics poses difficulties. To flush out whether antibiotics are the source of the increased risk and not the infections they are used to treat, healthy people would have to be given antibiotics. Because antibiotics pose other known health risks, a study like that would probably never be approved. I recommend taking antibiotics only when absolutely necessary and avoiding them whenever possible.

icals in your brain. These brain chemicals can also be positively influenced by many natural, nonpharmaceutical approaches. For instance, several studies have documented that regular exercise combats depression, as well as many commonly prescribed pharmaceutical antidepressants. Researchers have also found that yoga, certain types of meditation, acupuncture, music therapy, and *panchakarma* all effectively relieve depression.

A variety of herbs and supplements are very beneficial for improving this common condition: omega-3 fatty acids, B vitamins, S-adenosylmethionine (SAM-e), dehydroepiandrosterone (DHEA), tyrosine, DL-phenylalanine, 5-hydroxytryptophan (5-HTP), and the herbs St. John's wort and holy basil. Eating a diet high in fresh organic fruits, vegetables, and whole grains, and avoiding sugar, refined carbohydrates, caffeine, and alcohol can stabilize and lift your mood. Supplying your body with the right nutrients and avoiding the wrong ones brings balance to both your body and your mind.

If you suffer from depression, work with your doctor if you decide to try any of these natural approaches. You may find that you need less medication or a different, less harmful medication. You may even discover that some of these natural techniques work so effectively for you that you no longer require any medication at all. A warning, however: Don't go off your medication without your doctor's consent and don't take any of these supplements without getting your doctor's approval. Toxic side effects may occur if you take an herb such as St. John's wort with an antidepressant drug such as Prozac. Depression is a very dangerous condition, so be sure to work carefully with your doctor.

BE AWARE, ASK QUESTIONS

Pharmaceutical medications have their place in restoring health when necessary, but be aware that many prescription drugs, especially when taken long term, may have serious side effects. Take the time to find out the possible side effects of your medications. Make sure that *if* you have a choice in the medications you take, you choose the one with the lowest risks.

For virtually any chronic condition, there are usually safe, natural alternative approaches that can be very effective. With the resurgence of *Ayurveda,* we have regained a wealth of knowledge about how to detect, prevent, treat, reverse, and even cure chronic disease conditions. Built on a different and highly effective paradigm of health care, *Ayurveda* teaches you how to achieve an extraordinary state of health. This ancient system holds tremendous knowledge about the normal rhythms and processes of life—what strips you of your health and what helps to enhance it and keep you well. If symptoms arise, for example, during menopause, *Ayurveda* teaches that they are due to imbalances from improper diet or from a lifestyle that works against the laws of Nature. By simply making better diet and lifestyle choices, balance is gently restored and symptoms can be alleviated.

Sometimes it's necessary to take pharmaceutical medications. But you should also make every effort to restore balance to your body at the same time by stopping those things that helped to initiate and aggravate your condition and by starting those things that will help to protect and promote your health.

You can mop up the water on the floor, but unless you
turn off the faucet, you'll never get the floor dry.

—Author unknown

If you take on healthy habits and stop the unhealthy ones that are contributing to your illness, the number and dose of medications you require may drop significantly, even to the point where you can stop taking them. Reversals and cures of chronic conditions are often possible. Remember, however, always work with your doctor when adjusting your medications.

Chapter 21

Portrait of an Assassin

Pesticides and Other Hidden Toxins

*P*icture an assassin. His task depends on his ability to make himself invisible and remain undetected until the last possible moment. He studies his targets to find their weaknesses. As he silently positions himself for the kill, his victims don't have even the slightest hint of what's to come. He patiently waits for just the right moment. The instant his target becomes vulnerable, he strikes.

This portrait of an assassin describes the behavior of all the toxins in your environment. These toxins are in your food and water, your home and workplace, and the products you use. You aren't aware of them, but they are there, hidden in the shadows. They find a weakness in your body and start their infiltration. When your body becomes vulnerable due to stress, fatigue, or an emotional crisis, they move in for the kill.

Unfortunately, we all live in an extremely toxic world that's teeming with assassins. Fortunately, there are many ways to avoid toxins, reduce your exposure to them, and drive them out of your home and body.

THE CHEMICAL REVOLUTION

Chemical manufacturing began in the early 1900s, mostly with good intentions. (Remember that old expression, "The road to hell is paved with good intentions"?) The chemists thought that they were helping to make the world a better and safer place and that these chemicals would make our lives easier. For instance, some chemicals were developed to improve the efficiency of large-scale manufacturing plants to increase the productive output. Some chemicals were intended to increase crop production; others were created to help protect us from disease-carrying insects and pests. But what the chemists didn't know was that many of these chemicals would turn out to be extremely dangerous to our health and the environment.

A good example of a dangerous chemical created with good intentions is dichlorodiphenyltrichloroethane (DDT). This chemical, along with thousands of others, doesn't break down easily and, therefore, persists in our environment. The chemical architects didn't realize that their creations would contribute to the toxic soup overtaking our planet. They didn't know they were helping to turn Earth into a place where people, even in the most remote areas of the world, would suffer from the fallout of these toxins.

There are now toxins *everywhere*—in or over every square inch of this planet: in our water, air, soil, food, clothes, furnishings, dry cleaning, personal-care products, and cleaning products. Many of these toxins have been linked to a variety of health problems, including cancer. But the chemical assault doesn't stop there. There are also toxins in lawn and garden products, insect repellants, flea collars, paints, wallpaper, joint compound, sealers, insulation, carpet, tile, cabinets, woodwork, and, of course, home pesticides. There's not a baby born anywhere in America who doesn't have synthetic toxic chemicals in his or her body. As Bill Moyers discovered while creating his PBS documentary *Trade Secrets,* which aired on March 26, 2001, the average adult—including himself—has hundreds of different synthetic chemicals in his or her blood and fat.

Our homes, structures originally designed to provide shelter from storms and beasts, have now *become* the storms and beasts. The air in the average American home is *four times* more polluted than the air outdoors!

The number of chemical assassins in our world is overwhelming. Why? Largely because our government does a very poor job of regulating their safety. Today, more than 75,000 chemicals are registered with the Environmental Protection Agency (EPA), and only about 600 of them have been tested for safety. The government leaves the question of a chemical's safety up to the company that manufactured it. The EPA allows any new chemical to go on the market as long as the manufacturer "thinks" it's safe. Its safety may be questioned only *after* the chemical is linked to serious health problems or significant damage to the environment and wildlife. Usually, a huge public outcry is required before any serious testing is done. Many animals or people must die or be seriously injured before a chemical is pulled from the market.

Of those 600 chemicals that the EPA has tested, many have been found to be carcinogens or suspected carcinogens. Some can disrupt your endocrine system, which is made up of the glands that produce hormones, such as estrogen. Some endocrine disrupters mimic the estrogen molecule. They are called "chem-

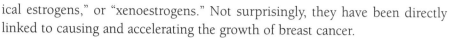

ical estrogens," or "xenoestrogens." Not surprisingly, they have been directly linked to causing and accelerating the growth of breast cancer.

Many other chemicals are toxic in other ways. They damage your nervous, reproductive, or immune system. Although they may not be carcinogens, they can weaken your body and make it more susceptible to cancer development and growth. Despite knowing this, many Americans use these chemicals anyway for convenience sake.

Organochlorines, as well as most other pesticides and chemicals, are concentrated and stored in the body fat of the animals you eat. Not surprisingly, poultry, beef, pork, fish and other seafood, dairy, and animal-derived oils have the highest concentrations of pesticides. But don't be fooled into thinking that the amount of pesticides on fruits and vegetables is small. A sample of conventionally grown celery was found to have *seventeen* different pesticide residues, ten of which were carcinogenic. The average apple may have the residue of as many as five to ten carcinogenic pesticides! This is another reason why it's so important to eat organically grown produce.

RESEARCH FROM AROUND THE WORLD

Whether or not chemical estrogens, or xenoestrogens, can initiate and promote breast cancer has been hotly debated for years. Some studies have found a link; others haven't. Based on the most recent research, however, there is little doubt that xenoestrogens do contribute to promoting breast cancer.

Israel

During the 1970s, Israeli women, particularly young women, were found to have a much higher incidence of breast cancer than women in other countries. Given all the known risk factors at the time, their rate of breast cancer was twice as high as would be expected. In the search to find out why, it was discovered that the milk from cows raised in Israel had some of the highest pesticide levels in the world. Pesticides, such as DDT and benzene hexachloride (BHC), were found to be 5 to 100 times greater in concentration in cow's milk from Israel than in milk from the United States.

The Israeli women were also found to have high levels of insecticides in their breast milk. In 1978 there was a public outcry. The government responded by banning BHC and DDT. The levels of these pesticides in cow's milk began to decline rapidly. By 1980, they had dropped 98 percent. The incidence of breast cancer in young women dropped significantly, too. Within a few short years, the number of premenopausal women diagnosed with breast cancer fell 30 percent.

Denmark

Several studies from Denmark show a very strong *direct* correlation between estrogen-mimicking pesticides and breast cancer. In a study published in the journal *Cancer Causes and Control* in 2000, researchers found that Danish women with high serum concentrations of the organochlorine DDT had a 300 percent increased risk of breast cancer. The higher the concentrations of DDT that were found in the women, the higher their incidence of breast cancer was. The researchers also found that another toxin, polychlorinated bipheyls (PCBs; for more information, see the inset "What Are PCBs?" on page 74), also significantly raised the risk of breast cancer.

A second Danish study published in 2000 in the *Journal of Clinical Epidemiology* found that another type of organochlorine called "dieldrin" also significantly increased the risk of breast cancer. The study found that as the concentration of this pesticide increased in women, so did their incidence of breast cancer. The women with the highest levels of dieldrin had twice the risk.

A third study from Denmark published in the *Journal of Clinical Epidemiology* in 2000 measured the concentration of this same organochlorine, dieldrin, in the blood of breast cancer patients and compared it to their survival rate. Researchers found a direct correlation: The higher the level of dieldrin in the blood, the worse the chances were of the patient's surviving. Their conclusion was that dieldrin raises the risk of breast cancer and lowers the chance of surviving the disease.

Germany

In 1998, a German study published in the *Journal of Steroid Biochemistry & Molecular Biology* found that organochlorine pesticides (DDT and hexachlorobenzine [HCB]) and PCBs are associated with an increased risk of breast cancer. In the study, the German women with breast cancer had higher levels of DDT and PCBs in their breast tissue. DDT was found in concentrations an average of 62 percent higher than those found in the women without breast cancer. PCBs were found to be 25 percent higher in the breast cancer patients.

DDT DETOX

A 2001 study from Westchester Medical Center in New York presented various ways in which you can lower the amounts and effects of organochlorines, such as DDT, in your body. Here are their recommendations:

1. **Eat phytoestrogen-rich food, such as soy.** The phytoestrogens found in plants such as soybeans compete with organochlorines for estrogen receptors. They can actually block the pesticides from attaching to the estrogen receptor.

2. **Eat the spice turmeric.** Turmeric can inhibit the estrogenic effect of pesticides. It also has a synergistic effect with phytoestrogens. It increases the power of phytoestrogens to block pesticides from attaching to estrogen receptors.

3. **Eat cruciferous vegetables.** Estrogenic pesticides cause the production of more of the "bad" type of estrogen. The phytochemical found in cruciferous vegetables, indole-3 carbinol, reverses that effect by stimulating the production of more of the "good" kind of estrogen.

4. **Keep your body weight down.** Since pesticides accumulate in body fat, the less body fat you have, the fewer pesticides your body can store.

5. **Low-fat and reduced-calorie diets may be beneficial.** If you eat less animal fat, you will consume smaller amounts of the toxins that concentrate in it. Also, if you eat less food in general, you'll also consume fewer toxins.

Eating only organically grown foods is the best way to prevent yourself from consuming additional doses of pesticides. Don't use home pesticides or other toxic household products, either. In Chapter 22, you'll find a table that lists non-

---

Breastfeeding Concerns

When a woman breastfeeds, pesticides are flushed out of the breast tissue, thereby significantly lowering the pesticide levels in her breasts. While it's true that the breastfeeding baby ingests these pesticides, research clearly shows that the protective benefits of breastfeeding far outweigh any negative effects on the baby's health. In fact, women who were breastfed as infants have a significantly lower risk of breast cancer than their formula-fed counterparts.

You can limit the amount of toxins your future baby will ingest by taking some precautions. For starters, *Ayurveda* recommends going through the purification procedure *panchakarma* before you get pregnant. (*Panchakarma* is discussed in detail in Chapter 23.) If you are unable to go to a *panchakarma* clinic, you can follow a modified detoxification program at home. Although you may not get the full benefit of *panchakarma* by taking this route, any toxins you manage to clear from your body will be beneficial.

Whether or not you choose to detoxify before you conceive, you can help to reduce your baby's exposure to pesticides by eating only organically produced foods and using only nontoxic products before, during, and after pregnancy.

toxic alternatives for standard toxic household products. (A list of companies that produce nontoxic products along with their websites can be found in the Resources section.)

CHEMICAL ESTROGENS

Many chemicals—not just pesticides—can act as estrogen mimickers, or xeno-estrogens. These include heavy metals, household products, and even pharmaceuticals. Table 21.1 below lists some of the major estrogen mimickers. Many of these chemical estrogens are also known to cause excessive weight gain. And, as you know, obesity increases the risk of breast cancer. (See Chapter 17 for more information on chemical elements involved in weight gain.) While all of these estrogen mimickers are of concern, a few discussions of specific chemicals follow the table.

TABLE 21.1. CHEMICALS THAT MIMIC ESTROGEN

Types of Chemicals	Specific Chemicals
Fungicides	benomyl, mancozeb, tributyl tin
Heavy Metals	cadmium, lead, mercury
Herbicides	alachlor, atrazine, nitrofen
Household Products (breakdown products of detergents and surfactants)	nonylphenol, octylphenol
Industrial Chemicals	benzopyrene, dioxin, PCBs
Insecticides	chlordane, dieldrin, methoxychlor, DDT, endosulfan, toxaphene dicofol, kepone
Nematocides	aldicarb, dibromochloropropane
Pharmaceutical Drugs	birth control pills, cimitidine (Tagamet), diethylstilbestrol (DES), HRT
Plastics	bisphenol A, phthalates

Beware of Bisphenol A!

In 1987, researchers at Tufts University in Boston accidentally discovered a substance in plastic that mimics estrogen and accelerates the growth of breast cancer. Alarmingly, this substance, bisphenol A, can leech out of plastic when it comes in contact with food or liquid. This endocrine-disrupting substance has been found in plastic-bottled drinking water; in canned foods (more than 85 percent of the food cans in the United States are plastic-lined); in foods stored in plastic containers or wrapped in plastic food wrap; in the saliva of patients whose teeth have been treated with dental sealant and composites; and in rivers, since this chemical is also a breakdown product of detergents.

When food is heated or cooked in a microwave in plastic containers that are not "microwave safe," bisphenol A pours out of them and into your food. So, to keep your foods free of bisphenol A, don't store or cook your food in plastic containers and avoid plastic wrap.

Concerns about Cadmium

Cadmium is a heavy metal commonly found in pigments, alloys, batteries, soldering processes, the air from burning fossil fuels, shellfish, animal livers and kidneys, and cigarette smoke (2–4 micrograms per pack). In the August 2003 issue of *The Journal of Nature Medicine,* cadmium was reported to have the remarkable ability to act like estrogen. The study found that even low-dose exposure to cadmium appears to increase the risk of breast cancer.

In this 2003 study by researcher B. Martin from Georgetown University, rats that had been exposed to cadmium while in the uterus reached puberty earlier than those rats that had not been exposed to this heavy metal. What does this mean to humans? Well, beginning menstruation at a young age increases the total number of periods over a woman's lifetime. The more periods she experiences, the more estrogen is released and the higher her risk of breast cancer is. And, in fact, this is what the study showed. In rats exposed to cadmium, breast cancer rates increased.

The World Health Organization (WHO) states that the maximum safe dose of cadmium for a human is 7 micrograms per kilogram (mcg/kg) per week. However, the rats in the study were only given 5 mcg/kg. This study raises the concern that low doses of cadmium may, in fact, *not* be safe as was previously thought. Additional studies are needed to more clearly define the safety and health risks associated with this and other heavy metals.

A Deadly Duo: Chlorine and Dioxin

The United States manufactures huge amounts of chlorine, an elemental gas rarely found in nature. It's used to bleach fabrics and papers to a pristine shade of white, making them appear clean and pure. We pay a big price for this illusion of purity. Chlorine is added to automatic-dishwashing detergent, bleach, disinfectant, mildew remover, toilet-bowl cleaner, laundry detergent, and swimming pools. Chlorine is an irritating, corrosive, hazardous pollutant that damages the Earth's ozone layer. In fact, it is one of the main contributors to the destruction of the ozone layer.

But the dangers of chlorine don't stop there. When chlorine is released into the environment, it reacts with organic materials and creates new toxins. Some of these toxins include chloroform and organochlorines (pesticides), which can damage your reproductive, endocrine, and immune systems. One type of organochlorine, called dioxin, is formed during chlorine processing. Dioxins are released into the environment from chlorine-processing plants. They enter the air, the water, the soil . . . and then your food and, ultimately, your body.

Dioxins are deadly. They are believed to be *the most* carcinogenic chemical known. The EPA has found dioxins to be 300,000 times more potent as a carcinogen than DDT. Recent research has shown a clear link between dioxins and cancer, suppression of the immune system, reproductive disorders in adults, and developmental disorders and deformities in children.

Don't despair—there are nontoxic alternative products for virtually everything. You'll learn that it's possible to minimize your exposure to toxins in your home, car, and workplace, and to rid your body of toxins that have already found their way into your body. So, rest assured—you *do* have the power and ability to protect yourself from these deadly foes. Read on to learn how.

Part Five

Preventing the Birth of the Enemy

Tips and Tools Against Toxins

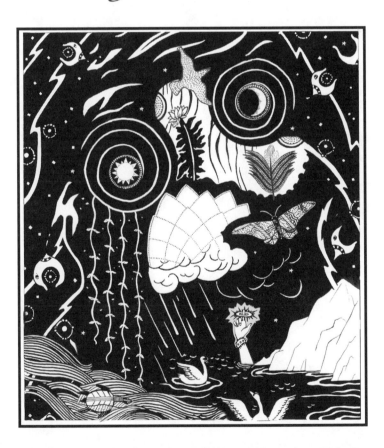

Chapter 22

Invite Friends,
Not Foes

A Treasure Chest
of Nontoxic Solutions

*T*he best way to battle the chemical assassins discussed in the previous chapters is to avoid them as much as possible. Don't invite them home, and don't allow them into your body through food or drink. Begin by assuming that they're in everything out there. Purchase only foods and products that are labeled by the U.S. Department of Agriculture (USDA) as "certified organic" or by reputable manufacturers as "toxin-free."

In the early 1970s, a few people began to blow the whistle on some chemical assassins, exposing their identity, their hideouts, and their normal routes of entry. A large, informal intelligence network sprang up, revealing more and more of them. Then, some people really got smart. They created companies that offered toxin-free products. Now, hundreds—if not thousands—of companies make nontoxic products and offer nontoxic solutions for just about everything.

I live my life based on one primary assumption: Everything is toxic unless proven otherwise. Unfortunately, that's not too far from the truth. It's helpful to assume that everything is toxic. It keeps you aware and searching for nontoxic alternatives. Fortunately, there are nontoxic products and solutions for just about everything.

Table 22.1 on the next page lists the major categories of common toxin-containing products, the toxins of most concern contained in those products, and nontoxic alternatives, which sometimes include the manufacturer's name. (For a more expanded list of organic- and nontoxic-product manufacturers, see the Resources section.)

TABLE 22.1. TOXINS AND NONTOXIC ALTERNATIVES

Categories	Toxins	Nontoxic Alternatives
Bedding	flame retardants formaldehyde petroleum-based pillows	Organic cotton and wool box springs and mattresses, organic cotton linens
Cabinets	formaldehyde glues particleboard plywood	Medite II, wheat grass, solid untreated wood
Carpet, carpet pads	ethylene glycol glues petrochemicals styrene butadiene urethane foam volatile organic (carbon-based) compounds (VOCs)	Natural-fiber carpets (wool, cotton, jute, goat hair), wool carpet pads
Cars using internal combustion engines	carbon monoxide lead nitrogen dioxide ozone particulate matter sulfur dioxide	Hybrid electric vehicles, electric cars, fuel-cell cars, natural gas, walking, bicycles
Caulking and sealers	ethylene dichloride synthetic plastic resins toluene xylene	AMF Safecoat nontoxic caulking and natural sealers, alternative housing construction (adobe, rammed earth)
Clothing	formaldehyde hydrocarbons	Rayon, hemp, linen, organic cotton, wool, and silk
Conventionally grown foods	chemical fertilizers fungicides herbicides pesticides	Organically grown foods
Cosmetics and personal-care products	formaldehyde petroleum toluene	Burt's Bees and other natural product lines
Dry cleaning	perchloroethylene (Perc)	Professional wet clean, machine wash, steam clean, hand wash, carbon dioxide (CO_2) gas

Categories	Toxins	Nontoxic Alternatives
Flea and tick collars	neurotoxins	Herb collars, herb baths, penny royal, eucalyptus, brewers yeast, garlic
Floor polishes	phenol	Natural oils, AMF Safecoat
Furniture	Same as above; fabrics may be treated with fire retardants, stain resistants, fungicides	Untreated natural-wood furniture, organic cotton or silk fabrics
Glues and adhesives	VOCs	Auro natural glue
Home pesticides	multitude of toxic chemicals	Nontoxic pest control, beneficial insects, Arbico
Household cleaners	chlorine phenols phosphates	Nontoxic cleaning supplies and detergents by Seventh Generation, E-cover, Country Save, Earth Friendly, Planet
Insect repellant	diethylmetatoluamide (DEET)	Neem, citronella, thyme, lemon grass, turmeric, geranium, Burt's Bees, All Terraine
Insulation	asbestos chlorofluorocarbons (CFCs) fiberglass particles formaldehyde polyurethane	Cellulose, icynene, denim
Joint compound (drywall mud)	antifungals binders dryers formaldehyde solvents (benzene)	Merco joint compound
Lawn-care products	chemical fertilizers herbicides	Organic lawn-care products (for example, Garden's Alive, Arbico)
Municipal water	benzene chlorine fluoride heavy metals pesticides	Whole-house water filters, carbon filters, distilled water, reverse osmosis, micropore filters
Paint thinners and strippers	methylene chloride solvents	Turpentine; Levos and Bioshield citrus thinners
Paints	binders solvents VOCs	Organic paints made by Livos, Bioshield, and Auro; "No-VOC" paints

Categories	Toxins	Nontoxic Alternatives
Paper	chlorine bleach	Tree-free paper, kanef, rice, other plant fibers, recycled paper
Paper towels, toilet paper	chlorine bleach	Recycled, unbleached paper (for example, Seventh Generation)
Particleboard, Oriented Strand Board (OSB), plywood	formaldehyde fungicides glues	Seal with AMF Safecoat, Safeseal
Resilient flooring, tile	polyvinyl chlorides (PVCs)	Linoleum, cork, bamboo, recycled rubber
Sealers and varnishes	Urethane	Natural varnishes made from oils and resins, Bioshield hard oil, AMF Safecoat, Oscolor
Wallpaper, especially those made from vinyl	petroleum-based adhesives PVCs	Untreated natural wall coverings, linens, plant fibers, cork, gypsum-coated fabric, pure-glass yarns by Innovative Wall Coverings, Maya Romanoff
Wood decks and deck furniture	arsenic fungicides polychlorinated biphenyls (PCBs)	Borax, salvage woods (redwood, cypress), nontoxic sealers

LIVING SAFELY WITH TOXINS

You may be concerned about all the toxic products in your home that you can't do anything about—especially the building products, such as insulation. First, be aware that building products, furniture, and carpets "outgas" immediately. This means that they release most of their toxins right away. Over time, although they continue to outgas, the rate and volume at which they do is so much smaller. If you live in an older home, these sources of toxins usually aren't much of an issue anymore. If you live in a new home, they are. You can purchase air filters to help remove the volatile organic (carbon-based) compounds (VOCs) from the air in your home, office, or car. A few examples of excellent portable air-filtration systems are listed below.

• Blueair HEPA Air Filters 501 and 402

• Healthmate HEPA Air Filter

• SilentAir 4000

• Desktop Air Filters

- UV Air Purifier (uses high-efficiency particulate air [HEPA], carbon, ultraviolet light, and ionization)

- Car ionizer (available at www.gaiam.com)

Ventilate your home well by keeping the windows open as often as possible. Don't let the temperature in your home get too warm, because heat increases the amount of toxic outgassing. If you do any type of remodeling in the future, such as painting or carpeting, be sure to use only nontoxic products.

Another way to cut down on the toxins released in a new home is to apply a product to your furniture, cabinets, or anything made with particleboard that seals the toxins in. AFM Safecoat SafeSeal is an excellent sealer; I used it when I built my home and found it to be simple to apply and very effective.

Green Builders

If you are considering purchasing a new home or if you are thinking of remodeling the home you're already in, I highly recommend that you speak with a specialist in the "green" building industry. Green builders are committed to building homes that are resource efficient and environmentally safe. There are several organizations in the United States that can put you in touch with green builders, as well as with distributors of nontoxic products for home improvements. When I built my home, I worked with several extremely helpful green builders to make my home and all its occupants as safe from toxins as possible.

Chapter 23

Cellular
Housecleaning
The Power of Purification

*C*hances are you're feeling a little nervous right about now because you realize that, for most of your life, you've been unknowingly inviting toxic assassins into your home and into your body. You know that, more than likely, your body is filled with assassins just waiting to go for the kill. But just like in every Indiana Jones movie, there is a way out of this seemingly hopeless situation. You can give your body's natural detoxification system a huge boost by using the ancient purifying technique from *Ayurveda* that I've mentioned several times earlier in the book. This technique is known as *panchakarma*. Current research shows that it's very effective at getting toxins out quickly—even those that have been stored in your fat for years. It's not painful or unpleasant—quite the opposite. In fact, it's one of my all-time favorite, personal pampering experiences.

Panchakarma literally means "five actions." It is an integrated precise sequence of soothing treatments done in a spa-like setting with medical supervision over the course of several days. The treatments are gentle and deceptively simple, but their effects are remarkably powerful. The healing intelligence of the body is given such a boost through the techniques of *panchakarma* that it's capable of triggering phenomenal purification and healing.

Think of it this way: There are few things in life that Goddesses enjoy more than going to the spa. Taking time off from all your duties and responsibilities to go to a peaceful and relaxing place, free from any demands, with nothing to do but soak up the healing offerings is the essence of joy. Although spending the day at the spa may seem on the surface to be nothing more than a luxurious day of pampering, it can actually be profoundly rejuvenating and fundamental to maintaining your health and beauty. Take the revitalizing, health-promoting effects of a typical day at a spa, multiply it exponentially, and you have an inkling of the restorative effects of *panchakarma*.

DISLODGING IMPURITIES AND TOXINS

Panchakarma is especially effective at dislodging impurities and toxins and flushing them from your body. Research shows that it does this extraordinarily well. A study published by Bob Heron and John Fagen in 2002 in the journal *Alternative Therapies in Health and Medicine* found that, in test subjects, the levels of polychlorinated biphenyls (PCBs) and pesticides, including DDT, dropped by 50 percent after just one five-day series of treatments. Dr. Heron also tested subjects who had gone through *panchakarma* an average of twice a year for more than nine years. Every toxin the subjects were tested for came back negative. In other words, no toxins were present in levels high enough to be detected. The researchers concluded that regular *panchakarma* treatments are effective at removing toxins from your body and keeping your toxin load extremely low. In fact, research shows that the *only* known effective therapy that rids body fat of toxic chemicals is *panchakarma*.

As you know, your body accumulates and stores hundreds of toxins from the environment and the foods you eat. You also accumulate impurities from the waste products that are created by normal cellular metabolism. In *Ayurveda,* all toxins in the body form *ama.* Too much *ama* leads to disease. According to *Ayurveda,* one of the main purposes of *panchakarma* is to get the *ama* out.

Panchakarma also profoundly balances the mind/body and prevents or reverses the development of disease. Preliminary research indicates that it may slow the aging process, too. The first time I went through this series of gentle but powerful techniques, within forty-eight hours I looked ten years younger and had never felt better in my life! That experience made me a believer in the power of *Ayurveda.*

THE STEPS OF *PANCHAKARMA*

The majority of *panchakarma* is done in a medical spa-like setting over a period of time of between several days and several weeks. For the best results, you should go for a minimum of three days and ideally stay five to seven days. But before you arrive at the spa, you begin the initial steps of *panchakarma* at home. "Home prep" is designed to begin the process of softening the impurities and toxins, and mobilizing them from your fat.

1. Home Prep: Internal Oleation

This first phase of *panchakarma* is technically called "internal oleation." Oleation means saturating your body with oils. The oil used in home prep is *ghee,* or clarified butter. *Ghee* is made by boiling butter until all the milk solids precipitate out (always use organic butter). In other words, butter without milk solids and water is *ghee*. The spa you choose will give you specifics on how to make *ghee*, how much to take, and when to take it.

Ghee has very different properties from butter. First, it stays solid at room temperature and never needs to be refrigerated. Second, it lasts virtually forever without going bad. In India you can purchase 100-year-old *ghee*. Third, unlike butter, *ghee* doesn't raise your cholesterol or promote hardening of the arteries. *Ayurveda* considers *ghee* to be an extraordinarily powerful medicine that, according to ancient texts, soothes all the *doshas* (properties found in all living things— *vata* governs movement; *pitta,* metabolism and transformation; and *kapha,* structure). It improves memory and mental function, strengthens the body, promotes longevity and beauty, and protects the body from various diseases. You can purchase organic ghee in some health food stores.

During home prep, *ghee* is taken in increasing amounts every day for four days. Instead of drinking melted *ghee* straight, which can be a bit challenging, I mix it with one-quarter to one-half cup of heated soy milk to make it more palatable. The purpose of drinking *ghee* is to raise the level of fat or lipids in your blood to form a "concentration gradient" between the stored toxins in the fat cells in your body and the pure fat (*ghee*) in your blood. You may recall from high school biology that a concentration gradient is produced anytime there is more of a particular substance on one side of a semipermeable membrane than on the other. A law of physics dictates that the concentration of molecules on one side of a semipermeable membrane must be equal to the other. So, molecules on the side with the higher concentration will pass through the membrane to the side with the lower concentration until the amounts are equal on both sides of the membrane.

Here's how *panchakarma* uses the concentration gradient to get toxins out: During the home-prep portion of *panchakarma,* you also consume a low-calorie diet. The fat stored in your fat cells is used for energy. Your fat cells become smaller as more fat is used. The amount of space for toxins in your fat cells lessens, so the toxins become more concentrated. The pure organic *ghee* you consume contains no toxins. By introducing large amounts of toxin-free fat into the blood, you create a concentration gradient between toxin-filled fat in the body and toxin-free fat in the blood—a physiological condition that isn't normally present. The concentrated toxins will flow out of your fat into the pure *ghee* in your blood until the concentration of toxins is equal in your fat and blood. According to physics, a 50-percent reduction in the amount of toxins in your body would be expected. This is exactly what Bob Heron's research showed.

After the internal-oleation phase of *panchakarma* is completed, you should take a twenty-minute hot bath. The heat increases blood flow and the delivery of toxins to the intestines. Due to the relatively large amount of *ghee* that is ingested during home prep, not all of it will be digested. The undigested *ghee* stays in the intestines. This again sets up a concentration gradient, and toxins and impurities are drawn into the intestines. Following the bath, a mild laxative, such as castor oil, senna tea, or a special herbal mixture, is taken to eliminate the toxins in the intestines.

2. Pulse Diagnosis: Detecting Imbalances

After completing the first phase of *panchakarma,* you are ready for the relaxing and enjoyable part: the in-residence treatments at an *Ayurvedic* medical spa. When you arrive at the clinic, an *Ayurvedic* physician, called a *vaidya,* takes your pulse and asks you a series of questions. The *vaidya* picks up a lot more information from your pulse than just your heart rate. In fact, an expert in pulse diagnosis can feel, with remarkable precision and accuracy, the state of balance and imbalance in all your body systems and tissues. It may seem like magic, but the explanation for how a *vaidya* is able to do this is quite simple. Quantum physics tells us that the fundamental structure of the universe is nothing more than vibration. Every structure in your body vibrates. Blood flows through blood vessels and comes into contact with every cell in your body. The vibration that each cell emits reflects its state of health. The vibrational information from every cell in the body is transmitted to and then carried by the blood. *Ayurvedic* physicians, as well as experts in traditional Chinese medicine (TCM) and several other ancient holistic forms of medicine, are trained to "feel" and interpret this information.

A *vaidya* can also determine your body type or "constitution" from your pulse. Based on all the information from the pulse, the *vaidya* prescribes a specific series of *panchakarma* treatments customized to your current state of health. The *vaidya* has many treatments to choose from, each with its own special benefits and purposes, but all with the ultimate purpose of restoring balance.

3. Massage: Moving Toxins and Inducing Balance

The prescribed series of *panchakarma* treatments usually begins with a special procedure called *abhyanga*—an herbalized, sesame-oil massage. Two technicians apply warm oil simultaneously to each side of your body using synchronized movements designed to facilitate getting the toxins out while soothing and balancing the nervous system. The pressure is soft, and the movements are extremely relaxing.

When both sides of your body are stimulated in the same way at the exact same time, the brainwaves in the two hemispheres of your brain will synchronize. This brainwave phenomenon is also seen during the practice of Transcendental Meditation (see Chapter 27). Not surprisingly, people who practice this highly effective form of meditation report the experience of "transcending" during *abhyanga.*

Researchers have observed that there is a strong correlation between the synchronicity of brainwaves and depression. Depression is characterized by very asynchronous brainwave patterns, meaning that the brainwave patterns emitted by one hemisphere of the brain are very different from those emitted by the other side. Researchers have found that when a person experiences relief from depression, his or her brainwave patterns become more synchronized. *Panchakarma* synchronizes your brainwaves. Researchers think that this may be why it's so effective at easing depression.

Because sesame oil is the most penetrating of all the oils, it is the preferred type of oil used for *abhyanga,* as well as for many other techniques in *panchakarma.* Sesame oil is absorbed through the skin and appears in the blood within minutes. It contributes to the blood-lipid/body-fat concentration gradient, helping to flush toxins out of the body.

Herbs with special medicinal properties are usually mixed in the oil. Up to seventy-five different herbs may be added. Sesame oil, with its incredible absorptive qualities, acts as a carrier to deliver medicinal herbs into the body. Delivering medicinal herbs through the skin may seem like an unusual practice, but it's not. Western pharmaceutical companies use this route, too. Many types of medications are designed to be administered topically in patches—for example, nicotine, nitroglycerin, and estrogen. The medications are absorbed through the skin where a network of blood vessels under the skin picks them up and transports them to the rest of the body.

Research has found that sesame oil also has several other beneficial effects, including anticancer properties. It can inhibit the growth of melanoma and colon cancer cells. It also contains antioxidants. If the oil is heated, the antioxidant activity increases. That's one of the reasons why the oil is always heated during *panchakarma.*

Two other toxin-releasing, coherence-building, whole-body massage techniques may also be prescribed based on a person's specific health needs: *udvartana* and *garshan. Udvartana* is performed using a paste made of ground grains. This technique cleans the skin, increases circulation, and promotes weight loss. *Garshan* is performed using raw-silk or wool gloves to create friction, thus stimulating circulation and helping to promote weight loss.

Nasya

This technique purifies the structures in your head and powerfully balances and enhances your five senses. *Nasya* improves mental clarity and stabilizes the mind. It's especially good for people with sinus problems and headaches. The technique of *nasya* is performed by one technician. A luxurious head and shoulder massage is given while you sit in a chair. Following the massage, you gently inhale herbalized steam. Then, lying down on a bed with your head slightly tilted back, the technician places a series of drops of herbalized sesame oil in your nose. The sesame oil soothes your sinuses and helps to facilitate the release of any congestion.

Shirodhara

This procedure is designed to relax your mind, soothe and nourish your nervous system, and detoxify your body. A gentle stream of slightly warm herbalized sesame oil is applied to your forehead. *Shirodhara* is actually considered a cooling treatment. Your eyes are covered with cotton balls and a washcloth. A soft roll is placed under your neck so that your head is tilted slightly backward. The technician applies a very slow stream of sesame oil back and forth across your forehead in an infinity (or figure-eight) pattern. Most people experience deep relaxation and an expanded state of consciousness when undergoing this procedure.

Shirodhara is particularly good for alleviating anxiety, insomnia, nervousness, and worry. It also improves malaise and stabilizes the mind. And it's beneficial for your skin, too. Many people notice a distinct glow to their complexion following a soothing, relaxing, peaceful session of *shirodhara*.

4. Heat Treatments: Melting the Impurities

The next major step of *panchakarma* uses a group of heat treatments to dilate the channels in your body and increase circulation, which facilitates the flow of toxins and impurities into your intestines where they can be eliminated. Also, toxins can be removed from your body through your sweat.

There are three main heat treatments in *panchakarma: swedana, pizzichilli,* and *pinda swedana*.

Swedana

Swedana is a traditional herbalized steam treatment. It's like a steam sauna, but with a few important differences. Instead of sitting on a bench as you would in a sauna, you lie on your back in a cedar cabinet with your head *outside* the cabinet. *Ayurveda* does not advise overheating your head. To keep your head cool and comfortable, a frozen cube of coconut oil is gently applied to your head and face during the treatment. It's remarkably soothing and refreshing. To keep you well hydrated, the technician gives you frequent sips of cool water.

Pizzichilli

This is my personal favorite of all the treatments. It's considered a royal treatment, and it's easy to understand why. Imagine lying on a table while two technicians massage your body as they use a hose to continuously pour thick streams of soothingly warm sesame oil over you. The first time I experienced the sensation of the warm oil cascading in waves over my body, I actually moaned out loud. It felt like warm melting butterscotch. After the treatment, I felt deeply relaxed and I glowed from head to toe.

Pinda Swedana

The third heat treatment, *pinda swedana,* is performed by two technicians who massage your body using quick long strokes with boluses of precooked herbs and hot medicated oils in soft, smooth cloth packs. *Pinda swedana* is designed to soothe any kind of musculoskeletal problems, especially arthritis. It's also said to nourish the body, enhancing its vitality.

5. Cleansing: The Final Stage

External oleation and heat treatments are performed each day to help lift the impurities and toxins out of the tissues and transport them into the intestines. Once in the intestines, it's very important to get them out. This is facilitated by a simple procedure called a *basti,* which is a gentle internal cleansing of the colon with either herbalized water or oils. The oil-based *basti* and the water-based *basti* are administered on alternating days. You can think of a *basti* as a very gentle herbalized colonic. Getting the toxins out of the colon quickly is powerful medicine, so some people find it to be a little uncomfortable. *Ayurveda* says that the *basti* treatment is so important that it alone could cure 50 percent of illnesses.

IMMEDIATE AND LONG-TERM BENEFITS

After completing *panchakarma,* people report having greater energy, clarity of mind, and a sense of well-being. They also report relief of symptoms and improvements in disorders of both the mind and body. Research on the effects of *panchakarma* shows that it rebalances physiology and significantly reduces oxygen free radicals.

Oxygen free radicals increase your risk of cancer and other degenerative disorders and accelerate aging. In 1993 in the *Journal of Research and Education in Indian Medicine,* Hari Sharma, M.D., documented that patients doing *panchakarma* had an initial rise in lipid peroxidase, an enzyme that goes up in the presence of oxygen free radicals. But following therapy, lipid-peroxidase levels fell way below pretreatment levels. These findings correspond to the rise of toxins in the blood as they are mobilized during treatment and to the fall of toxins after they are eliminated from the body.

Researchers have also found psychological improvements in patients following *panchakarma*. Standard psychological tests show that these people are less anxious, less depressed, less distressed, and less fatigued. In 1988, researcher Rainer Waldschütz used the Freiburg Personality Inventory, a standardized test that measures twelve different personality scales, to evaluate patients who had just finished *panchakarma* treatments. These post-*panchakarma* patients showed improvements in six of the twelve scales: decreased body complaints, reduced irritability, less bodily strain, fewer psychological inhibitions, more openness, and greater emotional stability.

Panchakarma also significantly improves several cardiac risk factors. Blood samples taken from patients shortly after they completed *panchakarma* showed many beneficial changes. For example, vasoactive intestinal peptide (VIP)—a substance that dilates coronary arteries—increased by 80 percent. The "good" kind of cholesterol (high-density lipoproteins; HDL) increased by 75 percent, and total serum cholesterol decreased.

Nothing is more powerful than this special series of techniques for eliminating the impurities that obstruct your full strength; nothing surpasses the balancing and healing effects; nothing centers you more; and nothing recharges you more. Think of it this way, after a week of *panchakarma*, the unobstructed flow of your Warrior Goddess's cosmic intelligence becomes so powerful and so intense that you positively glow with self-luminescence and beauty.

If you cannot go to a *panchakarma* clinic, you can detoxify at home. Although home detoxification programs are not as powerful as *panchakarma*, they can effectively remove toxins. Simply begin with the home-prep program for *panchakarma* described above. Then, for two weeks following the prep, take herbs that detoxify the liver, kidneys, and colon. You can work with a knowledgeable herbalist to determine which herbs to take and the dosages, or you can purchase a detoxification kit, such as Whole Body Cleanse from Enzymatic Therapy, from your local health food store. Also, follow a pure diet—lightly cooked fresh organic fruits, vegetables, and whole grains. Be sure to avoid alcohol, sugar, chocolate, cold foods, meat, drugs, cigarettes, and canned, preserved, and processed foods.

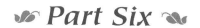 *Part Six*

Balancing Rest and Activity

Protection Against Breast Cancer

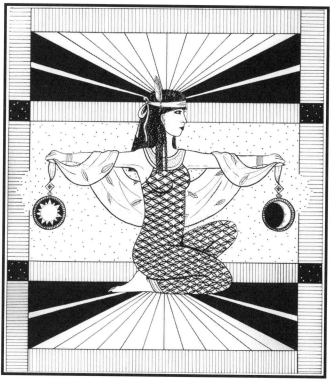

Goddess of Balance

Chapter 24

Healing Nectars of the Night
Melatonin and Other Bodyguards

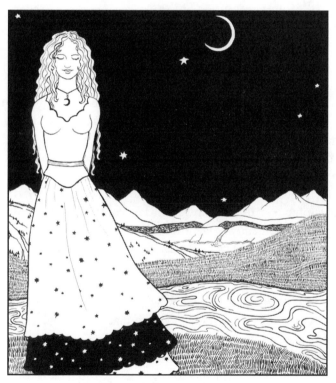

Goddess of Sleep and Dreams

Lack of knowledge is darker than the night.

—AFRICAN PROVERB

*I*t's a timeless *Ayurvedic* principle that *proper sleep and rest are fundamental to good health. Activity must be balanced with rest.* Think about a time when you have gone to bed early and enjoyed a peaceful rejuvenating night of sleep. You woke feeling fresh and full of energy, optimistic, and upbeat. When you looked in the mirror, the youthful and radiant face looking back at you took you by surprise. What you saw was the end result—the gift of proper sleep—of a multitude of complex biological processes designed by Nature to keep you healthy. When you follow the laws of Nature, these are the results you can expect to achieve. Proper sleep and rest are of supreme importance to your Warrior Goddess's health, strength, vitality, and beauty.

THE NECTAR OF SLEEP

When you sleep, your Warrior Goddess orders the nocturnal repair and purification of your mind/body to begin. She commands your mind/body to produce medicinal potions and nectars with truly magical healing properties. In scientific terms, they are known as chemicals and hormones.

The nectar of sleep is the hormone melatonin. Several years ago, researchers discovered some of melatonin's remarkable effects. This hormone subsequently received a lot of media attention, mainly for two reasons: 1) melatonin supplements can help relieve or quicken recovery from jet lag, and 2) they are safe, natural alternatives to sleeping pills. While these effects can be quite helpful, there's so much more to know about melatonin than the media shared.

When darkness falls, the pineal gland in your brain increases its production of melatonin. In other words, as soon as the sun sets, your Warrior Goddess calls for melatonin to start flowing. As the level of this hormone rises, you start to feel sleepy. The moment you fall asleep, it starts to flow even faster. The faster it flows, the greater its power becomes. If it flows to its highest potential, its power becomes so great that it becomes a raging river of cancer protection.

Melatonin mirrors the attributes of a goddess; it gently but powerfully seduces you into sleep, but while you're asleep, it acts as a great warrior on your behalf. It provides powerful protection from many of the factors that increase your risk of breast cancer.

This hormone is a very potent antioxidant, and, as you know, antioxidants are powerful defenders against the attack of oxygen free radicals. They disarm oxygen free radicals, rendering them incapable of damaging your cells and DNA, damage that could lead to cancer. Melatonin slows down the production of estrogen, prevents its overproduction, and blocks its stimulatory effects on breast cells. But melatonin's defenses don't stop there. It blocks two other threats that can increase cell division in the breast—the hormone prolactin, and the growth factor known as "epidermal growth factor."

Melatonin also enhances the tumor-fighting power of vitamin D and increases this vitamin's ability to stop tumor growth. In fact, it makes vitamin D's tumor-fighting abilities 20 to 100 times stronger! All of melatonin's various breast cancer–fighting capabilities can be summed up in three big points:

1. Melatonin prevents the initiation of breast cancer.

2. Melatonin slows down tumor growth.

3. Melatonin prevents metastasis.

The only thing you really need to remember about melatonin is this: It's a powerful weapon against breast cancer.

A Comrade to Chemotherapy

Taking supplemental melatonin can enhance the effectiveness of chemotherapy by increasing its ability to kill tumors. A 1999 study from Italy, reported in the *European Journal of Cancer,* found that breast cancer patients treated with chemotherapy lived longer if they were also given supplemental melatonin. In scientific terms, these patients increased their survival by one year. In other words, more women were alive one year following the diagnosis and treatment of their breast cancer than would normally have been expected to be. When melatonin supplements were given in addition to chemotherapy, the size of the tumors decreased significantly more than when chemotherapy was given alone.

Melatonin can also provide protection from many of the harmful side effects of chemotherapy. Chemotherapy is commonly toxic to several components in the blood. Platelets, which have an important role in blood clotting, are particularly vulnerable. Chemotherapy usually reduces the number of platelets in the blood, thereby increasing the risk of bleeding problems. Melatonin protects the platelets and keeps their numbers up. Researchers found that when melatonin was given to patients on chemotherapy, the number of platelets in their blood remained normal. These patients also had fewer toxic side effects from the drugs, including less damage to their nervous systems and hearts, and fewer mouth ulcers.

THE RHYTHMS OF NATURE

Whether you honor them or not, your mind/body is ruled by the natural cycles and rhythms of Nature. In other words, your Warrior Goddess has a schedule that she likes to keep to stay strong and balanced. She is very particular about the number of hours she sleeps, what time she goes to bed, and many other details. When you live in harmony with her cycles and rhythms, you enhance her strength. When she is strong and empowered, she expresses that power by increasing your body's natural healing capabilities—its inner healing intelligence. This principle is beautifully demonstrated by the profound effects that respecting or disrespecting these rhythms has on how melatonin expresses itself.

If you followed the natural rhythms of the sun, you would go to bed shortly after it sets. Research indicates that there is tremendous health value in following the cycles of the sun. Research shows that if you go to bed early, before 10:00 P.M., your melatonin levels rise to their highest possible and most medicinal levels during sleep. If you go to bed late, around 12:00 A.M. for instance, you are working against the natural rhythms of Nature and obstructing the flow of healing intelligence. Melatonin levels don't rise as high in this case, and you lose its full medicinal power. If you severely disrespect Nature's rhythms, you seriously impede the healing intelligence of your mind/body, and your Warrior Goddess loses her balance, becoming dull and weak. She can no longer protect you with brilliance, discriminating intelligence, and strength.

If you keep an extreme schedule that assaults the natural laws and rhythms of Nature (for example, if you work all night and sleep all day), the deleterious health consequences are spectacular. Your inner healing intelligence is dramatically weakened. For instance, researchers found that nurses who worked the night shift had a 50 percent higher risk of breast cancer. The longer they worked the night shift—that is, the longer they worked against the laws of Nature—the higher their risk of breast cancer became. Other researchers found that breast cancer tumors grew seven times faster in animals exposed to constant light.

When you sleep, your melatonin level rises, but melatonin responds to more than just your change in consciousness. Melatonin is a nocturnal nectar. It loves the darkness. The darker the environment is, the better it flows. Even though you don't consciously *see* when you sleep, your eyes perceive the light. Melatonin is as repelled by light as Count Dracula is. It shies away from even the faintest glimmers of light. Any light at night—even a soft nightlight or the glow of a full moon—will prevent your melatonin from rising to its full potential. Bright city lights burning continuously through the night may be one reason for the more common incidence of breast cancer in industrialized regions.

The darker it is, the more your melatonin responds and the more freely it flows. Melatonin loves the darkness so much that it seems to prefer blindness. In women who are blind, this natural medicinal hormone expresses its protective might in full glory. Blind women have half the incidence of breast cancer that women with normal eyesight have.

If you can't make your bedroom totally dark, I highly recommend that you wear an eye mask when you sleep.

Sleep Creates Immune Ammo

Melatonin is only part of the cancer protection that you gain during sleep. Your sleep patterns govern changes in the strength of your immune system that also affect your risk of cancer. Your Warrior Goddess, empowered by sleep at the proper time, can command more immune protection. She orders your immune system to produce a powerful cancer-fighting substance called "tumor-necrosis factor," a natural biological weapon that destroys tumors.

Your immune system takes the nighttime order very seriously. When your Warrior Goddess says, "jump," your immune system jumps. It creates ten times more tumor-necrosis factor when you're asleep than when you're awake. During sleep, another cancer-fighting weapon is also called forth from your immune system—natural killer (NK) cells. You can think of these cells as gladiators who kill tumor cells and any other undesirable cells that invade your body. But if you don't get enough sleep or don't sleep during the best times, your immune system won't respond to the command to make more NK cells. Researchers have found that without enough sleep, the number of your NK cells goes down significantly.

> *There is a time for many words,*
> *and there is also a time for sleep.*
>
> —HOMER, *THE ODYSSEY*, 800–700 B.C.E.

Natural Law

Five thousand years before Ben Franklin said, "Early to bed and early to rise makes a man healthy, wealthy, and wise," *Ayurveda* understood and taught people the natural laws governing sleep. Ben Franklin was right. His astute observations are in alignment with those natural laws—laws that never change. They are true, always have been true, and always will be true. According to ancient *Ayurvedic* texts, it is a law of Nature that when human beings *go to bed before 10:00 P.M. and get up by 6:00 A.M.*, they experience the most balancing and healing effects of sleep.

Modern research supports this 5,000-year-old recommendation. Scientists have found that you experience deeper stages of sleep when you go to bed by 10:00 P.M. This is partly due to the greater rise in melatonin and other hormone responses. When you get up before 6:00 A.M., you will probably notice that you feel more awake, less groggy, and more energetic than if you sleep later. Try it and see.

Sleep Is a Pillar of Health

Of all the thousands of natural laws governing your health, there are three that are considered the most important. They are described as the "three pillars" of *Ayurveda*. Proper sleep is one of those pillars. The other two are proper diet and lifestyle. This recommendation, *Go to bed before 10:00 P.M., and get up by 6:00 A.M.,* like most *Ayurvedic* recommendations, sounds simple but has profound health benefits. It's especially important when it comes to your risk of breast cancer. The study of night-shift nurses, mentioned earlier, found that if you sleep during these recommended hours, your risk of breast cancer is 50 percent lower than if you don't.

When you don't get enough sleep, it drastically weakens your Warrior Goddess. In fact, it diminishes her power more than almost anything else. Without enough sleep, she quickly falls apart, loses her coordination, and becomes less alert and discriminative. Her reaction times slow down. It becomes impossible for her to manage all the tasks and demands placed on her—and it shows. Without proper sleep, she is too weak to protect you from making mistakes that could cost you your life.

For example, when workers are fatigued because of lack of proper sleep, the risk of on-the-job errors and accidents is much higher. Worker fatigue is credited for such major accidents as the Chernobyl nuclear meltdown and the Exxon Valdez oil spill. Research shows that 60 percent of road accidents are caused by fatigue due to lack of sleep. In one study, drivers who stayed awake for more than seventeen hours had significantly impaired coordination, reaction time, and judgment. Even more frightening, these sleep-deprived drivers were found to be *more severely impaired than drivers who are legally drunk*! The moral of the story? Without proper sleep, your inner intelligence becomes dangerously weakened, and your risk of serious accidents goes up.

If you continually get less than the ideal amount of sleep, the hard fact is, you'll take years off your life. Sleep is so important that even one hour less of it each night can cut your life short. Research shows that people who sleep less than six hours a night don't live as long as those who sleep seven or eight hours.

The magnificent multitasking intelligence that manages your mind/body— your Warrior Goddess—needs rest to properly perform all the tasks she needs to carry out to keep you balanced and healthy. If you sleep fewer than four hours a night, she can't do her job, and diseases begin to manifest. Your risk of diabetes, high blood pressure, and weight gain increases.

Researchers have found that when you sleep only a few hours, glucose (blood sugar) is metabolized 30 percent less efficiently, and the stress hormone cortisol rises higher than if you'd gotten an adequate amount of sleep. When cortisol goes up, it causes your blood pressure to rise. It makes you more resistant to insulin, which increases your risk of diabetes. Not getting enough sleep is also associated with chronic fatigue, depression, and even divorce.

Too Much Sleep Isn't Good Either

As you have seen, natural law says that your mind/body does its best when you retire by 10:00 P.M. and rise by 6:00 A.M. This also means that sleeping too much—sleeping beyond these recommended hours—can throw you out of balance. Although your Warrior Goddess enjoys her sleep, she has a lot of things to accomplish during the day to help protect you. When it comes to sleep, there are optimum times and amounts. Sleeping too much makes her dull and unable to function well, so much so that fatal diseases may form.

Research has found that people who sleep more than nine hours a night have an increased risk of heart disease. A Japanese study, reported in *The New York Times* on February 10, 2004, surveyed the health and sleep habits of more than 100,000 people for ten years. This study found that people who slept eight hours a night had a higher mortality rate than those who slept seven hours a night. The longer the study participants slept, the higher their risk of dying became. The researchers haven't yet determined how sleep and mortality are linked. One possible explanation for their findings is that people with serious health problems tend to sleep more than healthy individuals.

Do Not Disturb

Sleeping at the wrong times isn't the only thing that can disturb the proper flow of melatonin. A study published in October 2001 in the *American Journal of Epidemiology* found several other factors that can lower melatonin levels: daylight, a high BMI (body mass index; see page 140), alcohol consumption, and the use of certain medications, including beta-blockers, calcium-channel blockers, and psychotropics.

If you drink alcohol, your Warrior Goddess won't demand as much melatonin as she normally would. In a study from the University of Connecticut, published in *Epidemiology* in November 2000, researchers found that the more alcohol a woman consumed in a twenty-four-hour period, the lower her melatonin level was. One alcoholic drink didn't have any effect, but two drinks caused a 9 percent reduction in the level of melatonin, and three drinks dropped the level by 15 percent. This may be another reason why alcohol increases the risk of breast cancer.

THE DANGERS OF ELECTROMAGNETIC FIELDS (EMFS)

An electromagnetic field (EMF) is an invisible electric field that is produced when an electrical current runs through a wire. EMFs are also a natural product of the Earth's magnetic field. Your Warrior Goddess doesn't like mechanically created EMFs, because they interfere with your mind/body, especially with your melatonin levels. Therefore, the effects of man-made EMFs can be very disruptive to your health—particularly your breast health. Even EMFs that seem innocuous, like those created by the wires and appliances in your home, can disturb your melatonin levels. Researchers have found that residential 60-Hz magnetic fields caused by normal electrical house wiring and equipment (such as clock radios, electric blankets, and televisions) depress melatonin levels.

In a comprehensive review of all the published studies on EMF exposure and breast cancer, a definite link between the two was found, and so we can say with certainty that EMF exposure contributes to breast cancer. In many studies, even male electricians showed an increased risk of the disease.

In eleven occupational studies, a statistically significant increased risk of breast cancer was found in several categories. Overall, the risk of breast cancer doubled in premenopausal women who had jobs with significant EMF exposure. These jobs included telephone-line installers, repairers, and line workers. The risk was 65 percent higher for system analysts and programmers and 40 percent higher for telegraph and radio operators.

A German study published in *Cancer Research* in 2002 found that 50-Hz EMFs caused breast tumors to start growing *and* accelerated their growth—but, in this study, melatonin levels remained normal. These researchers concluded that EMFs may disrupt the body some other way. Regardless of the specific disturbance that EMFs cause in the balance of your body, we know one thing for certain: Exposure to EMFs *can* cause breast cancer and accelerate its growth.

Fortunately, you can take steps to protect yourself from EMFs. For example, if you're building a new house or rewiring your existing one, have your electrician install a master switch in your bedroom. Turning this switch off at bedtime will cut off all the power and, therefore, any EMFs in your bedroom. Your electrician can also use "BX electrical cable" when wiring your home. This twisted wire doesn't produce significant EMFs.

Also, simply standing a few feet away from most electrical appliances reduces your EMF exposure to nearly zero. Whenever you use an appliance, such as a microwave, toaster, or blender, step a few feet away from it while it is operating. Another good way to reduce your EMF exposure is to purchase EMF shields for your cell phone and computer.

Of all the common electrical household appliances, hairdryers produce the strongest EMFs. Fortunately, some companies manufacture low-EMF hairdryers. So, if this is something you use daily, consider purchasing one (see the Resources section).

Understanding EMFs on a Quantum Level

The mind/body at its most finite level is nothing more than intelligent vibrations. Quantum physics has shown us this universal truth for all living matter. Cosmic intelligence organizes all these vibrations, which contain the intelligence to manifest everything in your physical structure. Some external influences are harmonious with this intelligence and support its full expression; others disrupt it and hinder its flow.

This intelligent vibration creates a measurable EMF around your mind/body. If you're exposed to an outside EMF, it can interact with yours. When the external EMF is out of harmony with your own, it creates imbalances in your field and obstructs the flow of its intelligence. When this intelligence is interrupted, the different parts of your mind/body don't all function properly, and diseases, such as cancer, can result.

HONORING THE NIGHT

The rhythms of Nature have created the night as a time of rest. It's a time when your mind/body undergoes magical repair, rejuvenation, and purification. The power and magnificence of your Warrior Goddess's healing protective powers depend upon your honoring all her desires. When you do, her ability to keep you well and balanced is extraordinary. When you don't honor her, she is weakened and loses the ability to keep you well. Honor and respect her ability to protect you by following Nature's rhythms and natural laws, and she will reward you with a great treasure—good health.

Chapter 25

The Medicine of Movement

How Exercise Lowers Your Risk of Breast Cancer

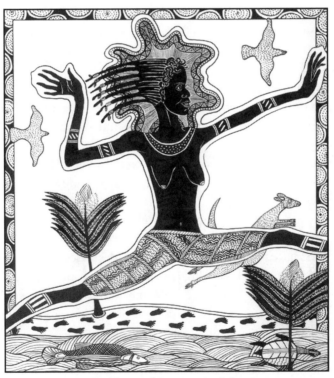

Goddess of Joyous Activity

To dance is to give oneself up to the rhythms of life.

—Dr. Maya Patel

To Live is to Dance—to Dance is to Live.

—Snoopy

S noopy is right. The natural rhythms of life are a harmonious balance of activity and rest. When you dance with those rhythms, you can experience life to its fullest. The degree to which you respect those rhythms plays a huge role in your risk of developing or surviving breast cancer. Resting and sleeping at the proper times have powerful medicinal effects. The right type of activity at the proper times of the day is also very powerful medicine. It produces an array of health-protecting potions: magical chemicals and hormones, each expressing its own healing intelligence. When you work in harmony with Nature's rhythms, your inner intelligence is powerfully strengthened to ward off the development and progression of breast cancer in many ways.

Regular invigorating aerobic movement decreases your risk of a multitude of disorders. It also has a huge effect on lowering your risk of breast cancer. Research shows that any type of aerobic movement for just thirty minutes, three to five times a week, decreases your risk of breast cancer by 30 to 50 percent. Vigorous activity also has lasting protective benefits. If you were very active as a teenager, your risk of breast cancer may be as much as 30 percent lower than that of more sedentary teens.

Your Warrior Goddess thrives on regular movement that elevates your heart rate. It enlivens and expands her intelligence, and endows her with balance, strength, and stamina. Those gifts she then bestows on you. She becomes masterful at balancing your female hormones and regulating your menstrual cycles in a way that enhances your protection from breast cancer.

Researchers have found that aerobic exercise decreases estrogen levels. It also causes your menstrual cycles to lengthen. The longer your menstrual cycles are, the fewer of them you'll have over a lifetime. In other words, you'll produce much less estrogen. Invigorating movement also produces hormonal changes that boost your immune system, making it stronger and more effective at fighting disease and getting rid of cancer cells.

Regular invigorating movement also helps to keep your weight down. That's important when it comes to your risk of breast cancer. People who are obese have twice the risk of breast cancer as those who are of normal weight do (see Chapter 17). Weight gain during early adulthood is thought to be a major contributor to approximately one in every three cases of breast cancer diagnosed after menopause. The main reason for this is that fat creates estrogen. After menopause, your fat becomes an estrogen factory. So, if you include lively physical activity in your daily routine, you can keep both your fat stores and your risk of breast cancer to a minimum.

MENDING MATTERS OF THE HEART

Your heart beats about 100,000 times a day and about 35 million times every year. It circulates six quarts of life-giving blood to all the cells in your body three times every minute. But it is far more than just a pump. *Ayurveda* considers the heart to be the seat of your mind and consciousness. Of all the sacred spaces within your mind/body, your Warrior Goddess is most fond of your heart. It's where she communicates with you through your feelings.

When you show devotion to your Warrior Goddess by moving every day in ways that stimulate this sacred space, she expresses her gratitude by creating a powerful medicinal tonic that protects and strengthens your heart. It helps to keep your cardiovascular system strong, cuts many of the risk factors associated with heart disease and stroke, and lowers blood sugar, cholesterol, and triglycerides. It makes the good kind of cholesterol (high-density lipoproteins; HDL) go up and the bad kind (low-density lipoproteins; LDL) go down.

> *While I dance, I cannot judge, I cannot hate.*
> *I cannot separate myself from life.*
> *I can only be joyful and whole.*
> *That is why I dance.*
>
> —Hans Bos

Emotions are felt in the heart. *Ayurveda* says that the heart is the organ of emotion. *Ayurvedic* physicians always consider emotional causes first when they are evaluating patients with heart disease. Positive emotions can strengthen your heart, and negative emotions can weaken it. Research shows that if you have repressed anger and feelings of hostility, your risk of heart disease is higher.

Stimulating movements can help to soothe your emotions, too. A study published in the *Mayo Clinic Proceedings* in 1999 found that patients who participated in a cardiac-rehabilitation program within a month of having a heart attack showed significant improvements in feelings of hostility, anxiety, and depression. These patients also had a higher appreciation of the quality of their life. That's important when it comes to your risk of breast cancer, because research shows that depressed women are much more likely to develop this disease.

AEROBIC EXERCISE

Brisk revitalizing activities are so stimulating to your Warrior Goddess that they enable her to bless you with a wide spectrum of protection. They lower your risk of type 2 diabetes and of developing cancers of the colon, ovary, uterus, and pancreas. If you smoke cigarettes—something extremely frustrating to her cosmic intelligence—exercise encourages her to forgive you somewhat by lowering your risk of lung cancer. Exercise will also reduce your risk of certain conditions, including asthma, mild emphysema, back problems, arthritis, glaucoma, and neurodegenerative diseases, such as Alzheimer's disease and senile dementia. Exercise can even help you to live longer.

The right types of movement provide your Warrior Goddess with a natural pharmacy of healing chemicals called neuropeptides, which are produced by your brain. Neuropeptides relieve stress and reduce the risk of all stress-related illnesses including peptic ulcers. Research also shows that neuropeptides soothe your emotions and decrease depression as effectively as many popular antidepressant medications.

There are shortcuts to happiness, and dancing is one of them.

—VICKIE BAUM

Your Warrior Goddess is just waiting for you to start your sacred dance with her. She wants you to find some form of invigorating movement that speaks to you and expresses your soul. It may be dancing, bicycling, rowing, running, or a team sport. When you begin to increase your heart rate through an activity of your choosing, she will encourage you to continue. She is so grateful to you for this powerful form of protection that she will order pleasure-inducing endorphins—your body's natural morphine—to be released from your brain in return. Endorphins lift your spirits and give you a natural high. It's a great natural reward for the effort and dedication to your health.

Your schedule may be tight, but when you move your body with intentional vigor, even briefly, she loves the strength that she receives from it so much that she's willing to work around your schedule. She bestows the same protection on you no matter how you divide up the time you spend on aerobic activities. A study from the Department of Epidemiology at the Harvard School of Public Health published in 2000 found that it didn't matter whether you exercised for a long continuous period or broke it up into multiple shorter sessions. For instance, ten minutes of exercise three times a day is just as effective as one thirty-minute session.

Your Warrior Goddess appreciates every little bit of your effort. You can honor her by getting up and doing something during commercials if you're watching television. Park your car at the far end of the parking lot, and walk briskly to your destination. Get up from your desk for a few minutes every couple of hours, and climb a few flights of stairs. Remember, it all adds up. If your boss asks what you're doing, explain that you're taking a few minutes to make yourself more productive, decrease your number of sick days, and lower the company's healthcare costs! I doubt you'll hear any complaints.

STRENGTH TRAINING

Aerobic exercise isn't the only type of exercise that lowers your risk of breast cancer. Strength training with weights works, too. First, it increases muscle mass, and muscle uses more energy than fat. Therefore, your metabolism speeds up and that helps you lose even more weight. Second, strength training has been found to lower insulin-like growth factor-1 (IGF-1) levels by 15 percent. As you may recall, IGF-1 is a strong stimulator of breast cancer, so anything you do to lower the amount of it in your body will make a big difference in your risk of breast cancer.

Strength training is also the best thing you can do for your bones. It keeps them strong and lowers your risk of osteoporosis. A study conducted by Oregon State University published in 2001 followed postmenopausal women who did specific weight-bearing exercises for five years. The women had no decline in their bone density at the end of the study. Those women who didn't exercise lost density. Researchers feel that the best form of exercise for your overall health is a combination of aerobics and strength training.

ANCIENT *AYURVEDIC* WISDOM

Ayurveda has recognized the importance of regular exercise for more than 5,000 years. It recommends that you participate in "medicinal movements" every day. But it also recognizes that too much of the wrong kind of exercise for your body type can have the opposite effect. It puts a strain on your body and can cause injuries and imbalances that increase your risk of disease. For instance, putting too much force into invigorating activities causes the release of oxygen free radicals, and that raises your risk of cancer. Extremely heavy exercise may make your muscles stronger, but the body, as a whole, may become weaker.

Ayurvedic Exercise Recommendations

1. **Exercise to 50 percent of your capacity.** If you follow this advice, you'll never overstrain your body, and it will gradually become stronger. You'll feel exhilarated and energized instead of drained. You'll be able to exercise every

day instead of needing to take days off to recover. For example, if the most weight you can bench-press is 50 pounds for ten reps, do five reps instead.

2. **Exercise in the morning.** Different types of energy govern different times of the day.

Between 6:00 A.M. and 10:00 A.M. is *kapha* time when your energy tends to be settled and slow. If you exercise during this time, you stimulate yourself out of any sluggishness, and you will feel energized all day. Incidentally, waking up in *kapha* time can make you feel lethargic when you get up. That's why *Ayurveda* recommends waking up before 6:00 A.M.

Between 10:00 A.M. and 2:00 P.M. is *pitta* time. *Pitta* is associated with heat and digestion, and, therefore, *pitta* time is considered the worst time to exercise. When the sun is at its peak, you can easily become overheated by exercise. This is also the time of day when your digestion is at its peak. During this time you should eat your largest meal of the day, not exercise.

Between 2:00 P.M. and 6:00 P.M. is *vata* time; *vata* governs movement. This is an acceptable time to exercise (although morning is considered best). The cycles then repeat. *Kapha* time is from 6:00 P.M. until 10:00 P.M. Only light exercise, such as walking, is recommended during this time. You should use this time to slow down and get ready to go to sleep. Vigorous activity during these hours is too stimulating and may cause you to have difficulty falling asleep.

3. **Choose movements that are right for your type.** *Ayurveda* recognizes that each of us is different. Different activities are recommended depending on your body type. Just as there are *vata, pitta,* and *kapha* times of day, there are *vata, pitta,* and *kapha* kinds of people.

Vata people are thin and prone to anxiety and nervousness; they are usually cold and do everything fast. If this is you, slow-paced light exercises such as swimming, walking, and yoga are recommended.

If you have a medium build, are usually hot, and have a quick temper and sharp intelligence, you are a *pitta* type. Moderate exercises such as brisk walking, cross-country skiing, swimming, cycling, weightlifting, and tennis are good for you.

If you have a tendency to be overweight, are easygoing and reliable—but possibly a little lazy—you are a *kapha* type. You need to get up and get moving as much as possible. Vigorous exercise, such as jogging, more intense weightlifting, and aerobics, is excellent for you.

4. **Perform special movements to facilitate the union of your mind/body and breath.** If you have ever wondered where yoga originated, wonder no more. Yoga got its start as unique postures prescribed by *Ayurveda.* In addition to

regular exercise, *Ayurveda* recommends that you do yoga, too. The word "yoga" means union. The purpose of the exercises is to bring union to the mind and body, creating balance and promoting health. Yoga also helps to increase flexibility. Normally, you lose flexibility as you age. Yoga has been found to reduce anxiety, fatigue, tension, and stress and to improve mental function.

A Japanese study published in June 2000 in the journal *Perceptual and Motor Skills* examined the brainwave activity, as well as the level of the stress hormone cortisol, in yoga instructors during their practice of yoga. Researchers found that alpha brainwaves increased. Alpha waves correspond to a state of restful alertness. They are also the type of brainwaves found during the practice of Transcendental Meditation (TM). In addition, researchers found that blood-cortisol levels decreased during the practice of yoga. Cortisol levels go up in response to stress and go down when stress is relieved. As you can see, yoga has several powerful health-enhancing effects—especially reducing stress. According to studies at the National Institutes of Health (NIH), stress causes or aggravates approximately *90 percent* of all illnesses, including cancer, so reducing stress is *very* important.

5. **Wait at least two hours after a full meal to exercise.** It takes about two hours for your stomach to empty after a full meal. During this time, blood flow is increased to the digestive tract to facilitate digestion. If you exercise too soon after eating a full meal, you will divert the blood flow from your digestive tract to your muscles and impede the digestive process.

6. **Wait at least thirty minutes after you exercise before you eat.** When you exercise, blood flow increases to your muscles and is shunted away from your digestive tract. Therefore, if you eat while exercising, or too soon afterward, there won't be enough blood available for your digestive tract to function properly. After about thirty minutes of rest, your muscles no longer need additional blood so your digestive tract can get all the blood it needs without any interference.

7. **Don't strain when you exercise. Cut back if you start to breathe heavily through your mouth.** Research shows that overexercising can actually be detrimental to your health. It depresses your immune system and increases free-radical production. So it's important not to stress yourself too much during exercise. Just like medications, herbs, foods, or anything else that's good for your health, there's a proper amount to take; too much or too little of these things can create imbalances that lead to disease.

8. **If you meditate, practice yoga before meditation and your conventional exercises afterward.** Yoga helps to center and relax the body and mind and

prepare it for meditation. On the other hand, stimulating exercise activates the body and mind—the opposite of the effect required to foster meditation.

> Everything in the universe has rhythm—everything dances.
>
> —MAYA ANGELOU

FINDING YOUR OWN MOVEMENT

If you have never experienced a form of movement that expresses your soul, keep looking; you'll find it. You were designed to enjoy moving with vigor and dynamism. Nature created special neuropeptides to reward you with bliss when you dance and move to the individual expression of your soul. These magical molecules of movement create a feeling of exhilaration and make you naturally high on life.

There are so many different ways that you can express yourself in movement. No matter what your personal preferences are or what your physical condition is, you can find something that resonates with your soul. Consider biking, jogging, or brisk walking; you can do these activities solo or with a friend. If you like to have company when you exercise, find a partner for a two-person sport such as tennis, racquetball, or one-on-one basketball. Or you may simply want to find a buddy to work out with at the gym. If you discover that you enjoy working out at the gym but you need a more structured format to keep you motivated, make a series of appointments with a personal trainer. Last, if you like to be part of a group that meets regularly, take an exercise class. You can find a class for just about anything: aerobics, cycling, kickboxing, martial arts, dancing, rowing—you name it.

Even if you are obese and haven't exercised in years, it's never too late to start. However, be sure to speak with your doctor before you begin any exercise program. Walking is a great activity for just about anyone who wants to begin exercising. Each day, choose a destination that's a little farther away or simply pick up the pace at which you walk. Beginner's yoga is another good starting point. Try out different activities to find the one that's fun for you and suits you best.

> To dance is to be out of yourself, larger, more powerful,
> more beautiful. This is power. It is glory on Earth,
> and it is yours for the taking.
>
> —AGNES DE MILLE

Chapter 26

Emotional Healing

Using Your Emotions
for Your Benefit

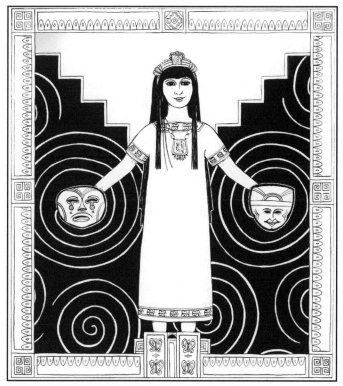

Goddess of Emotional Choice

A merry heart does good like medicine.

—PROVERBS 17:27

*E*ach feeling that you have creates a biochemical reaction in your body. When you feel up and positive, your mind/body produces the chemicals and hormones that enhance your inner healing intelligence, stimulate your immune system, and strengthen your health. When you feel depressed or angry, your mind/body produces other hormones and chemicals that obstruct your healing intelligence, depress your immune system, and weaken your health. In other words, positive emotions stimulate a surge of powerful natural chemicals that magnify your Warrior Goddess's healing might. Negative emotions and stress have the opposite effect; they depress your Warrior Goddess, dampen her brilliance, and diminish her ability to defend and protect. It's no wonder researchers have found that the chemicals released in response to your emotions can affect your risk of breast cancer.

EMOTION MOLECULES

Every emotion you feel is packaged in molecules that spread throughout your body. These molecules of emotion, in turn, cause the release of other chemicals and hormones or may stimulate impulses in your nervous system. When you feel positive and upbeat, healing chemicals are released that help to keep you strong and healthy. When you feel down and depressed, stress hormones and other chemicals that impair your immune system and your health become abundant. Negative emotions, unresolved anger, repressed and suppressed emotions, and stress can take a big toll on your health. But there are many techniques that you can use to process your emotions effectively and reduce how much your mind/body reacts to stressful situations.

In her book *Molecules of Emotion,* Candice Pert, Ph.D., documented that every thought you think, every emotion you express, triggers the release of neurotransmitter molecules that spread throughout your body. If you've ever questioned the mind/body connection, think back to a time when you just missed hitting another car or almost fell down the stairs. Your heart started racing, your breathing increased, a prickly sensation may have rushed through your body, you felt a little lightheaded, had a sinking feeling in your stomach, and maybe even started trembling. When you become angry or upset, your face turns red, your blood pressure goes up, and your skin may break out in hives. In these situations, your body is reacting to a flood of chemicals released by your brain and nervous system. The connection between mind and body is clearly an intimate one; you can't separate them.

One of the most fascinating studies I've ever read dramatically proves the point of the union between mind and body. It's a study of heart transplant donors and recipients published in the journal *Integrative Medicine* in March

2000. Researchers observed as many as five donor characteristics in a recipient after transplant.

In one case, a fifty-six-year-old heart transplant recipient began having flashbacks of seeing a Jesus-like image followed by a flash of light. He then experienced an intense burning sensation over his face. The organ donor had been a thirty-four-year-old policeman who died after being shot in the face by a drug dealer who allegedly looked like Jesus.

In another case, the donor was an eighteen-year-old introverted male who wrote poetry and music. The recipient was an eighteen-year-old female who, according to her father, had been "wild." After her transplant, she started playing the guitar and writing songs and became quiet and reserved like the donor.

Other examples include a militant gay woman who chose a heterosexual lifestyle after receiving the heart of a heterosexual woman; a five-year-old child who recognized the never-before-seen father of the donor in a crowd, ran up to him, climbed into his lap, and called him "Daddy"; and a male recipient who loved meat before the transplant, but became nauseated by it after receiving the heart of a female vegetarian.

The Science of How Emotions Affect Our Immune System

When you feel an emotion, scientists say that it's processed through the brain's limbic system and the hypothalamus. The hypothalamus releases neuropeptides, which then stimulate the pituitary gland to release hormones. All the endocrine glands, especially the adrenals, react to these hormones by producing other hormones that can weaken or strengthen the function of the immune system. Certain immune-system cells called "lymphocytes" have receptors that receive messages from the molecules released by thoughts and feelings. The hypothalamus also has receptors for peptides released by the immune system's lymphocytes.

A two-way communication takes place between your emotional center and your immune system. Anger, fear, and rage produce neurochemicals that strain your body and can damage your organs. On the other hand, laughter reduces levels of cortisol and epinephrine, stress hormones that are released by the adrenal glands. Laughter also stimulates the activity of the immune system. In a study published in *Alternative Therapies in Health & Medicine* in March 2002, researchers found that laughter increased natural killer (NK) cell function, as well as that of many other types of immune-system cells. These immune-boosting effects lasted for twelve hours after "humor intervention." Depression and suppression of strong emotions can generate such a blow to your immune system that it nearly stops functioning. Depressed women are nearly four times more likely to get breast cancer than those who have never been depressed, according to researchers at the University of Pennsylvania.

Time spent laughing is time spent with the gods.

—A JAPANESE PROVERB

To Be Human Is to Be Emotional

We are spiritual beings having a human experience. The human experience involves a wide range of feelings and emotions—from sadness, resentfulness, and hatred, to compassion, forgiveness, and love. As human beings, it is part of our journey to continually feel and process emotions. Imagine if you felt nothing—no compassion, no desire, no joy, no sense of accomplishment, no pride, no pleasure, no pain. Nothing could move you to tears—not the most exquisite beauty of Nature, not the birth of your child, not the atrocities of war. Nothing! It's hard to even imagine. Feelings and emotions were designed for a reason: They give purpose to life.

The Energy Center of Emotion

The ancient *Ayurvedic* texts describe energy centers called *chakras*, which are located in different areas of the body. The heart *chakra* is referred to as the fourth *chakra*. In Sanskrit, it's called the *Anahata chakra*. It's said to be the energy center that enables you to feel higher emotions, such as love, compassion, forgiveness, tolerance, happiness, and joy. Your heart is what allows you to "feel," according to *Ayurveda*. It is the center of your emotions and the home of your consciousness. Activating and balancing the heart expands your consciousness. The heart *chakra* is considered to be the fundamental center for your growth as a human being.

Dr. Caroline Myss, medical intuitive and author of *Anatomy of the Spirit: The Seven States of Power and Healing* and *Why People Don't Heal and How They Can*, says that the fourth *chakra* focuses on your feelings about your internal world. Your emotional responses to your own thoughts, ideas, attitudes, and inspirations, as well as the attention you give to your emotional needs, are all contained within this *chakra*. Anatomically, the fourth *chakra* is located right over your heart and breasts. Energetically speaking, everything you feel with your heart also affects your breasts.

According to Dr. Myss, breast cancer is a fourth *chakra* issue. The fourth *chakra* has to do with how you express the emotions that you feel and your capacity to form mutually beneficial, balanced relationships with others and with yourself. In Dr. Myss's experience, women who develop breast cancer have issues with hope and trust. They often suffer from hurt, sorrow, and unfinished business. In a 1995 study, women who had suffered a major loss such as divorce, loss of a job, or some other stressful trauma within the past five years were twelve times more likely to have breast cancer than those who hadn't had one. According to Christiane Northrup, M.D., in her book *Women's Bodies, Women's Wisdom,* studies that look at the different personality patterns of women with different types of cancers found some statistically significant common patterns in women with breast cancer. For example, they tended to have emotionally distant fathers; they had a greater tendency to stay in loveless marriages; and during their childhood, they most likely had the responsibility of caring for their younger siblings. These women also had a greater probability of not taking care of their own physical needs and getting proper medical care.

Behavioral studies show that women who develop breast cancer have a tendency to be caregivers. They take care of everyone else's needs before they take care of their own. Take a look at your life, and make sure you're taking care of your own needs. Don't sacrifice what you need to do to take care of yourself in order to take care of other people. Nurture yourself by doing things that make you feel good. As a very wise friend of mine says, "The best way to take care of other people is to take care of *yourself* first."

Managing our emotions increases intuition and clarity.
It helps us self-regulate our brain chemicals and internal hormones.
It gives us natural highs, the real fountain of youth we've been
searching for. It enables us to drink from elixirs locked within
our cells, just waiting for us to discover them.

—Doc Childre

LEARNING TO COPE WITH STRESS

Arriving home from a rough day at the office, you open the door. The kids are shouting, the house is a mess, the dog ran away, and everyone wants to know what's for supper. Yes, you know what stress feels like, but do you really know the magnitude of destruction that this level of chronic stress can have on you? According to studies at the National Institutes of Health (NIH), *approximately 90 percent of all illnesses—mental and physical—are caused by or aggravated by stress!*

Dr. Hans Seyle, a pioneering stress researcher, defines stress as a psychophysiological (mind/body) event that takes place when your system is overwhelmed by any experience: physical, mental, or emotional. Stress isn't something *out there;* it's completely subjective and internal. It is a mind/body reaction.

Researchers have found that stress causes a cascade of neurochemical reactions that can lead to disease. In stressful situations, the adrenal glands release cortisol, epinephrine, and norepinephrine, otherwise known as the *stress hormones.* The pituitary releases more stress-related hormones, and as a result, the sympathetic branch of the autonomic nervous system "revs" up. The response is known as *fight or flight.* It's very useful—even essential—in an emergency, because it gives you the ability to respond quickly for your safety, for example, jumping out of the way of a New York City taxicab.

However, that fight-or-flight response is neither necessary nor appropriate if, for instance, you're at work and you receive an e-mail from your significant other saying that he wants to date other people. You can neither engage in a fight nor take off in flight under the circumstances.

The subsequent psycho-physiological response leaves behind a soup of chemicals that stick around and wreak havoc on your system. They can cause high blood pressure, insomnia, anxiety, depression, frustration, anger, and tension; they can increase risk factors for heart disease, diabetes, and stomach ulcers; they can depress your immune system; and they can even enlarge your waistline. Stress reactions also cause an increase in oxygen free radicals, which are linked to most degenerative diseases including accelerated aging, wrinkles, and cancer.

As I was reflecting on stress and its effects on the body, I came to the conclusion that stress, in one form or another, is responsible for the origin of *all* disease. *Ayurveda* describes five disease stages, and the first stage begins with an imbalance. According to *Ayurveda, perfect health is all about the perfect balance of mind and body.* So, when something takes your system out of balance, it creates stress in your body, and that stress initiates disease.

You're probably familiar with the list of big stressors: death of a loved one, divorce, moving, and loss of a job. But what you may not have considered is that just about anything can create stress in your body. Too much or too little of things that are considered good for you—or even essential—can do it: good food, rest, exercise, a vacation, or any sensory stimulus. Of course, traditionally bad-for-you things can cause it, too, like eating the wrong food, eating too late at night, staying up too late, watching too much TV, or watching a violent movie. Other big stressors can be war, a drop in the stock market, toxins in your environment, a strained relationship, traffic, loud noises, and the challenges of travel. Anything can induce a stress reaction if you don't receive it in the proper way at the right time in the correct amount.

According to *Ayurveda,* the best way to prevent stress is to live life in a way that keeps your body in perfect balance. This is precisely what the techniques and recommendations of *Ayurveda* are designed to do. The most precise way to do this is to see an *Ayurvedic* physician (a *vaidya*) who will determine your physiological type (*vata, pitta, kapha,* or a mixed blend of two of these types) and prescribe the proper foods, exercises, and routines you need to keep your specific physiology in balance. Keep in mind that what brings one person into balance may induce stress in another. However, despite individual differences, there are many things that are effective at reducing stress or, at least, at decreasing your physiological response to it.

10 STRESS-REDUCING TECHNIQUES

1. **Get enough sleep at the proper times.** This topic is covered in Chapter 24.

2. **Eat primarily fresh organic fruits, vegetables, and grains.** Hundreds, if not thousands of studies, show that a plant-based diet—especially when the plants are organically grown, whole, fresh, and unprocessed—is loaded with protective nutrients, like antioxidants, that guard against stress and disease. Conventionally grown foods (grown with pesticides and other chemicals), red meat, processed foods, leftovers, and frozen or canned foods all have lower nutritional values, increase oxygen free radicals, and are generally toxic to your body. Chapter 5 deals with this subject.

3. **Practice an effective, stress-reducing meditation.** More than 500 research studies have shown that Transcendental Meditation (TM) is more effective at reducing the signs and symptoms of stress than any other meditation or stress-reducing technique, including biofeedback and progressive muscle relaxation. TM significantly lessens anxiety, depression, insomnia, digestive disturbances, neurotic tendencies, physical complaints, and psychosomatic problems. This mental technique also decreases the risk of being admitted to the hospital for any reason—physical or mental—by more than 50 percent. Chapter 27 contains a full discussion on the benefits of TM.

4. **Avoid assaults to your senses.** Any strong, prolonged, or otherwise caustic stimulus to your senses can induce stress: loud noises, certain forms of music (for me, the worst is the heavy-metal, head-banging, homicidal/suicidal variety), strong unpleasant odors, hot spices, watching TV or sitting at a computer too long, or exposure to extreme temperatures.

5. **Listen to relaxing music.** Studies show that classical music or any other soothing music of your choice can cause a significant relaxation response.

6. **Get a massage, or give yourself one.** Massage has been found to release many hormones associated with relaxation, and it boosts the immune system. The effects are enhanced when a good penetrating oil, like sesame oil, is used.

7. **Have fun.** Don't let your life become all about work and getting things done on your to-do list. Make sure you balance things out by regularly including some of your favorite activities. Frequently participate in activities that are fun and joyful for you, such as getting out in Nature, riding your bike, going to a play, singing, playing with your kids, enjoying a day at the spa, spending time with friends, dancing, or soaking in the bathtub with a good book. Make a habit of doing something that brings you joy every day.

8. **Take an antioxidant supplement.** The many benefits of taking a good antioxidant are discussed in Chapter 13. A stress reaction creates excess oxygen free radicals, which have been linked to most chronic degenerative disorders including Alzheimer's disease, cancer, and accelerated aging. Some good antioxidants are vitamin C, vitamin E, selenium, and CoQ_{10}. The *Ayurvedic* herbal mixture *Amrit Kalash,* according to research, may be the best antioxidant of all. Dr. Yukie Niwa, a Japanese researcher, studied more than 500 different antioxidants over a period of thirty years. He found that the most powerful and effective antioxidant of all those tested was Maharishi *Amrit Kalash.*

9. **Take an herbal supplement.** Certain herbs have been shown to effectively reduce the stress response through a variety of mechanisms. They are called "adaptogens" because they help us adapt to stress. For example, research shows that an *Ayurvedic* herb called holy basil, which has a 5,000-year-plus history of use, protects against and reduces stress. It decreases the release of the stress hormone cortisol. It also enhances stamina and endurance, increases the body's effective use of oxygen, and boosts the immune system when you're under stress. In addition, it slows aging and provides a rich supply of antioxidants, as well as a multitude of other benefits.

10. **Exercise regularly.** In many studies, regular aerobic exercise has been found to be *as effective* in relieving depression as pharmaceutical medications.

Some of these stress-reducing techniques are what *Ayurveda* would call "behavioral *rasayanas.*" As you may recall, *rasayana* is "that which negates old age and disease." *Ayurveda* recommends certain behaviors to negate old age and disease. Molecular studies have shown that uplifting activities and emotions produce molecules (neuropeptides) that strengthen your immune system and overall health. The behavioral *rasayanas* to practice, according to *Ayurveda*, are *respect, love, compassion, uplifting speech, cleanliness, charity and regular donations, religious observances, being positive, moderation,* and *simplicity.* The behaviors to avoid are *anger, violence, harsh or hurtful speech, speaking ill of others, egotism, dishonesty,* and *jealousy.*

> *Why not learn to enjoy the little things—*
> *there are so many of them.*
>
> —AUTHOR UNKNOWN

Ayurveda also says that to reduce stress you should *pay attention to the rhythms of the day, week, month, and year.* If you attune yourself to the rhythms of Nature and adjust your activities accordingly, you will strengthen your immune system and enhance your health. If you keep unnatural routines, you will weaken your immune system.

Modern science has documented daily fluctuations in hormones and biorhythms. There are better times during the day for some activities than for others. The most obvious one is sleep (see Chapter 24). If you sleep during the "wrong" hours, your risk of breast cancer can increase by as much as 50 percent.

IDEAL *AYURVEDIC* DAILY ROUTINE

- Rise before 6:00 A.M.
- Use the bathroom.
- Give yourself a sesame-oil massage.
- Wait twenty minutes, and take a warm shower.
- Practice yoga for at least fifteen minutes.
- Practice breathing exercises (*pranayama*; see page 210) for about ten to fifteen minutes.
- Meditate for twenty minutes or longer.
- Exercise for about a half hour (see Chapter 25 for more details).
- Eat a light breakfast of cooked fruits.
- Go to work.
- Eat your main meal at noon.
- Rest for ten minutes after your meal.

- Go back to work.

- Do your evening meditation program: yoga, breathing, and meditation.

- Eat a light dinner.

- Walk after dinner.

- Read something pleasant, enjoy pleasant conversation, or listen to soothing music.

- Go to bed by 10:00 P.M.

> *Slow down and everything you are chasing*
> *will come around and catch you.*
>
> —JOHN DE PAOLA

PRANAYAMA—USING YOUR BREATH

Breathing is synonymous with life. If you stop breathing, you stop living. But breathing has many finer aspects than the black and white of life and death. The way you breathe can affect your health for better or worse. *Ayurveda* uses a set of breathing techniques called "*pranayama*" to enhance health and lower stress.

Prana is a Sanskrit word that means "breath," but its full meaning goes way beyond that. In *Ayurveda, prana* is known as "life energy," paralleling the ancient notion of "*chi*" energy in China, "vital force" for the ancient Greeks, and "*ki*" in ancient Japanese medicine. *Prana* is the life force that governs all bodily functions and influences your mind, memory, thought, and emotions. By breathing with the techniques of *pranayama, Ayurveda* says you can strengthen your life force and induce balance, which enhances your health and lowers your risk of disease.

Pranayama literally means "regulating the breath." The techniques of *pranayama* are numerous but usually involve breathing through alternating nostrils. The technique of breathing through alternating nostrils is said to create balance in the physiology, improve the function of the nervous system, and benefit many specific organs.

Research has documented that the regular practice of *pranayama* increases the depth and the length of time that you're able to hold your breath and enlarges the vital capacity of your lungs. It improves stress-hormone balance and decreases pulse rate, blood pressure, and blood fats such as cholesterol. *Pranayama* can also be extremely beneficial in treating asthma.

One *Pranayama* Technique

Pranayama is usually practiced just before meditation to settle the body and mind and facilitate transcending (see Chapter 27). You can also use *pranayama* to help calm yourself whenever you are upset. Here's a simple way to practice:

1. Sit upright, and close your eyes.

2. Use your right thumb to gently close your right nostril.

3. Breathe out through your left nostril slowly and naturally until you breathe your breath completely out. Don't force it.

4. Breathe slowly back in the same (left) nostril.

5. Close your left nostril with the long finger or ring finger on your right hand.

6. Release your thumb on your right nostril, and breathe out slowly and easily.

7. Breathe back in through the same (right) nostril.

Repeat this process for about five to ten minutes. You should notice an almost immediate calming effect.

There is more to life than increasing its speed.

—MOHANDAS K. GANDHI

CHANGING YOUR REACTION

Life is stressful. Many events take place every day that are beyond your control. You can't prevent them from happening, but you can change how you react to them. Remember, stress isn't something *out there*. It's purely subjective and an *internal* reaction. You can decrease the severity of your stress response by getting enough sleep at the proper times, respecting the rhythms of Nature, eating a healthy diet, avoiding assaults on your senses, participating regularly in activities that bring you joy, taking care of yourself by getting regular massages, listening to relaxing music, exercising daily, and remembering to breathe (especially using the techniques of *pranayama*). Finally, one of the most powerful techniques you can use to protect your health from the damaging effects of stress is the daily practice of an effective meditation—the topic of the next chapter.

Tension is who you think you should be.
Relaxation is who you are.

—CHINESE PROVERB

Chapter 27

Turning Inward

Cranking Up the Volume
of Balance

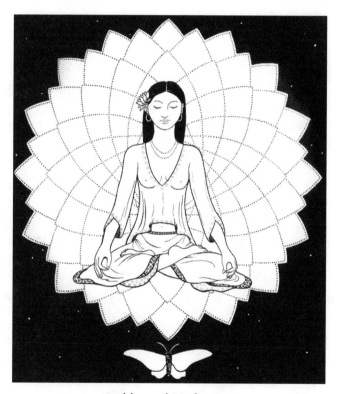

Goddess of Meditation

If the inner mind is not deluded,
the outer actions will not be wrong.

—Proverb of Tibet

*T*urning inward to reach that quiet part of yourself is one of the simplest and most effective things you can do to rebalance and recharge your health. At the center of each of us is our soul and spirit—the part of ourselves that is connected to all other people and all other things. It is our *true* Self. But in this plane of existence, we are often so caught up with surface activities and concerns that we forget where our true Self lies—deep within. When we take the time to quiet our mind and reconnect with our Self, we are also tapping into universal energy, because at the finest level, *that's* who we are. Uniting with the Source is like touching Nature's tuning fork—we start to vibrate with tremendous calming, rebalancing, and healing energy.

The most effective way to turn inward is through the practice of meditation. While you sleep, your Warrior Goddess—although replenished by your rest— is still actively managing all the critical purification and rejuvenation events that take place within your body. But when you meditate, your Warrior Goddess soaks much more deeply in a soothing bath of pure relaxation. She stays with you, but she also goes home to her Source. Each time you reunite with your Self, your Warrior Goddess experiences rebirth and emerges with immense strength. When you make it a daily practice to go within and reunite with your Source, your Warrior Goddess's power to keep you balanced, whole, and well becomes so vast that she remains virtually invincible.

Transcendental Meditation® (TM)

Research shows that the most effective stress-relieving, anxiety-reducing, and health-promoting form of meditation is Transcendental Meditation (TM). *Ayurveda* considers TM to be the single most important modality for inducing balance, integrating the mind and body, preventing disease, and restoring health.

THE FOURTH STATE OF CONSCIOUSNESS

To meditate means to think, contemplate, or concentrate on something. *To transcend* means to go beyond. During the practice of TM, a unique state of consciousness is reached by transcending thought. It is characterized by a state of restful alertness and deep silence. Typically, the only states of consciousness you routinely experience are waking, sleeping, and dreaming.

When you practice TM, your mind goes to a fourth distinct state of consciousness, appropriately named "transcendental consciousness," or pure consciousness. Brainwave recordings, called electroencephalographs (EEGs), reveal that this special state of consciousness produces patterns completely different from those seen when you are awake, dreaming, or sleeping. For instance, the left and right hemispheres of the brain are normally asynchronous, which means that they have very different rhythms in their brainwave patterns. During transcendental consciousness, the two hemispheres begin to synchronize and alpha waves predominate. Alpha waves are generally associated with a state of restful alertness. Practitioners of this type of meditation report that when they "transcend," they experience feelings of rest, relaxation, calmness, peace, expansiveness, and unity with the world. In essence, this mental technique is a powerful behavioral *rasayana*—"that which negates old age and disease."

Quantum Physics and Consciousness

Quantum physics has shown us that the world we perceive, the material world, is just an illusion. An atom—the smallest particle of an element—is made up of more space than matter. So, what appears solid, such as a table, is actually mostly empty space. According to quantum physicists, underlying all the diversity of the material world is the real world: a homogeneous, nonchanging, unified field composed of nothing but small vibrating strings. If you're interested in reading more about this, I recommend a wonderful book that beautifully explains the "superstring theory" called *The Elegant Universe* by quantum physicist Brian Greene.

What lies beyond these strings? What controls the vibration of all these strings and how they manifest the diversity of the material world? According to scientists (and logic), there *must* be an underlying field of intelligence or consciousness that manages these strings. Scientists have called this field of intelligence the "unified field of intelligence," or the "unified field of consciousness." This field holds the power to orchestrate Nature; therefore, it contains all the laws of Nature.

When you experience transcendental consciousness, your mind merges with this unified field of consciousness. This merging powerfully establishes balance in your mind/body. In other words, when you tap into the Source that holds the knowledge of all the things you need to do to keep your body in perfect balance and perfect health (the laws of Nature), you are immersed in this knowledge and at the same time soothed and healed by its balancing effects. Not surprisingly, when people first connect with this Source of knowledge, they discover that they spontaneously start making choices in alignment with good health. For example, their yearning to smoke cigarettes, drink alcohol, and partake in other disease-promoting activities decreases, and their desire to eat nourishing foods and engage in healthy activities increases. That's why research shows that regularly experiencing this unified field of consciousness produces powerful health benefits in mind, body, spirit, and emotions.

TM's Mind/Body Health Benefits

More than 500 studies have been conducted on TM at 200-plus independent institutions and universities in more than thirty different countries. These studies show that the health benefits of experiencing transcendental consciousness daily are nothing short of miraculous. It dramatically reduces stress and anxiety and promotes good health. (For more information on the background of TM, see the inset "The History of TM" below.)

As you may recall, according to the National Institutes of Health (NIH), stress is the cause of, or a major contributing factor in, more than 90 percent of all illnesses. Because TM radically lowers stress, it also substantially lowers the risk of most diseases. For example, research shows that people who practice this form of meditation daily have 56 percent fewer hospital admissions for all diag-

---

The History of Transcendental Meditation

Transcendental meditation is not a new technique. In India, it was passed on from teacher (yogi) to student for thousands of years. It remained unavailable to the general public until the late 1950s when concern over the deteriorating health and collective consciousness of the world's people drove one yogi into action. Maharishi Mahesh Yogi adopted the task of teaching this technique to the public. He and his lineage of masters knew that the simple mental practice of TM was so powerful that if enough people were taught how to do it, it could substantially improve health, calm the collective consciousness, and promote world peace.

In the mid-twentieth century, the practice of meditation was radically foreign to most people in the West. In order to gain widespread acceptance and to encourage as many people as possible to learn it, a focus was also placed on research to prove and document TM's many astounding benefits. Studies were initiated all over the world. Today, thanks to the proliferation of studies that show that TM is a remarkably effective approach for boosting and fostering health and peace, millions of people throughout the world have learned this technique and practice it daily.

noses, including cancer and accidents, and 87 percent fewer admissions for cardiovascular diseases, including heart disease.

The research-proven health benefits of the regular daily practice of TM are numerous, diverse, and impressive. They include lower blood pressure, reversal of coronary artery disease, better mental capacity with improved academic performance, enhanced creativity, and improved verbal and analytical thinking. TM is also associated with less worry, depression, and anxiety, as well as with fewer emotional disturbances, better relationships, enhanced job performance, and increased satisfaction.

TM and Addictions

For many people, overcoming health-destroying addictions is one of the most difficult challenges they will face in their lifetime. Standard treatment programs are very successful for some, but for others, especially over the long term, they are not. Researchers have found that people have greater success in overcoming addictions if they replace a health-destroying habit with another habit—ideally one that is health-supporting, such as the practice of an effective stress-reducing meditation. A meta-analysis of 198 independent treatment outcomes for drug, alcohol, and cigarette addictions found that the daily practice of TM was more effective in helping people overcome these addictions than any of the standard treatment programs.

TM and Aging

One of the most astonishing findings about the regular practice of TM is that it can *reverse* the aging process. Research shows that individuals who have meditated for more than five years are physiologically about twelve years younger than those who haven't. These conclusions were based on measurements of near-point vision, hearing, and systolic blood pressure—all of which predictably worsen with age.

As you age, the levels of hormones in your body also change. For example, you produce much less of the hormone dehydroepiandrosterone sulfate (DHEA)—the most abundant hormone found in young adults. DHEA has many positive roles in the body, one of which is to help in the production of lean muscle mass. By the time you reach your mid-thirties, you start losing lean muscle mass, and declining DHEA levels are thought to be largely responsible for this phenomenon. Research shows that you can slow down the rate at which DHEA levels drop and stay physiologically younger by exercising and practicing TM. In general, the level of DHEA in TM practitioners is the same as that normally found in people five to ten years younger.

As a woman, maintaining youthful DHEA levels is especially important since this hormone also has a protective role against breast cancer and osteoporosis. Studies show that women with high DHEA levels have lower risks of these diseases.

Please note that I don't recommend taking supplemental DHEA because its long-term safety has not been adequately evaluated and there is some cause for concern. Raising and maintaining your DHEA levels naturally seems to have a far different effect on your body than taking supplemental DHEA. DHEA is a steroid-type molecule that is converted to testosterone and estrogen in the body. Taking supplemental DHEA may abnormally raise the levels of these hormones and has been reported to cause unwanted hair growth, acne, and mood swings. Of even greater concern is that it may also increase the risk and accelerate the growth of breast and prostate cancer. If you have breast cancer, you definitely should not take supplemental DHEA.

Learning TM

You can't learn TM from a book. As my good friend and long-time teacher of this technique says, "Think of it like flying a plane." You would never try to fly a plane if your only experience came from reading a flight-instruction manual. There are many variables and subtle nuances that can make the difference in a safe flight. Similarly, awareness of the refined subtleties of TM can make all the difference in successful practice. If you don't practice TM properly, you will not reap the full health benefits.

Like flight instructors, certified teachers of TM have gone through a long, rigorous training course to become proficient at teaching this technique. To locate a certified teacher in your area, call 1-800-LEARN-TM. The Transcendental Meditation program is taught in seven steps over four days.

There are a couple of common concerns people have that interfere with learning and practicing this technique. The first is time. When will they find time in their already overloaded day to meditate? Rest assured, TM is practiced for only twenty minutes, twice a day. Anyone can squeeze two twenty-minute sessions into their day with relative ease. Here's how: Wake up twenty minutes earlier than you usually do, or meditate on your way to work if you take mass transit, or skip one half-hour television show in the evening and meditate, instead.

Another common concern that people have is that learning to meditate is difficult because you must force your mind to stop thinking. People who believe this fear that they won't be able to meditate successfully because their mind is always racing. The TM technique is a simple, effortless, natural process that your mind easily follows. You don't have to *try* to do anything. There's no forcing, no concentrating, and no effort required.

Taking the time to learn and practice TM is one of the best gifts you can give your Warrior Goddess. There's nothing more powerful that you can do to improve your overall health and decrease your risk of disease. Practicing TM will also help you to specifically reduce your risk of breast cancer by decreasing stress, promoting hormones that reduce your risk, and helping you to make spontaneous choices that are better for your health. If you smoke or drink alcohol—two risk factors for breast cancer—TM can also help you break your addictions to these substances by reducing your desire for them.

OTHER FORMS OF MEDITATION

Learning TM is expensive, and unfortunately teachers are becoming more difficult to find. So, if you cannot arrange to learn TM, consider learning another form of meditation. Although other forms of meditation may not be as effective as TM, they certainly have their benefits. Be sure to research various techniques to find one that works for you. Certain types of concentration meditation may actually increase anxiety, so be careful in your choice of technique. Other good stress-reducing and health-promoting practices, such as yoga or the breathing technique *pranayama,* can provide you with excellent health benefits.

Part Seven

Putting It All Together

The Plan of Attack

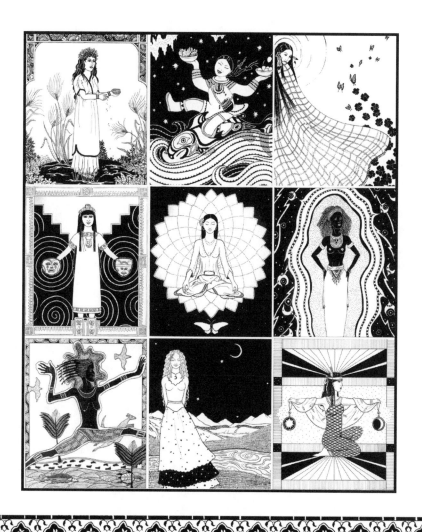

Chapter 28

Dr. Christine Horner's 30-Step Program

How to Protect Against and Fight Breast Cancer

*I*f nothing else, know this: You are far from powerless when it comes to your health and your risk of breast cancer. You have the ability to enormously lower your chances of getting this disease. And if you already have breast cancer, you can significantly improve your chances of surviving it, preventing a recurrence, and living a long and healthy life.

Okay, you're ready to begin the program! Don't let any of the information you read in the previous chapters overwhelm you. There's no need to make many radical changes all at once. Be gentle with yourself. While it's important that you eventually adopt all of the techniques and recommendations presented in this book to maximally protect your health, you don't have to implement them all at once. You don't have to start them all today or tomorrow or this week. Change your life gradually so that making these lifetime changes isn't stressful. Start with one change, one new "custom," at a time; then, when you're ready, add another. Soon, you'll be doing everything you can to enhance your inner healing intelligence and to keep your body strong and vibrantly healthy.

The only thing that has to be finished by next Tuesday is next Monday.

—JENNIFER YANE

This program was designed to give you a simple—yet inspiring—step-by-step approach to help you successfully make all the health-promoting changes discussed in this book. It's structured to be easy and stress-free. There's no *right* way to do the program, nor is there an advantage if you do the program in the order it's presented. So, if you want to mix up the order of the steps, that's perfectly fine. The first few steps aren't any more or less important or powerful than the last few steps. You may want to choose the steps that come most easily and naturally to you first, and, later, choose the more personally challenging ones—or vice versa.

It's important that you choose a comfortable pace. People are usually better at sticking with a program if it is time-sensitive. So, select a time schedule, and then follow it as closely as you can. For instance, you can opt to implement a new change every day for thirty days, or each week for thirty weeks, or every month for thirty months. Although the schedule is flexible, the end result is not. You'll eventually need to make most of these changes. Making only some of them will not give you enough protection..

> Don't let the fear of the time it will take to accomplish something
> stand in the way of your doing it. The time will pass anyway;
> we might just as well put that passing time to the best possible use.
>
> —EARL NIGHTINGALE

> Be not afraid of going slowly; be afraid only of standing still.
>
> —CHINESE PROVERB

Just for fun, let's imagine that you've transported yourself 100 years into the future. The culture and its customs and habits are radically different from the place you left behind. The world is far more advanced and enlightened now, and all of the ideas in this program are part of this culture's tradition. All women—all people—here experience perfect health. Now, you must fit yourself into this world. This is your guidebook. Follow it and share it so that we can make this future world a reality.

Learning these new customs will take you on a wondrous, magical adventure that will make you feel better than you've ever felt; it will slow down your aging and nurture and protect your health. These customs will take you to a land of Warrior Goddesses, where the Goddess in every woman shines! Let's begin the adventure. . . .

> Yesterday is a dream, tomorrow but a vision. But today well-lived
> makes every yesterday a dream of happiness, and every tomorrow
> a vision of hope. Look well, therefore, to this day.
>
> —SANSKRIT PROVERB

Friendship & Support

A great way to begin this program is to invite a group of supportive friends to join you on your new health adventure. Be creative, and make it fun. For instance, you could start your own Warrior Goddess group. Structure it any way you like. I recommend monthly meetings—or even weekly meetings, if time permits. At each meeting, the members of the group implement one new custom. You can share your experiences, encourage one another, and explore new and exciting ways to integrate each step of the program into your lives. Some ideas for meetings include preparing creative vegetarian dishes highlighting a new medicinal food or spice; taking yoga or exercise classes together; hiking in Nature or taking trips to a spa; forming a community-sponsored agriculture (CSA) group; creating a buyers' group to get discount prices on supplements and herbs; and so on. The possibilities are endless.

If you or other group members have teenage daughters, invite them to do the program with you, too. Remember, teenagers have immature breast tissue that is more susceptible to toxins in the environment. Research shows that what you do during the teenage years is so important that it has lasting lifetime effects. If your teenager regularly exercises, doesn't smoke, and has healthy eating habits, her risk of breast cancer will be 30 to 50 percent lower for the rest of her life, regardless of her diet or habits later in life! But you'll want to encourage your daughter to maintain these habits. If she does, her risk of breast cancer and most other chronic diseases will be even lower.

TODAY IS THE DAY

Today is the day that you've decided to begin a new relationship with yourself. It is a sacred moment. As Antoine de Saint-Exupery said, "A single event can awaken within us a stranger totally unknown to us. To live is to be slowly born." This day is an event that will begin to awaken within you something you may not have been aware of—the extraordinary power of your inner healing intelligence—your Warrior Goddess. It is the moment of conception for the birth of a new you, an even more extraordinary woman than you already are, a woman with deep understanding and reverence for her body, a woman who experiences and honors her body's profound intelligence, a woman who possesses remarkable wisdom and knowledge about how to harness the power of Nature to achieve balance and an excellent state of health. You are becoming a woman who is not a victim to fluctuating states of health but is, instead, a powerful master of balance.

According to an old English proverb, the first step is usually the hardest. But once you commit yourself to living a life that supports your health in every way, you'll find that a universe of support will flow your way.

> Begin to weave, and God will give you the thread.
>
> —GERMAN PROVERB

DR. CHRISTINE HORNER'S 30-STEP PROGRAM

As mentioned previously, the steps in this program do not have to be done in order. In fact, as you've probably already noticed, I don't even refer to them as "steps." Instead, I present them as new customs to implement into your daily life. Unlike carrying out a step and then moving on to the next step, you will be acquiring and maintaining a healthy habit each time you move forward in the program—you'll leave nothing behind. By the time you've completed the program, you will have acquired thirty new customs that will arm your Warrior Goddess with all the ammunition she needs to keep you safe.

CUSTOM #1

**Eat fresh, organically grown fruits and vegetables every day.
Include cruciferous vegetables at least three or four times a week.**

This is the day that you will discover and experience the amazing medicines of organically grown fresh fruits and vegetables. Remember that they contain extraordinary intelligence and a phenomenal, natural anticancer pharmacy. Let their healing flavors explode in your mouth. As you look at their vibrant colors, remind yourself that each color is actually a potent natural medicine. Feel the nourishment of these foods gently flooding your body. Give thanks for the bounty of divine healing that Nature provides. Give thanks for the farmers who have devoted themselves to growing this food, devoid of toxic chemicals, and with consciousness of and respect for the Earth and the mind/body.

Before you can prepare your first meal of organic vegetables and fruits (be sure to feature a cruciferous vegetable—see page 45 for a list), you must first find a good source for organic produce. A great place to find organic produce is at your local health food store or at a larger chain store catering to organic products, such as Wild Oats or Whole Foods (see the Resources section). If you don't have any of these stores nearby, find out if there's a local farmers' market or an individual farmer who sells seasonal organic fruits and vegetables. If there isn't such a market or farmer close to where you live, don't despair. There are many other creative ways to keep your kitchen filled with affordable organic produce.

For instance, you could start a community-sponsored agriculture (CSA) group (see the Resources section), which is simply a group of friends or neighbors who hire a farmer to grow organic foods for them on a plot of his or her land. Everyone shares in the cost of growing the food. What you pay for CSA organically grown produce is usually less than what you would pay for the same food in a grocery store. Another wonderful benefit of participating in a CSA is that your food is locally grown. That means it will be fresher and richer in nutrients than the food in grocery stores. Plants start to lose nutrients as soon as they are picked, so the fresher they are, the more nutrients they have. Often the organic food in stores has traveled long distances, and by the time you buy it and eat it, it is several weeks old and has lost many of its nutrients.

If you enjoy gardening, consider growing your own food organically. There are many books on organic gardening, so you can easily learn how to do it. Companies that specialize in organic lawn and garden care, such as Garden's Alive! or Arbico Organics (see the Resources section), are also great resources for tips and supplies for organic gardening. These companies have very knowledgeable people on staff who can help you get started and answer your questions.

The Internet makes it possible for you to get organic foods no matter where you live. Several companies offer an organic food–delivery service if you simply order from them on their Internet site (see the Resources section).

Remember that how you eat is just as important as what you eat. Review the *Ayurvedic* recommendations for enhancing digestion (see The Top 12 Aids to Digestion on page 41), and try to follow them as much as possible. By optimizing your digestion, you can substantially improve the value you get from your food.

The first step binds one to the second.

—FRENCH PROVERB

CUSTOM #1—POINTS TO REMEMBER

• Organically grown produce is grown without harmful chemical pesticides, herbicides, fertilizers, or genetic modifications. Studies show that it has a higher nutritional value and is much more supportive of your health and the environment than conventionally grown food.

• Organic fruits and vegetables are low in fat and calories and high in fiber, antioxidants, and vitamins.

• Organic produce contains a virtual anticancer pharmacy that includes hundreds of phytochemicals, including carotenoids, which are potent cancer and disease fighters.

• Cruciferous vegetables are particularly adept at reducing the risk of breast cancer as a result of three beneficial substances: indole-3 carbinol, sulforaphane, and D-glucaric acid.

■ Indole-3 carbinol fights breast cancer by forcing estrogen to break down into a protective, non-cancer-promoting type of estrogen. It also activates a tumor-suppression gene.

■ Sulforaphane stimulates enzymes in the liver to deactivate carcinogens.

■ D-glucaric acid supports a process in the liver that eliminates toxins and estrogen from your body.

• Women who eat the most cruciferous vegetables have a 40 percent lower risk of breast cancer.

• Vegetarians have a 50 percent lower incidence of most chronic disorders, including breast cancer.

Life is either a daring adventure, or it is nothing.

—HELEN KELLER

CUSTOM #2

Eat organic whole grains every day.

In the last century, it became popular to process grains to produce an ostensibly desirable white color for bread and rice. But this misguided practice also strips grains of many of their nutrients, especially B vitamins and fiber. That's why *whole* grains are so much better than processed grains for supporting your health and helping you to resist cancer.

Because whole grains are conspicuously absent from the traditional American diet, most of us are unfamiliar with the marvelous diversity of delectable grains. Based on our customs, you might think that the only way to eat whole grains is in cereal or bread. But whole grains can also be used to make delicious appetizers, side dishes, main courses, and even desserts. Look through a few cookbooks to find recipes that include whole grains. I recommend the excellent cookbook *Heaven's Banquet: Vegetarian Cooking for Lifelong Health the Ayurveda Way* by Miriam Kasin Hospodar. Not only does this book have wonderful recipes, but it also includes detailed information about each food: what it is, how to measure and cook it, its history, its nutritional and medicinal benefits, and how *Ayurveda* uses it as a medicine—all interlaced with beautiful quotes and entertaining stories.

Be exotic and try highly nutritious grains, such as amaranth and quinoa. Amaranth, an important food to the Aztec Indians of Mexico centuries ago, is a tiny grain that is high in protein and calcium. Quinoa, its South American cousin and former staple of the ancient Incan diet, is also very high in protein. In fact, quinoa is the only grain that is a complete protein, meaning that it contains all the essential amino acids. Other savory grains that you can find at most grocery stores are barley, brown rice, buckwheat (kasha), millet, oats, spelt, rye, and kamut (a type of high-protein, hypoallergenic wheat).

Remember that each plant contains its own blend of unique medicines. The larger the medicine chest that you give to your body, the greater its ability is to keep you healthy. Big medicine chests come from eating a wide diversity of foods. Don't let the thought of cooking with new and unfamiliar foods intimidate you. With the help of a good cookbook, you'll find that creating new dishes with these nourishing foods is easy and fun.

Most health food stores or grocery stores specializing in organic foods stock grains in bulk bins at discount prices. There's also a list of Internet sites in the Resources section that sell organic grains. If you have one of these stores in your area, go there to see what types of organic grains they carry. Purchase a small amount of several different types of grains, and give each one a try. If you find that you don't like the taste of a certain type of grain, try it in at least three different recipes before you pass judgment and cross it off your list. With the right spices or combination of other ingredients, you will more than likely find a way that you *do* enjoy it. Remember, the more diverse the foods that you eat are, the wider the spectrum of healing nutrients you make available to your body.

If you have formed a Warrior Goddess group, have each member choose a different grain, create a soup, salad, main course, side dish, or dessert with it, and bring it to the meeting. Again, be creative, and have fun. Find an unusual recipe in a cookbook or invent your own. Great recipes don't have to be complex or require a lot of time. For instance, some grains are extremely tasty simply boiled in water and then tossed with sautéed spices. If you find a recipe—or make one up—that turns out to be great, please share it on my website at www.drchristinehorner.com.

The responsibility for change . . . lies within us. We must begin
with ourselves, teaching ourselves not to close our minds
prematurely to the novel, the surprising, the seemingly radical.

—ALVIN TOEFFLER

CUSTOM #2—POINTS TO REMEMBER

• Whole grains are rich in antioxidants, vitamins, trace minerals, fiber, and lignans.

• Soluble fiber deactivates carcinogens in the colon.

• Insoluble fiber absorbs water, dilutes carcinogens, binds estrogen and eliminates it, regulates insulin and glucose, promotes weight loss, lowers blood fats (lipids), and adds bulk to the stool.

• Women who eat a high-fiber diet have a 54 percent lower risk of breast cancer.

CUSTOM #3

Avoid all health-destroying fats.
Consume health-promoting fats every day.

Remember that there are both poisonous and protective fats. To nurture your health, avoid "bad" fats and consume "good" fats. If you don't already read food labels, start now. If a food contains trans fats, hydrogenated fats, or partially hydrogenated fats, don't buy it and don't eat it. These are the most dangerous types of fat for your health. Check all the foods you already have at home. If you find anything that contains these disease-promoting fats, throw it out!

Use organic olive or macadamia nut oil for sautéing and for any other recipe that requires cooking oil. They are considered two of the best oils for these purposes, because they tolerate heat so well. Heating any oil—even olive oil—on high heat can destroy its antioxidants and create trans fats. So, when you cook with these oils, always use lower temperatures.

The most health-preserving and cancer-hindering type of fats you can eat are omega-3 fatty acids found in organic flaxseeds. These are so beneficial for your health that you should make it a point to consume at least 1 tablespoon of fresh, organic flax oil every day. Some people have no problem at all swallowing flax oil without mixing it with something—I'm not one of them, and you may not be either. Flax oil can be added to a smoothie or a protein shake. It also makes an excellent salad dressing. Keep in mind that you are on a fun adventure, so be imaginative and share your ingenuity with your friends.

If you have started a Warrior Goddess group, you can add to the fun by giving an award, such as a gift certificate for a massage or any other stress-reducing service, to the person who comes up with the tastiest recipe. There's only one rule you should remember about using flax oil: *Do not heat it.* Heat destroys many of its healing properties.

Conjugated linoleic acid (CLA) is another type of health-promoting fat that also thwarts breast cancer. It's not possible to consume enough CLA from food, so you must take it as a supplement. CLA comes in soft-gel capsules and is found in health food stores or stores that specialize in supplements for body-builders. Research shows that taking about 3,000 milligrams (mg) a day is enough to lower your risk of breast cancer. CLA is best taken in divided doses, usually 1,000 mg with each meal. (See the Resources section for sources for organic flax oil, organic olive oil, and CLAs.)

We cannot do everything at once, but we can do something at once.

—CALVIN COOLIDGE

CUSTOM #3—POINTS TO REMEMBER

- Fat is important for the proper functioning of your body.

- Some types of fat support health, while others destroy it.

- High-fat diets may increase your risk of breast cancer by as much as 50 percent.

- Saturated animal fats increase insulin resistance and, therefore, insulin levels in the blood. Women with high insulin levels have a 283 percent greater risk of breast cancer.

- Saturated animal fats concentrate toxic chemicals, including pesticides that are known to increase the risk of breast cancer.

- Insulin-like growth factor-1 (IGF-1), the most potent stimulator of breast cancer known, is found in high amounts in nonorganic whole-fat dairy products.

- Trans fats, partially hydrogenated fats, and hydrogenated fats are chemically altered fats that are very dangerous to your health because they promote inflammation and oxygen free radicals.

- Women who have the highest amounts of trans fats in their body have a 40 percent increased risk of breast cancer.

- The best ratio of omega-6 fatty acids to omega-3 fatty acids to consume is between 1:1 and 4:1. Americans typically eat an extremely unhealthy ratio of these fats—about 20:1.

- Women with the highest amounts of omega-6 fatty acids in their bodies have a 69 percent increased risk of breast cancer.

- Omega-3 fatty acids are the healthiest types of fat you can eat.

- The best plant source of omega-3 fatty acids is flaxseeds.

- Women with breast cancer who have high levels of omega-3 fatty acids in their bodies have a 50 percent lower incidence of metastasis.

- Omega-9 fatty acids, which are abundant in olive oil, have a neutral effect in the breast. But because they block bad fats, eating this type of fat lowers your risk of breast cancer.

- CLAs are a unique mixture of omega-6 fatty acids that lower the risk of breast cancer.

CUSTOM #4

Eat 2–3 tablespoons of flaxseeds every day.

Shoot for the moon. Even if you miss, you'll land among the stars.

—LES BROWN

Remember that when it comes to lowering your risk of breast cancer and improving your chances of surviving it, research shows that flaxseeds are one of the most powerful medicinal foods you can eat. These tiny seeds provide a fortress of protection of such magnitude that you will want to make sure you consume them in some form every day.

To eat fresh organically grown flaxseeds, grind a few tablespoons in a coffee grinder until they become the consistency of a fine powder. Then sprinkle the delicious nutty flax powder over fruit, add it to a vegetable dish, stir it into a smoothie, or if you make your own bread or muffins, simply mix some of it into the dough before baking. Just like soy, there are many ways to enjoy flaxseeds, so I recommend getting a cookbook that specializes in recipes using flax.

If you have formed a Warrior Goddess group, have each member bring a different dish that incorporates flaxseeds to this meeting. Depending on how innovative and industrious you want to be, your group could make up new recipes, vote on the best ones, write them down, and create your own cookbook. Please share your recipes with me on my website at www.drchristinehorner.com.

Eating ground flaxseeds every day can be difficult, especially if you travel. You can also get the powerful anticancer substances in flax, called lignans, by taking a supplement called Brevail. One capsule of Brevail contains the same amount of lignans as about 4 tablespoons of flaxseeds. Health food stores usually carry all these items. (Sources for flaxseeds and Brevail are listed in the Resources section.)

Sow a thought, and you reap an act; sow an act, and you reap a habit;
sow a habit, and you reap a character; sow a character, and you reap a destiny.

—CHARLES READE

CUSTOM #4—POINTS TO REMEMBER

- Flaxseeds are one of the most powerful foods known to protect against and fight breast cancer.

- The richest plant source of omega-3 fatty acids is the flaxseed.

- Flaxseeds are high in fiber.

- The seeds of the flax plant contain 100 times more lignans than any other known edible plant.

- Lignans are powerful anticancer substances that are able to arrest and deter the growth of breast cancer in at least a dozen different ways.

- You can also get the daily recommended amount of flax lignans by taking one capsule of a supplement called Brevail.

CUSTOM #5

Eat soy-based whole-food products several times a week.

A vision must be followed by the venture.
It is not enough to stare up the steps—we must step up the stairs.

—VANCE HAVNER

Research shows that whole soy foods are highly protective against breast cancer. In fact, women who eat the largest amounts of soy foods have the lowest risk of breast cancer. Begin by making a vegetarian dish that features a delicious, organically produced, soy-based whole-foods product such as natto, tofu, tempeh, fresh cooked soybeans, or miso, and make it at least three to four times a week. It's particularly important to buy soy foods that have been organically produced because most soybeans grown in the United States are genetically altered. Since the long-term consequences of eating genetically modified foods aren't known, you definitely want to avoid them as much as possible.

I recommend getting a good tofu or soy cookbook. You'll be amazed at all the creative, diverse, and surprisingly tasty dishes you can create using soy. For instance, you can craft fabulous salad dressings, dips, drinks, main meals, and desserts with tofu. Don't forget that roasted soy nuts make a delicious and healthy snack food. They are low in fat and are one of the best sources of the protective qualities of soy.

Remember to avoid genistein supplements isolated from soy, because studies show that genistein, without all the other substances in whole soy foods to interact with it, may not be protective and, in fact, may be harmful.

If you have formed a Warrior Goddess group, have each member bring something made with soy to this meeting. You might want each person to choose a different course or a different form of soy so you get a good sampling of the many ways to enjoy this wonderful food. (You'll find a list of companies that offer a large variety of soy foods in the Resources section.)

CUSTOM #5—POINTS TO REMEMBER

• Soy contains phytoestrogens, which act as weak estrogens that block stronger estrogens from attaching to estrogen receptors in the breast.

• The three major phytoestrogens in soy are genistein, daidzein, and glycitein.

• Turmeric enhances the estrogen-blocking abilities of soy.

• Don't take isolated genistein supplements because they may stimulate the growth of breast cells.

• Eat a wide variety of soy foods, but don't make your diet all about soy. Remember that food diversity is important.

• Women who eat the most whole soy foods have a 30 to 50 percent lower risk of breast cancer than women who don't.

CUSTOM #6

Eat exotic Asian foods such as maitake mushrooms often.

Asian women have a much lower incidence of breast cancer than American women do, and a large part of the reason is the foods they eat and don't eat. Asian cuisine is high in soy, but soy foods aren't the only types of Asian foods that ward off breast cancer. There are many others. (See Chapter 11 for a reminder.)

One special type of mushroom, the maitake mushroom, has been part of Japanese medicine for thousands of years and contains an armory of therapeutic weapons against breast cancer. Maitake mushrooms are considered a gour-

Trying to eat all the beneficial foods that defend against breast cancer every day isn't realistic. Taking supplements is sometimes an excellent alternative. If you decide to go this route on occasion, be sure to purchase only quality supplements from reputable companies. To make supplementation more convenient and affordable for women and to ensure excellent quality, I collaborated with the highly reputable company Enzymatic Therapy to create a supplement called Protective Breast Formula (PBF). PBF contains a combination of seven different supplements, each with powerful effects against breast cancer. This formulation includes indolplex 25% DIM (derived from indole-3-carbinol), calcium-D-glucarate, turmeric, green tea extract, maitake mushroom D-fraction, grape seed extract, and vitamin D_3. (See the Resources section or visit www.protective breast.com for more information.)

met food in America. They come fresh or dried and can be found in the gourmet section of some grocery stores and at Asian markets. They are also available as a supplement—either in capsules or in a liquid extract. You can order maitake mushrooms or supplements over the Internet (see the Resources section). The recommended daily dose is 3–5 grams, or 10–30 drops of the liquid extract, three times a day.

There are no shortcuts to any place worth going.

—BEVERLY SILLS

CUSTOM #6—POINTS TO REMEMBER

• Maitake mushrooms stop tumor growth, cause tumors to shrink, and prevent them from spreading to other areas of the body.

• Maitake mushrooms stimulate the immune system.

• Maitake mushrooms can kill 95 percent of prostate cancer cells in twenty-four hours.

• Of those women with stage-2 to stage-4 breast cancers who were given maitake mushrooms, 68.8 percent experienced a reduction in tumor size and an improvement in symptoms.

The road to success is dotted with
many tempting parking places.

—AUTHOR UNKNOWN

CUSTOM #7

Drink green tea every day.

Drinking eight to ten cups of green tea each day can significantly lower your risk of breast cancer, and if you already have breast cancer, it may extend your life. Eight to ten cups a day may seem like a lot of green tea, but it's easy to drink that much if you sip it throughout the day. However, if you try to drink this much and find that you simply can't do it, just drink as much as you comfortably can.

If you don't like the taste of traditional green tea, you may like one of the flavored varieties. I've found organic green teas in many tantalizing flavors such as strawberry rose, mint, mango, Mandarin orange, cinnamon apple, and jasmine. If drinking tea just isn't your cup of tea, you can get the benefits of green tea by taking supplements. Two 250-mg capsules a day is recommended. (See the Resources section for a list of companies that make organic green tea and green-tea supplements.) You can also get your suggested daily intake of green tea by taking Protective Breast Formula (see the Resources section).

If you've formed a Warrior Goddess group, have a tea party. Have everyone bring a different flavor of green tea and an appetizer that includes a medicinal food, such as maitake mushroom puffs, tofu dip, fresh broccoli and cauliflower, and flax muffins.

CUSTOM #7—POINTS TO REMEMBER

• Green tea is considered the number-one anticancer beverage.

• Green tea contains powerful anti-inflammatories and antioxidants.

• Women who drink the most green tea have a lower risk of breast cancer and live much longer if they develop breast cancer than women who don't drink it.

• Green tea stops tumors from growing back, inhibits the growth of breast cancer, and decreases the incidence of tumors metastasizing to the lung.

• Always buy organic green tea because some nonorganic brands have been found to contain the pesticide DDT.

CUSTOM #8

Consume turmeric every day.

Turmeric is so extraordinary at protecting against and fighting breast cancer, as well as several other types of cancer, that it's considered the number-one anticancer spice. Turmeric inhibits cancer in several ways, including blocking all the powerful cancer-promoting actions of the inflammatory COX-2 enzyme.

Turmeric is a traditional spice used in Indian cooking, but you can use it in any dish of any ethnic origin. It's responsible for the intense bright yellow-orange color in curry, so you can either cook with turmeric or with a curry that contains turmeric.

Cooking with turmeric or curry is easy. *Ayurveda* recommends adding turmeric near the end of cooking because its healing properties are most powerful if it's lightly cooked. About one-fourth teaspoon of dried powdered turmeric should be added for each serving.

Adding turmeric to soy foods produces an especially potent medicine. Remember that turmeric enhances the estrogen-blocking capabilities of the phytoestrogens in soy. Combining turmeric and green tea also creates a phenomenal anticancer alchemy. Turmeric makes green tea's anticancer ability eight times stronger, and green tea enhances turmeric's by three times. So, if you want to get the most potent medicinal effects from turmeric, add this remarkable spice to your soy dish and serve it with a cup of green tea!

Turmeric comes as a dried powder and can be found in the spice section of any grocery or health food store. Favor using organically grown turmeric to avoid pesticide residue. If you can't find organic turmeric in your store, you can order it on the Internet.

On the days you don't cook with turmeric, you can take it as a supplement. The recommended dose is two 500-mg capsules a day. (See the Resources section for a list of companies that make organic turmeric supplements.) You can also get the suggested daily dose of turmeric by taking Protective Breast Formula (see the Resources section).

If you've formed a Warrior Goddess group, have each member bring a dish made with turmeric or curry. Serve organic green tea as the beverage.

CUSTOM #8—POINTS TO REMEMBER

- Turmeric is considered the number-one anticancer spice.

- This beautiful spice is 300 times more powerful as an antioxidant than vitamin E.

- An extraordinary COX-2 inhibitor, turmeric also blocks the estrogenic effects of breast cancer-inducing pesticides.

- Turmeric and green tea enhance each other's anticancer effects.

- The estrogen-blocking capabilities of soy are increased when you add turmeric.

- Turmeric defends against breast cancer in a multitude of ways.

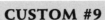

CUSTOM #9

Eat at least one clove of garlic several times a week.

A nickel will get you on the subway, but garlic will get you a seat.
—OLD NEW YORK PROVERB

Not only is garlic delicious, but it's also a powerful medicine against breast cancer. It is extremely high in antioxidants and selenium, boosts the immune system, lessens the formation of carcinogens in the breast, prevents toxins from binding to DNA, and stops breast tumors from growing and dividing. Research shows that eating just a few cloves of garlic a week can significantly lower your risk of breast cancer.

The healing powers of garlic are best if you eat it raw. Crush it, wait fifteen minutes for it to activate its enzymes, and then put it on your salad or vegetables. If you choose to cook garlic, make sure you don't overcook it because you will destroy most of its antioxidants. If you prefer not to eat garlic because you're concerned about the odor of garlic radiating from your body, you can take an aged, odorless garlic supplement instead—600–900 mg a day is recommended. (Check the Resources section for good brands.)

If you've formed a Warrior Goddess group, have each member bring a different garlic dish, for example, roasted elephant garlic with olive oil on fresh whole-grain bread, pickled garlic, or gazpacho soup with extra garlic.

CUSTOM #9—POINTS TO REMEMBER

- Women who eat as little as one clove of garlic a week have a statistically significant lower incidence of breast cancer.
- Garlic has more antioxidants than any other vegetable.
- This fragrant herb boosts the immune system.
- Garlic decreases the formation of carcinogens in breast tissue by 50 to 70 percent.
- You can take odorless garlic as a supplement to avoid the odor.

CUSTOM #10

Include wakame or mekabu seaweed in your diet.

Wakame and mekabu seaweeds are high in the mineral iodine, and research shows that they are at least as effective at killing breast cancer cells as many common chemotherapeutic drugs. These seaweeds can be found in the Asian section of grocery stores, health food stores, or Asian markets, or they can be ordered from the Internet (see the Resources section). Chop the seaweed up and add it to stir-fried vegetables, soups, grains, stews, or marinated dishes. Cooking instructions are usually on the package.

If you've formed a Warrior Goddess group, have each member bring a food to this session that features one of these seaweeds. You might also want to call a Japanese or Asian restaurant in your area to see if these items are included on their regular menu. If not, ask if they would be willing to order wakame or mekabu seaweed and prepare several dishes with it for your group.

Custom #10—Points to Remember

• Wakame and mekabu seaweeds are high in iodine, which suppresses breast cancer growth by causing cancer cells to die.

• These seaweeds can kill breast cancer cells and stop the growth of breast cancer more effectively than some common chemotherapeutic drugs.

• Iodine is taken up by breast cancer cells but not by normal cells. Scientists think that it may be possible to treat breast cancer in the future with radioactive iodine—a substance that is harmless to the body (except for the thyroid).

CUSTOM #11

Take a whole-foods vitamin every day.

Vitamins are micronutrients that are needed to assist many of the chemical reactions in your body. Your body can't make most vitamins, so you must get them from an outside source. It's difficult to get all the vitamins you need from your food because our soil is nutrient-depleted and because food loses many of its nutrients as it travels long distances to market, sits on the shelf, is processed, and is cooked. Research shows that supplemental amounts of certain vitamins—especially vitamin B_{12}, folate, vitamin D, and vitamin E—can lower your risk of breast cancer. Since we typically don't absorb synthetic vitamins very well, I recommend taking a vitamin supplement made from whole foods. (Check the Resources section for a list of companies that make them.)

Vitamin D is unique because, unlike other vitamins, you can make your own. Sunlight stimulates your body to produce vitamin D naturally, so you can simply take a walk in the sunshine for fifteen minutes a day to meet all your daily requirements for vitamin D. An early-morning or late-afternoon walk is ideal. If you live in a place with unusually inclement weather, especially during the cold winter months, you'll need to either eat foods fortified with vitamin D or take a supplement. If you have begun Custom #11 or if you are taking Protective Breast Formula, you are already getting all the vitamin D you need.

CUSTOM #11 — POINTS TO REMEMBER

• Vitamins assist your body's enzymes.

• Folic acid is crucial for making proteins and for constructing and repairing DNA.

• Alcohol, birth control pills, and nonsteroidal anti-inflammatory drugs (NSAIDs) cause folic acid levels to drop.

• Women who drink at least 15 grams a day of alcohol and have low folate levels have a very high risk of breast cancer.

• Vitamin B_{12} works with folate to make and repair DNA.

• Women with low B_{12} levels have high rates of breast cancer.

• Vitamin B_{12} applied directly to breast cancer cells stops them from growing.

• Vitamin D makes your breast cells more resistant to toxins, decreases the ability of breast cancer cells to grow and divide, stops tumor cells from growing, and boosts the immune system.

• You can make your own vitamin D through a chemical reaction in your skin that occurs when it is exposed to ultraviolet light.

• Just fifteen minutes a day of sunlight is all you need to make your daily requirement of vitamin D.

• Vitamin E is a powerful antioxidant.

• Vitamin E slows down tumor growth, promotes the death of tumor cells, and prevents new blood vessels from growing into tumors.

• You absorb vitamin E better from food than from supplemental vitamins—especially synthetic vitamins.

• Vitamin C and CoQ_{10} make the antitumor effects of vitamin E even stronger.

CUSTOM #12

Get adequate amounts of selenium every day.

Selenium is an essential part of one of your body's own powerful antioxidants, glutathione peroxidase. Remember that antioxidants eradicate excess oxygen free radicals—those tiny molecules of oxygen that ruthlessly attack your cells and

DNA, causing damage that can lead to cancer, as well as a host of other serious diseases. Selenium gives a tremendous boost to your body's healing intelligence, so much so that research shows as little as 200 micrograms (mcg) a day lowers your risk of breast cancer—and most other types of cancer—by 50 percent.

Plants are our major source of selenium, but because our soil is now selenium-deficient and nutrient-poor, most of us don't get enough selenium. However, one food that is always packed full of large amounts of selenium is the delicious Brazil nut. Just a few organically grown Brazil nuts every day will give you more than enough selenium to fulfill your daily requirements.

If you don't like the taste of Brazil nuts or if you're allergic to them, begin taking 200 mcg a day of a good selenium supplement. (See the Resources section for a list of companies.)

CUSTOM #12—POINTS TO REMEMBER

• Selenium is an essential part of your body's own potent antioxidant, glutathione peroxidase.

• Women with breast cancer have much lower levels of selenium than women who don't have cancer.

• Selenium also helps to fight cancer by preventing cancer cells from growing, causing cancer cells to die, stopping blood-vessel growth into tumors, and enhancing the immune system.

• Iodine makes selenium more effective.

• Taking 200 mcg a day of selenium can lower your risk of breast cancer and most other cancers by 35 to 50 percent. If you have cancer, selenium can decrease your odds of dying from it by 52 percent.

• Selenium is found in garlic, onions, leafy green vegetables, mushrooms, and whole grains.

• Don't take too much selenium; if you do, you can develop a condition called selenosis, which is characterized by hair loss, gastrointestinal upset, white blotchy nails, and nerve damage.

CUSTOM #13

If you are over age thirty-five, take supplemental coenzyme Q_{10} (CoQ_{10}) every day.

CoQ_{10} is a natural vitamin-like substance that is essential for the production of energy. It's also a powerful antioxidant. Researchers have found that supple-

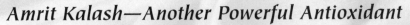

Amrit Kalash—Another Powerful Antioxidant

When certain plants are combined, they form synergies that exponentially increase their antioxidant power. The *Ayurvedic* herbal preparation *Amrit Kalash* is a combination of forty-four herbs, spices, and fruits. This beneficial blend is at least 25,000 times more powerful than vitamin E as an antioxidant. In fact, it has been found to be the strongest antioxidant ever tested. This preparation can help to prevent the formation of tumors, slow tumor growth, shrink tumors, and help to alleviate the side effects of chemotherapy without interfering with its effectiveness (see page 117). Moreover, *Amrit Kalash* may slow the aging process and even reverse it. (If you wish to obtain this magnificent antioxidant, see the Resources section.)

---

mental CoQ_{10} can stop the growth of breast cancer and dramatically shrink tumors.

CoQ_{10} comes in many different strengths and varieties. The recommended amount depends on the type of CoQ_{10} supplement. For instance, your body uses fermented CoQ_{10} far more efficiently than synthetic CoQ_{10}. So, you need far less of the fermented CoQ_{10} than the synthetic. About 22 mg of fermented CoQ_{10} is equivalent to 400 mg of the synthetic variety.

Custom #13—Points to Remember

- CoQ_{10} is essential for the production of energy.
- CoQ_{10} is a potent antioxidant.
- CoQ_{10} appears to be very effective at shrinking tumors, including metastatic tumors.
- CoQ_{10} prevents organ damage from chemotherapy.
- If you take medication for high blood pressure, cholesterol-lowering statin drugs, or red yeast rice, you should take supplemental CoQ_{10}.

CUSTOM #14

Take an herbal anti-inflammatory several times a week.

The so-called "secrets of success" will not work unless you do.

—Author unknown

Research shows that women who take an anti-inflammatory an average of three times a week, especially one that inhibits the COX-2 enzyme, have a 50 percent lower risk of breast cancer. Since pharmaceutical anti-inflammatories can have dangerous side effects, I recommend taking an herbal anti-inflammatory, particularly the potent herbal COX-2 inhibitor Zyflamend. This supplement is a combination of ten powerful herbs. Take two capsules of Zyflamend with a meal, several times a week. If you already have breast cancer, take two capsules every day.

CUSTOM #14—POINTS TO REMEMBER

• Chronic inflammation fuels the initiation and progression of many different types of cancer and chronic disorders.

• Chronic stress, some foods (such as refined carbohydrates and sugar), and certain fats (such as omega-6 fatty acids and trans fats) promote inflammation.

• The COX-2 enzyme, which is involved in the inflammatory process, also plays a key role in the initiation and progression of several types of cancer, including breast cancer.

• About 50 percent of all breast cancers overexpress the COX-2 enzyme.

• Research shows that taking a COX-2 anti-inflammatory at least three times a week can reduce the risk of breast cancer by 50 percent.

• Herbal COX-2 inhibitors may work just as well as the pharmaceutical ones, but without the potentially dangerous side effects.

• Cancer research is currently being conducted on the effectiveness of Zyflamend. So far, the results are impressive.

I'm a great believer in luck, and I find the harder I work,
the more I have of it.

—THOMAS JEFFERSON

CUSTOM #15

Do not eat red meat.

Eating red meat, especially large amounts of well-done or grilled meats, significantly increases the risk of many diseases. These diseases include such common deadly diseases as breast cancer, prostate cancer, colon cancer, gallbladder disease, heart disease, high blood pressure, and stroke.

If you don't want to completely give up red meat, at least cut way back on the amount of it that you eat. Don't eat it more than once or twice a month, and eat only meat from animals that have been organically raised. Organically raised animals aren't fed toxic chemicals or growth hormones, which increase your risk of breast cancer even further. Also, by selecting organic, you are choosing not to support the conventional meat industry—an industry that pumps animals full of toxins and keeps them in horrific, abusive conditions. Never eat well-done or grilled meat because these cooking methods create excessive amounts of heterocyclic amines, dangerous carcinogens.

If slaughterhouses had glass walls, everyone would be a vegetarian.

—PAUL MCCARTNEY

If you don't want to give up the flavor of red meat, the best choice you can make is to eat vegetable-based meat substitutes instead. For virtually any type of meat, there's a delicious alternative that closely mimics the flavor and texture of real meat without all the health hazards (see the Resources section for a list).

If you've formed a Warrior Goddess group, have each member bring a different type of meat substitute for everyone to sample.

CUSTOM #15—POINTS TO REMEMBER

- Women who eat the most red meat have an 88 to 330 percent higher risk of breast cancer.

- Cooking animal protein creates dangerous carcinogens, especially when grilling or cooking meats at high temperatures.

- The saturated fat in animals stores cancer-causing toxins from the environment and growth hormones and increases other cancer promoters: insulin, inflammation, and oxygen free radicals.

- There are many delicious meat substitutes that can satisfy your desire for the taste and texture of meat without damaging your health.

Famous Vegetarians

Here's a list of a few famous people and historical figures who made the wise choice not to eat meat: Pythagoras, Leonardo da Vinci, Benjamin Franklin, Albert Einstein, Mahatma Gandhi, George Bernard Shaw, Robert Louis Stevenson, Henry David Thoreau, and Paul and Linda McCartney.

CUSTOM #16

Avoid refined sugar. Use a natural sweetener such as Stevia instead.

One half of knowing what you want
is knowing what you must give up before you get it.

—SIDNEY HOWARD

Cancer loves sugar. Refined sugar is the preferred food of tumors. Refined carbohydrates and sugars also cause insulin levels to go up, and excess insulin is a powerful promoter of diseases such as breast cancer, diabetes, and obesity. If you have a sweet tooth, satiate your yearnings with fresh organic fruit. For example, organic dates will satisfy even the most intense sweet-tooth attack. Instead of sprinkling sugar on your cereal or adding it to your favorite beverage, use a natural product such as Stevia. The craving for sweets is actually an addiction that can be broken rather easily. Research shows that after only three weeks of avoiding sugar, you will lose your desire and taste for it. For instance, if you try a piece of candy after three weeks of consuming no sweets, it will taste so sweet to you that you won't like it.

If you've formed a Warrior Goddess group, have each member prepare a dessert or beverage sweetened with Stevia. Cooking with Stevia can be tricky, so I recommend getting a Stevia cookbook (see the Recommended Reading section). Support one another in breaking the sugar habit. Remember, all it usually takes is three weeks to lose your desire for sugar.

Bad habits are easier to abandon today than tomorrow.

—YIDDISH PROVERB

CUSTOM #16—POINTS TO REMEMBER

• Cancer loves sugar. The more you eat of this poison, the faster cancer will grow.

• Refined carbohydrates and sugars cause your pancreas to release high amounts of insulin.

• High insulin levels increase your risk of breast cancer by as much as 283 percent.

• Insulin causes cancer cells to divide and grow faster.

• Insulin lowers the number of protein binders in your blood and, thus, increases the amount of estrogen that can attach to your breast cells.

- After you eat sugar, your immune system becomes 50 to 94 percent less effective *for five hours.*
- Refined carbohydrates and sugars promote obesity.
- Stevia is a natural sweetener and a great sugar substitute with many health benefits.
- Artificial sweeteners may be damaging to your health, so avoid them.

CUSTOM #17

Keep your body-fat percentage low.

You cannot plough a field by turning it over in your mind.

—AUTHOR UNKNOWN

Keeping your body fat in check significantly lowers your risk of postmenopausal breast cancer. It also dramatically reduces your chances of developing diabetes, heart disease, and many other serious diseases. The Center for Disease Control (CDC) estimates that obesity-related health problems cause 300,000 deaths every year. If you have followed the program sequentially, you are already practicing many of the customs that will help you to lose and maintain a healthy weight—for example, eating fresh organic fruits, vegetables, and whole grains; avoiding red meat, processed foods, and sugar; taking flax oil or eating flaxseeds; and exercising every day.

If you find that you have frequent desires to snack, try this: Eat six small meals instead of three large meals, and plan what you're going to eat on a particular day the night before. Every three hours or so, eat a small portion of protein with a serving of vegetables. Include a serving of fresh fruit and whole grains in two of your meals. Eating planned, small, frequent meals will keep you from getting hungry, overeating, and having the compulsion to eat the wrong things.

If three meals a day works well for you, remember to eat your main meal at noon because that's when your digestion is strongest. In the evening when your digestion is much weaker, eat lightly. Make sure most of the foods you choose to eat are in alignment with the recommendations in this book, because what you eat and don't eat have a tremendous influence on your risk of breast cancer.

If you have a serious weight problem, joining a weight-loss program such as Weight Watchers can be very helpful. However, consult your doctor before starting a weight-loss program.

If you've formed a Warrior Goddess group, plan out how you are going to support each member to achieve and maintain a healthy weight. Perhaps you could go to a class together, help one another plan meals, exercise together, or create a buddy system for support.

No diet will remove all the fat from your body because the brain is entirely fat. Without a brain, you might look good, but all you could do is run for public office.

—George Bernard Shaw

I never worry about diets. The only "carrots" that interest me are the number you get in a diamond.

—Mae West

Custom #17—Points to Remember

- In the United States, 300,000 people die every year from obesity-related health problems.
- Obesity is thought to be responsible for 20 to 30 percent of all postmenopausal breast cancers.
- Fat cells manufacture estrogen, especially after menopause.
- Almost two-thirds of Americans are overweight or obese.
- Estimating your body-fat percentage is the best way to determine if you are overweight or obese.
- Toxins in the environment may contribute to obesity by disrupting our normal weight-control mechanisms; that's another reason to eat organic foods.

CUSTOM #18

Rarely, if ever, drink alcohol.

The best way out of a problem is through it.

—Author unknown

First you take a drink, then the drink takes a drink, then the drink takes you.

—F. Scott Fitzgerald

Even one drink of alcohol a day increases your risk of breast cancer, so it's best to avoid this dangerous beverage completely. If you enjoy the taste of wine, there are several companies that make delicious and satisfying nonalcoholic wines. If you have a serious drinking habit, now is the time to get help. You have taken the initiative to honor your body and mind by implementing many of the other customs, and this one is of utmost importance. Depending on the severity of your habit or addiction, you may need to enter an in-residence treatment program or participate in an excellent program such as Alcoholics Anonymous (AA). Alcohol can be very destructive to your health and your relationships, so make every effort to get it out of your life and keep it out. If it plays a big role in your life, now is the time to change that. Most people find that it's difficult or embarrassing to admit that they may have a drinking problem. But keep in mind that you're not alone. There are many wonderful programs and compassionate understanding people just waiting to help you.

If you've formed a Warrior Goddess group, have each member bring a nonalcoholic healthy beverage to this meeting. If you would like to try nonalcoholic wines, have each person bring a different brand and flavor to see if there is one you especially like. Remember that the potent antioxidant and cancer fighter resveratrol, which is responsible for many of the health benefits of red wine, is also found in grapes. So, try fresh grape juice made with a juicer or a blender such as Vita-Mix. (There's also a list of organic grape juices in the Resources section.) If you or any member of your group has a drinking problem, support one another by getting help.

You must do the thing you think you cannot do.

—Eleanor Roosevelt

Custom #18—Points to Remember

- Even one drink of alcohol a day increases the risk of breast cancer.
- The health detriments of alcohol far outweigh any health benefits.
- Alcohol increases estrogen and prolactin, both of which increase cell division in the breast.
- Grapes contain a substance called resveratrol, an antioxidant and COX-2 anti-inflammatory that research shows inhibits the formation and growth of breast cancer.
- Grape seeds also contain powerful antioxidants and can kill breast cancer cells and decrease the amount of estrogen your body produces.

• Overcoming a drinking problem can be difficult, so don't hesitate to seek help from one of the many excellent programs that are available.

CUSTOM #19

Never smoke tobacco products.

Smoking is one of the leading causes of statistics.

—Author unknown

Cigarettes are killers traveling in packs.

—Author unknown

Because of all the health problems caused by smoking tobacco products, including an increased risk of breast cancer, smoking is a bad habit that you never want to start. If you currently smoke, begin cutting back and choose a date when you will quit. Stopping this destructive habit is one of the most important things you can do for your health. As a fellow physician and former smoker said to me, "Smoking is a decision. You can decide not to smoke."

For some people, overcoming this addiction isn't that tough; but for others, it is extraordinarily difficult. Keep in mind that although breaking this habit may be very challenging, it's not impossible. You *can* do it. Most people need some support to be successful. Fortunately, there are many programs available to assist you. For example, research shows that the regular practice of Transcendental Meditation (TM) is one of the most successful approaches for helping you overcome any addiction. Make a plan, set goals and dates, find a program, enroll others to support you, and go for it.

If you've formed a Warrior Goddess group and any of your members smoke, everyone should offer their support to those members to help them stop. Be sure to let those who smoke tell you exactly what you can do to support them. Don't offer unrequested coaching or place unwanted demands on them. Allow them to direct and make choices for their own lives.

Men are made stronger on realization that the helping hand
they need is at the end of their own arm.

—Sidney Phillips

Forget past mistakes. Forget failures. Forget everything
except what you're going to do now and do it.

—WILL DURANT

CUSTOM #19—POINTS TO REMEMBER

• Smoking during adolescence can increase the risk of breast cancer by 50 percent.

• Women who either smoke or inhale passive smoke may have as much as a 60 percent increased risk of breast cancer.

• For some people, breaking the cigarette habit is extremely difficult. If you are one of these people, seek help and support yourself in every way possible so that you can be successful.

CUSTOM #20

Don't take birth control pills or hormone replacement therapy (HRT),
except in rare circumstances determined by your doctor
and only for a brief time.

If you have been taking birth control pills or HRT for several years, schedule an appointment with your doctor to come up with a plan to get you off these medications. If your gynecologist or family physician won't work with you to get off these medications, find a physician who will. There are many doctors who specialize in natural or integrative medicine, and you may be able to find one in your area.

Both birth control pills and HRT have been shown to significantly increase your risk of breast cancer, so you'll want to use alternative methods if you can. Sometimes, these medications are necessary for a short time, and when taken for brief periods, they will not have dire consequences to your health. If you find that

---

Be aware that certain heart medications and antidepressants can significantly increase the risk of breast cancer. If you are taking medication for depression or heart problems, find out what risks are associated with its use. If necessary, speak with your doctor about alternatives. Remember, both heart problems and depression have the potential to be extremely serious, so *never* discontinue medication without your doctor's approval and supervision.

you must take these medications, make sure that you're doing all the other steps in this program to minimize your risk. Remember that breast cancer isn't caused by one thing. It's the result of the balance of *everything* you do in your life. If you are doing enough to protect yourself, then the likelihood of one of these medications being able to tip the scale and cause breast cancer will be much lower.

In Chapter 20, I mentioned several very good books that provide excellent guidance on how to use natural approaches to restore balance to your body during menopause. These approaches, along with the use of a few herbs, may completely eliminate or significantly improve any uncomfortable symptoms you have during this natural transition of life. (These books are also listed in the Recommended Reading section.) You might find that the new customs that you're already practicing have created so much balance in your mind/body that your menopausal symptoms have gone away or have gotten much better.

If you are still of reproductive age, you don't have to rely on birth control pills to prevent pregnancy. There are many effective alternatives to choose from. If you are not monogamous, condoms are your best choice because they provide protection from sexually transmitted diseases (STDs), including HIV (the virus that causes AIDS). If you are in a monogamous relationship, try different methods of birth control until you find the one that works best for you and your partner.

Anytime you make a change, it may seem uncomfortable at first just because it's new and different. But give it a chance. Usually, you can adjust in a short time, and it will no longer seem awkward. If you don't want any more children, seriously consider permanent sterilization. Surgical sterilization means either a vasectomy for a man or a tubal ligation for a woman. Surgical sterilization is usually easier for men, because the operation is done under local anesthesia, the recovery is short, and the complication rate is low.

If you've formed a Warrior Goddess group—and only if you feel comfortable doing so—share with one another what works for you, including your experience with different birth control methods or the names of gynecologists who have experience with natural approaches to menopause.

The greatest wealth is health.

—VIRGIL

CUSTOM #20—POINTS TO REMEMBER

• Long-term use of birth control pills has been shown to increase the risk of breast cancer.

• Women who take the pill after age forty have a 50 percent higher risk of breast cancer.

• Women with a first-degree relative who has breast cancer and who take birth control pills long term have a significantly higher risk of breast cancer.

• Menopause is not a disease. It is a natural transition of life that's best approached naturally, if possible.

• Menopausal symptoms arise from imbalances that, when corrected, usually improve or completely resolve.

• HRT increases the risk of heart disease, strokes, blood clots, gallbladder disease, invasive breast cancer, endometrial cancer, and ovarian cancer.

• HRT may increase the risk of breast cancer by as much as 66 to 100 percent and raise the risk of dying from breast cancer by as much as 22 percent.

• Taking a combination of estrogen and progestin contributes more to your risk of breast cancer than taking estrogen alone.

Never, never, never give up.

—WINSTON CHURCHILL

CUSTOM #21

Use only nontoxic cleaning products in your home and office.

We cannot direct the wind but we can adjust the sails.

—AUTHOR UNKNOWN

Cleaning supplies are almost always filled with health-damaging toxins that you won't find listed on their labels. The federal government doesn't require that the ingredients in cleaning products be listed on the package. If a cleaning product isn't made by one of the companies that specifically make nontoxic cleaning products, you can bet it's got toxins in it. Throw it away. Buy only nontoxic cleaning products. (See the Resources section for a list of companies that make these products.) Most health food stores and some grocery stores carry nontoxic cleaning products. If your local store doesn't carry them, ask the manager to order them. These products are also available online and through certain catalogs, such as Harmony catalog sponsored by Gaiam.

If you've formed a Warrior Goddess group, have each member try a different nontoxic cleaning product, bring it to the meeting, and report what they liked or didn't like about it. There are many different companies that make non-toxic cleaning products, so if, for example, you don't like one company's glass cleaner, try another's. I have found good nontoxic products that work just as well as their toxic counterparts for *all* my cleaning needs. I'm sure you can, too.

CUSTOM #21—POINTS TO REMEMBER

• Manufacturers are not required to list the harmful chemicals contained in their cleaning products on the product's label.

• Most cleaning products contain toxic chemicals.

• There is an effective nontoxic cleaning product to replace every toxic one you currently use.

> *Most of us can read the writing on the wall;*
> *we just assume it's addressed to someone else.*
>
> —IVERN BALL

CUSTOM #22

Keep your home as toxin-free as possible.

In order to change, we must be sick and tired of being sick and tired.

—AUTHOR UNKNOWN

Cleaning products aren't the only sources of toxins in your home. They're everywhere! They are in your water, clothing, furnishings, construction materials, dry cleaning, personal-care products, lawn and garden products, insect repellant, flea collars, paints, wallpaper, carpet, tile, particleboard, and so on. Assume that everything is toxic. See Table 22.1 on page 168 for a reminder of the various sources of toxins in your home and their nontoxic alternatives.

Go through your house and find all the sources of possible toxins that you can easily do something about. For example, discard any pesticides or toxic lawn and garden products you have in your home, and research nontoxic ways to handle all your outdoor needs. Buy only chlorine-free paper products that are also labeled "tree-free," if possible. Use a water purifier, or buy purified drinking water (hard plastic bottles are safer than those that can be crushed easily). Purchase bed linens that are made of organic cotton when your old sheets are ready to be replaced. Likewise for your mattress. Whenever you do any home improvements, always choose nontoxic materials or use nontoxic sealers to prevent toxins from outgassing. (See the Resources section for companies that manufacture many of these products.)

If you live in an older home, the amount of toxins still outgassing from construction materials will be extremely low. However, if you live in a new home, it's a different story. If your house is fewer than two or three years old, the level of toxins in your home may be very high. Since heat causes the release of more toxins, keep your house on the cool side to keep the level of outgassing toxins lower. Keep your windows open as often as possible. It's also a good idea to buy a good air filter. Consider using a nontoxic sealer to trap the toxins. Certain houseplants, such as Boston ferns, English ivy, rubber plants, peace lilies, and bamboo, can absorb toxins from the air, so keep a few plants in each room.

Constantly be on the prowl to seek and avoid toxins. Develop an acute awareness of where toxins hide. Be aware of all the wonderful nontoxic alternatives, but don't feel that you must replace everything at once. For most, that's not practical or affordable. Don't stress over it. Move at a comfortable pace to gradually make your home as toxin-free as possible.

If you've formed a Warrior Goddess group, have each member investigate a nontoxic alternative for a common toxic item in the home and report what she discovers. If there's an organic lawn and garden service in your community, invite a representative to speak to your group.

Choices are the hinges of destiny.

—EDWIN MARKHAM

CUSTOM #22—POINTS TO REMEMBER

- Assume that everything is toxic unless specifically identified as nontoxic.

- Develop the habit of questioning the safety of a product and finding out if there's a nontoxic alternative.

- There are nontoxic alternatives to just about everything.

- You can prevent toxins from outgassing from particleboard, furniture, cabinets, and other construction materials in your home by using a nontoxic sealer.

- Organic lawn and garden companies have nontoxic solutions for all your needs, including pest problems.

• Don't stress over replacing everything in your home immediately. Make gradual changes.

• If you live in a new home, use an air filter, keep your house cool, and keep the windows open as often as possible.

CUSTOM #23

Purify your body several times a year.

If I'd known I was going to live so long, I'd have taken better care of myself.

—Leon Eldred

No matter how pure your diet and lifestyle are, you're constantly being bombarded by unavoidable environmental toxins. Some of these toxins, such as organochlorine pesticides, significantly increase your risk of breast cancer. So, it's important to take a week or two, once or twice a year, to purify your body and get some of these toxins out. Research shows that the *Ayurvedic* purification procedures known as *panchakarma* are extremely effective at eliminating toxins. In fact, just one five-day series can cut your load of toxins in half.

There are many clinics throughout the world that specialize in *panchakarma* treatments. In the United States, there are excellent clinics in Vedic City, Iowa, and Lancaster, Massachusetts. I've also located many other clinics in the United States that offer *panchakarma,* from Kauai, Hawaii, to Albuquerque, New Mexico, to Coral Springs, Florida. If you'd prefer to go to Europe, where the cost is usually much less, there are several clinics in countries such as Switzerland and Germany, or you could go to India.

If getting away to a clinic for a week isn't possible, you can detoxify at home. However, there's been no research on home-detoxification programs, so it's impossible to say exactly what percentage of toxins you can get rid of this way. But, you'll almost certainly be able to reduce some of your toxin load. There are many programs for detoxifying at home. One simple way is to follow the home-prep program for *panchakarma* (see Chapter 23), stay on a pure-foods diet for several weeks, and take herbs that help to purify your colon, liver, and kidneys. (Check the Resources section for websites that help with home detoxification.)

If you've formed a Warrior Goddess group, do something outlandish—go to a detox clinic together. Think outside the box; anything is possible. You could create a modified clinic at someone's home. For instance, invite massage therapists to come and give you sesame-oil massages or give them to one another. If someone has a sauna or has a membership at a gym that has one, you could all go there one day. Each member could volunteer to prepare vegetable juices or soups for everyone for one day of the week. Schedule colonics together—no kidding. Work together to create a detox program that everyone can do.

Limits exist only in your mind.

—AUTHOR UNKNOWN

CUSTOM #23—POINTS TO REMEMBER

• Toxins can be eliminated from your body using purification techniques.

• Research shows that just one five-day *panchakarma* treatment can cut your toxin load in half.

• *Panchakarma* treatments also create profound balance, relieve depression, and improve many chronic conditions.

• If you can't go to a clinic, do a home-purification program.

• Although there's no research documenting the amount of toxins you may get rid of on a home-detoxification program, you *will* be able to get rid of some.

CUSTOM #24

Go to bed by 10:00 P.M., and get up before 6:00 A.M.

A good laugh and a long sleep are the best cures in the doctor's book.

—IRISH PROVERB

When you go to bed by 10:00 P.M. and get up before 6:00 A.M., you are following the natural rhythms of Nature and your body produces the highest surge of the astoundingly protective hormone, melatonin. Most people notice that when they begin to consistently sleep during these hours, they suddenly feel much better, have more energy, think more clearly, and are far more productive—wonderful side benefits to a habit that profoundly lowers your risk of breast cancer. Remember also that melatonin shuns light and loves the darkest of the dark. So, be sure to shut off all the lights and close the blinds in your bedroom.

If you have a habit of going to bed much later than 10:00 P.M., you may find that it's virtually impossible for you to fall asleep before 10:00 P.M. Experts recommend that, each week, you go to bed thirty minutes earlier than you did the week before until you have adjusted to a 10:00 P.M. bedtime.

If you find you need some help getting to sleep while you are transitioning to an earlier bedtime, you might want to try supplemental melatonin. Research shows that melatonin supplements not only help you to sleep, but they may also provide additional protection against breast cancer. However, the safety of taking melatonin on a long-term basis hasn't been studied. Until there is research showing that long-term use of melatonin supplements is safe, limit your use of it to short periods. Be aware that if you use melatonin as a sleep aid every night for several weeks and then abruptly stop taking it, you may have difficulty falling asleep.

Studies show that supplemental melatonin usually produces a more restful sleep than pharmaceutical sleep aids, and it doesn't cause a "hangover." In my opinion, melatonin is safer than most pharmaceutical sleeping pills. So, if you occasionally have trouble sleeping and would like to take something to help, melatonin is an excellent option. However, if you frequently have trouble sleeping or know that you have a sleep disorder, see your physician.

If you've formed a Warrior Goddess group, discuss how each of you can complete your daily tasks and still get to bed by 10:00 P.M. Share your experiences with each other, especially concerning any emotional, physical, or spiritual changes you experience once you start this simple, yet powerful habit.

Some make it happen, some watch it happen,
and some say, "What happened?"

—AUTHOR UNKNOWN

CUSTOM #24—POINTS TO REMEMBER

• When you go to bed by 10:00 P.M. and get up before 6:00 A.M., you are following the natural rhythms of Nature. Hormonal fluctuations will be optimal, and the hormone melatonin will rise to its highest level.

• Melatonin is a powerful antioxidant and specifically arrests and deters breast cancer in many ways.

• Women who work the night shift produce far less melatonin and have a 50 percent higher risk of breast cancer.

• Melatonin supplements enhance the effectiveness of chemotherapy, protect against its damaging side effects, and improve your chances of survival from breast cancer.

- Melatonin is light sensitive. It needs complete darkness to rise to its highest level.

- Blind women have a 50 percent lower risk of breast cancer.

- Getting the proper amount of sleep at the right times is one of the most important things you can do to preserve and protect your health.

- Sleeping too many hours may actually increase your risk of illness.

- Alcohol and electromagnetic fields (EMFs) cause melatonin levels to drop.

CUSTOM #25

Minimize your exposure to electromagnetic fields (EMFs).

The impossible can always be broken down into possibilities.

—AUTHOR UNKNOWN

Electromagnetic fields (EMFs) emitted from common household appliances and wires have been shown to increase the risk of breast cancer. Go through your house and identify everything that might emit EMFs. Check your bedroom for electrical devices, such as clock radios, and move them at least several feet away from your head or consider replacing them with nonelectrical devices. For instance, change your clock radio to a battery-operated clock. The good news is that most of the EMF exposure you get from these devices becomes negligible when they are moved just a few feet away.

Microwave ovens produce significant EMFs. If you choose to use a microwave oven, avoid all the EMFs it emits simply by standing a few feet away or by going into another room while it's in use. (Incidentally, microwave cooking destroys most of the antioxidants in foods. Moreover, *Ayurvedic* physicians (*vaidyas*) say that microwave cooking changes the quality of the food so much that it creates imbalances in the body.)

Hair dryers produce more EMFs than any other appliance. If air-drying your hair isn't an option, purchase a low-EMF hair dryer (see the Resources section).

If you've formed a Warrior Goddess group, make a game of identifying sources of EMFs in each member's home. Then, design a plan for keeping EMF exposure low in each of your homes.

CUSTOM #25—POINTS TO REMEMBER

- Research shows a definite link between EMF exposure and breast cancer.

- All electrical appliances and wires produce EMF.

- Hair dryers produce more EMFs than any other household appliance.

- EMF emissions drop very rapidly a short distance from an appliance. Just standing a few feet away from most electrical devices and appliances is all you need to do to avoid the EMFs they produce.

- Just 50 Hz of EMFs causes breast cancer tumors to start growing and accelerates their growth.

- You can purchase EMF shields for your cell phone and computer.

CUSTOM #26

Embrace thirty minutes of aerobic activity every day.

*Those who think they have not time for bodily exercise
will sooner or later have to find time for illness.*

—EDWARD STANLEY

*Movement is medicine for creating change
in a person's physical, emotional, and mental states.*

—CAROL WELCH

This is the moment you've been waiting for. Now is the time you're going to begin an invigorating aerobic activity that raises your heart rate *every day*. First, check with your doctor before starting any exercise program. You must take your current state of health and aerobic condition into consideration when selecting the type of activity that best suits you. Usually, walking is an excellent choice for almost any beginner. If you haven't exercised in years, start walking at a comfortable pace, then gradually pick up the pace and increase your distance.

There's an endless list of activities that can improve and maintain your aerobic condition. Choose those that you enjoy because you are much more likely to continue doing something you like. Remember that exercising regularly is one of the most important things you can do to support your health. Not only does it lower your risk of breast cancer by 30 to 50 percent, but it also lowers your risk of many other diseases, including heart disease, colon cancer, diabetes, and obesity.

Review Chapter 25 for more suggestions about choosing an activity that elevates your heart rate. Remember to choose activities that bring you joy.

If you've formed a Warrior Goddess group, have one of the meetings at a fitness center and participate in an exercise class. Some members may buddy-up and take the class on a regular basis.

> Don't say you don't have enough time. You have exactly the
> same number of hours per day that were given to Helen Keller,
> Pasteur, Michelangelo, Mother Teresa, Leonardo da Vinci,
> Thomas Jefferson, and Albert Einstein.
>
> —LIFE'S LITTLE INSTRUCTION BOOK,
> COMPILED BY H. JACKSON BROWN, JR.

> I have to exercise in the morning
> before my brain figures out what I am doing.
>
> —MARSHA DOBLE

CUSTOM #26—POINTS TO REMEMBER

• Regular aerobic exercise produces a cascade of health-promoting chemicals and hormones that significantly decrease your risk of many diseases including breast cancer.

• Just thirty minutes of aerobic activity three to five times a week can lower your risk of breast cancer by 30 to 50 percent.

• Teenagers who exercise regularly can lower their risk of breast cancer for the rest of their lives.

• Exercise can alleviate depression as effectively as many common antidepressant medications.

• The best time of day to exercise is in the morning.

• Regular invigorating movements also reduce your risk of heart disease; type 2 diabetes; cancers of the lung, ovary, uterus, and pancreas; lung diseases, such as asthma and emphysema; arthritis; glaucoma; and neurodegenerative diseases, such as Alzheimer's disease and dementia.

> Stopping at third base adds no more runs than striking out.
>
> —AUTHOR UNKNOWN

CUSTOM #27

Practice a stress-reducing meditation every day.

*Too many people miss the silver lining
because they're expecting gold.*

—MAURICE SETTER

Practicing a research-proven stress-reducing meditation every day is so balancing to your mind/body that it can lower your risk of all diseases by as much as 50 percent. The most effective form of meditation for relieving stress and promoting health is Transcendental Meditation (TM). To find a teacher near you, call 1-800-LEARN-TM. Learning TM is relatively expensive, but its many health benefits make it worth the cost. If the cost is too much for your budget or there isn't a TM teacher in your area, begin another stress-reducing technique. Research shows that other techniques of meditation and relaxation may not be as effective as TM, but they *are* beneficial. Avoid techniques that require mental concentration because research shows they may actually increase stress.

You may find that listening to guided meditations or relaxing music on an audiotape or CD provides the stress reduction you need. If you're looking for more, yoga is a wonderful ancient practice you may want to consider. Research shows that it keeps the body supple, promotes balance, and reduces stress. There are many different types of yoga. Regardless of your physical condition, almost everyone can practice some form of yoga. Because of its wonderful health benefits, yoga has become very popular and is taught in most U.S. cities. You may want to purchase an instructional yoga videotape and practice it at home.

If you've formed a Warrior Goddess group, practice a relaxation technique at one of the meetings. Perhaps your group could sign up for yoga classes together, or you could create your own class with a few interested members.

CUSTOM #27—POINTS TO REMEMBER

• Stress plays a role in more than 90 percent of all illnesses, physical and mental.

• Women who have suffered a major stressful trauma have a twelve times greater risk of developing breast cancer within five years.

• Practicing a stress-reducing meditation every day can have profound beneficial effects on your mind, body, and spirit, and it can lower your risk of breast cancer.

• Research shows that TM is the most effective form of meditation in relieving stress and anxiety and in promoting health.

• People who practice this form of meditation have a 50 percent lower incidence of all diseases.

• Other stress-relieving techniques can have good health benefits, too; for example, *yoga* has been found to relieve stress and improve a variety of health conditions.

• Avoid meditation techniques that require mental concentration because they may actually increase anxiety.

CUSTOM #28

Practice stress-reducing breathing techniques every day.

The time to relax is when you don't have time for it.

—ATTRIBUTED TO BOTH JIM GOODWIN AND SYDNEY J. HARRIS

Stress has been found to contribute to about 90 percent of all illnesses, including breast cancer. So, practicing a daily stress-reducing technique, such as the simple breathing exercise called *pranayama,* can profoundly influence and support your health.

To perform *pranayama,* sit quietly where you won't be disturbed and begin breathing through alternating nostrils, as described under *Pranayama*—Using Your Breath on page 210. Notice how relaxed you feel afterward. The wonderful thing about *pranayama* is that it requires no equipment, special location, or expense. So, anyone can engage in this health-promoting technique anytime, anywhere. To achieve the greatest benefits from *pranayama,* practice it at least twice a day for five to ten minutes each time.

There are also many other techniques of *pranayama* that you could learn. The method I have described is one of the simpler, more basic ones. But if you're interested in learning other forms of *pranayama,* find out if there are any nearby classes available or research the other techniques (see the Resources section).

If you've formed a Warrior Goddess group, take a class together or have each member research a technique of *pranayama* and teach it to the other members. Practice each technique for five to ten minutes.

How beautiful it is to do nothing, and then rest afterward.

—SPANISH PROVERB

CUSTOM #28—POINTS TO REMEMBER

• *Pranayama* is a simple ancient practice of regulating the breath. It has profound health benefits.

• Research shows that the regular practice of *pranayama* increases the depth of your breath and your breath-holding capacity. It also improves stress-hormone balance, blood pressure, and heart rate, and it lowers cholesterol.

• Practicing *pranayama* is simple. It can be done anywhere, and it costs nothing.

CUSTOM #29

Take an herbal adaptogen every day
to lower your body's response to stress.

Herbal adaptogens have been found to lower your body's response to stress and protect against its damaging effects in a multitude of ways. Some of the best adaptogen herbs are ginseng and the *Ayurvedic* herbs *ashwagandha* and holy basil. These supplements are available from most health food stores, some grocery stores, and on the Internet. (Check the Resources section for listings.) The recommended daily dosage for *ashwagandha* is 1–2 tablespoons of root powder or 1–2 grams of root, or simply follow the direction on the supplement label. The recommended daily dosage for ginseng is 1–2 grams of root or 200–400 mg in standardized capsules. The recommended daily dosage for holy basil is 1–2 standardized capsules. I recommend holy basil by New Chapter.

> Following an ideal daily routine lowers stress and brings balance. See Ideal *Ayurvedic* Daily Routine on page 209.

CUSTOM #29—POINTS TO REMEMBER

• Herbal adaptogens are effective at lowering your physiological response to stress.

• Holy basil, for example, decreases cortisol and enhances stamina, endurance, and the body's effective use of oxygen under stress. It also protects and boosts the immune system during stress.

• Don't rely on an herb alone to protect you from stress; adopt as many stress-reducing habits and behaviors as possible.

CUSTOM #30

Take care of your needs.

There must be quite a few things a hot bath won't cure,
but I don't know many of them.

—SYLVIA PLATH, *THE BELL JAR*

Research shows that women who develop breast cancer are more likely to give too much at the expense of their own needs. Since our culture trains women to do this, we need to break this habit. Instead, we need to practice asking ourselves what serves us best and then do it. For instance, you may decide that a massage on a regular basis is something that supports you. Many women think that massages or other nurturing treatments are just frivolous pampering; they're wrong. Research shows that human touch is powerful medicine. Massage not only lessens muscular tension and discomfort, but it also stimulates the immune system and decreases depression—both of which have profound effects on keeping your body well and warding off disease. If you can't make it to a spa for a professional massage, request a massage from your significant other. Research shows that massage is beneficial to both the giver and the receiver. It's also a wonderful way to enhance intimacy with your partner. And nothing has been found to be more powerful in supporting health than the experience of love and intimacy. If you're not in an intimate relationship right now, massage yourself. In fact, self-massage contributes to good health so much that *Ayurveda* recommends daily sesame-oil self-massages as part of the ideal health routine.

Train yourself to listen to your needs. Nurture yourself like you would your children. As one of my good friends, a professional life coach, says, "The best way to take care of other people is to take care of you." You can't fully help others if you are stressed, exhausted, and emotionally spent. But if you keep yourself balanced, rested, and sourced, you can support those you love so much better. Nature gave each of us a miraculous mind/body and with it, the responsibility of taking care of it. No one else has been assigned to take care of your mind/body except you. It's your primary responsibility. If you don't accept this responsibility, you will become sick and then you won't be able to help those you love.

It is one of the most beautiful compensations of this life that
no man can sincerely try to help another without helping himself.

—RALPH WALDO EMERSON

The more you take care of yourself, the more likely you are to reach your full potential and *that* is the purpose of your life. You are here on a journey to experience the highest version of yourself and to contribute your unique gifts to the world. With few exceptions, you can only do that fully if you are healthy.

If you've formed a Warrior Goddess group, have each member reflect and share with the group a new practice she could start that takes care of her needs. Think about ways to support one another. For example, one member could baby-sit for another member's kids once a week for an hour or two. This will free up time for the other member to get a massage, go for a hike, read a book, or do whatever it is that takes care of her needs. Or, you could even free up time for *everyone* in the group by starting a dinner co-op. Each member takes a turn preparing large meals and sharing them with the other group members.

CUSTOM #30—POINTS TO REMEMBER

• Every emotion you feel creates a biochemical reaction in your body that affects your health.

• Negative emotions take a toll on your health, while positive emotions such as laughing stimulate your immune system and help to keep you healthy.

• It's important to feel all your emotions, but it's best to learn how to process your negative emotions so that they don't linger.

• Women with breast cancer tend to give too much at the expense of their own needs, stay in loveless relationships, have issues with hope and trust, and suffer from hurt, sorrow, and unfinished business.

When health is absent, wisdom cannot reveal itself,
art cannot become manifest, strength cannot be exerted,
wealth is useless, and reason is powerless.

—HEROPHILIES, 300 B.C.E.

The best way to predict your future is to create it.

—AUTHOR UNKNOWN

MISSION ACCOMPLISHED

That's it. You're now doing most everything we know of that will substantially lower your risk of breast cancer. If you haven't noticed her yet, look in the mirror. Look closely at your reflection. You should be able to see the Warrior Goddess within you shining in radiant health. Your new health-creating and health-preserving choices are contributing to making the enlightened culture of

Complete Grocery List

I recommend that you use the following list as a guide when you go to the health food store or the natural food section of your grocery store. These are all items that I've covered in this book, and if you can't find them locally, check the Internet. Remember to buy only organic, if you can!

- ❏ *Cruciferous vegetables: broccoli, cauliflower, kale, bok choy, or Brussels sprouts*
- ❏ *Brazil nuts*
- ❏ *Flaxseeds and flax oil*
- ❏ *Fruits: apples, apricots, oranges, berries, grapes, melon, and so on*
- ❏ *Garlic*
- ❏ *Green tea*
- ❏ *Olive oil*
- ❏ *Sesame oil*
- ❏ *Soy products: tofu, tempeh, miso, soy milk, or soy meat substitute*
- ❏ *Stevia*
- ❏ *Turmeric*
- ❏ *Vegetables: asparagus, beets, artichokes, garlic, spinach, and so on*
- ❏ *Wakame seaweed*
- ❏ *Whole grains: brown rice, quinoa, amaranth, or barley*

Supplement List

I recommended products made by Enzymatic Therapies, New Chapter, and Maharishi *Ayurvedic* Products International. These companies are highly reputable and put extremely careful thought into every step of creating each product. They principally use organically grown herbs or herbs grown and collected in the wild. They use no chemicals, pesticides, or harsh processing practices that could destroy the quality of the herbs. Generally, all the products are created from whole foods and are not synthetic. These companies make the highest quality products on the market, products that work in a manner most in harmony with your body.

- ❑ *Multivitamin*
- ❑ *Amrit Kalash*
- ❑ *CLA*
- ❑ *CoQ$_{10}$*
- ❑ *Holy basil*
- ❑ *Maitake mushrooms*
- ❑ *Protective Breast Formula*
- ❑ *Selenium*
- ❑ *Zyflamend*

the next century a reality today. You can play an even larger role in making this visionary culture real by sharing these new customs with your friends. The more of us there are who adopt these customs, the faster our world will change to one where good health is normal and chronic diseases such as cancer are rare.

Remember that the health benefits of all these customs or practices don't just add up, they multiply. So, the difference you're making in decreasing your risk of breast cancer is *huge*! Doing all these things won't give you a 100-percent guarantee that you'll never develop breast cancer. But your likelihood of getting this terrible disease will be very small. If you do get it, your chances of having a less aggressive tumor and surviving it are much greater. If you already have breast cancer, remember, all these things can help you, too.

Keep up the good work. It's important to keep all the customs you've adopted. Just doing a few things every once in a while won't give you the protection you really want. I do all these things. They can be done, and it's not hard. You just need to adjust to the changes, and you will. You should be feeling a lot better by now, too. Feeling better is good motivation. You will undoubtedly continue to feel better and better. Your energy levels should go up, and you will probably get sick less often. If you have other chronic disorders, you may notice an improvement in them, as well.

Nothing is more important than your health. Without it, you have nothing. Congratulations on completing the program! I'd love to hear from you to see what differences it has made in your life already. Please contact me through my website at www.drchristinehorner.com, or write to me at:

Dr. Christine Horner
P.O. Box 812
Taos, NM 87571

*May you live with perfect health and fulfillment
all the days you walk this earth.*

Thank you for allowing me to contribute to you.

Namasté

Resources

Contact information is subject to change.

AIR-FILTRATION SYSTEMS

Gaiam®, A Lifestyle Company
Website: www.gaiam.com
Blueair HEPA Air Filter 501 and 402;
Healthmate HEPA Air Filter; SilentAir 4000;
Desktop Air Filters; UV Air Purifier (uses
HEPA, carbon, UV light, and ionization); Car
Ionizer

AMRIT KALASH

Maharishi Ayurveda Products Int'l
P.O. Box 180
Avon Lake, OH 44012
Phone: 800-255-8332
Fax: 719-260-7400
E-mail: info@mapi.com
Website: www.mapi.com

ANTIOXIDANT SUPPLEMENTS

Enzymatic Therapy
825 Challenger Drive
Green Bay, WI 54311-8328
Phone: 800-783-2286
Fax: 888-570-6460
Website: www.eticonsumer.com

Maharishi Ayurveda Products International
P.O. Box 180
Avon Lake, OH 44012
Phone: 800-255-8332
Fax: 719-260-7400
E-mail: info@mapi.com
Website: www.mapi.com

New Chapter
22 High Street
Brattleboro, VT 05301
Phone: 800-543-7279
Fax: 800-470-0247
E-mail: info@new-chapter.com
Websites: www.new-chapter.com *or*
www.newchapter.info

AYURVEDIC HEALTH SPAS

The Ayurvedic Institutes
11311 Menave Blvd., N.E.
Albuquerque, NM 87112
Phone: 505-291-9698
Website: www.ayurveda.com
Offers panchakarma.

Maharishi Vedic Health Center
679 George Hill Road
Lancaster, MA 01523
Phone: 877-890-8600 or 978-365-4549
Website: www.Lancasterhealth.com
Offers panchakarma.

The Raj
1734 Jasmine Avenue
Fairfield, IA 52556
Phone: 800-248-9050, 641-472-9580
  (in IA)
E-mail: theraj@lisco.com
Websites: www.theraj.com
www.ayurvedamedgroup.com/meet-our-
  team.html
Offers panchakarma.

For European health spas that offer *panchakarma,* visit:
www.ayurveda.de/mag_forsch.htm
www.ayurveda-
  badems.de/english/haus/index.php
www.maharishi-european-
  sidhaland.org.uk/

BEDS, BEDDING, FURNITURE

Earthsake
1425 4th Street
Berkeley, CA 94710
Phone: 800-414-8074
Website: www.earthsake.com

Ecobaby Organics
332 Coogan Way
El Cajon, CA 92020
Phone: 800-596-7450
Website: www.purerest.com *or*
  www.ecobaby.com

Furnature
86 Coolidge Ave.
Watertown, MA 02472
Phone: 800-326-4895
Website: www.furnature.com

Tomorrow's World
9659 First View Street
Norfolk, VA 23503
Phone: 800-229-7571
Website: www.tomorrowsworld.com

BUILDING CONSULTANTS AND PRODUCTS

Shelter Ecology, Inc.
Website: www.shelterecology.com

Building for Health Materials Center
Website: buildingforhealth.com

Natural House Company
Website: www.naturalhouseco.com

CABINETS

Shelter Ecology, Inc.
Website: www.shelterecology.com

Nirvana Safe Haven
Website: www.nontoxic.com

Building for Health Materials Center
Website: www.buildingforhealth.com

CALCIUM D-GLUCARATE SUPPLEMENTS

Enzymatic Therapy
825 Challenger Drive
Green Bay, WI 54311
Phone: 800-783-2286
Fax: 888-570-6460
Website: www.eticonsumer.com
Available in Protective Breast Formula
(www.protectivebreast.com / 866-795-3517)

CARPETS AND FLOORING

Contempo Floor Coverings, Inc.
Phone: 310-837-8110

E-mail: contempocarpets@hotmail.com
Website: www.contempofloorcoverings.com

CLOTHING

Esperanza Threads
1160 Broadway Avenue
Bedford, OH 44146
Phone: 440-786-9009
Website: www.esperanzathreads.com
Organic apparel and goods.

Feeling Goods
5511 Keybridge Drive
Boise, ID 83703
Phone: 877-349-2102
Website: www.feelinggoods.com

Green Babies, Inc.
28 Spring Street
Tarrytown, NY 10591
Phone: 800-603-7508
Website: www.greenbabies.com

Under the Canopy
1141 South Rogers Circle
Boca Raton, FL 33487
Phone: 888-CANOPY-9 (888-226-6799)
Website: www.underthecanopy.com

Maggie's Functional Organics
306 West Cross Street
Ypsilanti, MI 48197
Phone: 800-609-8593
Fax: 734-482-4175
E-mail: maggies@organicclothes.com
Website: www.organicclothes.com

Webspirit Links Directory for Organic Clothing
Website: www.webspirit.com/Links/
organicclothing.html

COENZYME Q$_{10}$ SUPPLEMENTS

Enzymatic Therapy
825 Challenger Drive
Green Bay, WI 54311
Phone: 800-783-2286
Fax: 888-570-6460
Website: www.eticonsumer.com

New Chapter
22 High Street
Brattleboro, VT 05301
Phone: 800-543-7279
Fax: 800-470-0247
E-mail: info@new-chapter.com
Websites: www.new-chapter.com
www.newchapter.info

COMMUNITY-SPONSORED AGRICULTURE (CSA)

Alternative Farming Systems Information Center (AFSIC)
Websites: www.nal.usda.gov/afsic/csa/
www.nal.usda.gov/afsic/AFSIC_pubs/
at93-02.htm

CONJUGATED LINOLEIC ACID (CLA)

NOW Foods
Website: www.nowfoods.com

DIGESTIVE FORMULAS

Enzymatic Therapy
825 Challenger Drive
Green Bay, WI 54311
Phone: 800-783-2286
Fax: 888-570-6460
Website: www.eticonsumer.com

New Chapter
22 High Street
Brattleboro, VT 05301
Phone: 800-543-7279
Fax: 800-470-0247
E-mail: info@new-chapter.com
Websites: www.new-chapter.com *or*
www.newchapter.info

Maharishi Ayurveda Products Int'l
P.O. Box 180
Avon Lake, OH 44012
Phone: 800-255-8332
Fax: 719-260-7400
E-mail: info@mapi.com
Website: www.mapi.com

EDAMAME (SOYBEANS)

SeaPoint Farms
2183 Fairview Road
Costa Mesa, CA 92627
Phone: 888-722-7098
E-mail: info@seapointfarms.com
Website: www.seapointfarms.com

Cascadian Farms
Consumer Services
719 Metcalf Street
Sedro-Woolley, WA 98284
Phone: 800-624-4123
Website: www.cascadianfarm.com

Quality Natural Foods
P.O. Box 16391
Hooksett, NH 03106
Phone: 888-392-9237
E-mail: sales@qualitynaturalfoods.com
Website: www.qualitynaturalfoods.com/
shopnew/miso.html

ENVIRONMENTAL TOXINS (INFORMATION)

Scorecard (Environmental Defense)
Website: www.scorecard.org

U.S. Environmental Protection Agency
Website: www.epa.gov

FLAXSEEDS AND FLAX OIL

Barlean's Organic Oils
4936 Lake Terrell Road
Ferndale, WA 90278
Phone: 360-384-0485
Fax: 360-384-1746
Website: www.barleans.com

FOODS, ORGANIC

Amy's Kitchen, Inc.
2330 Northpoint Parkway
Santa Rosa, CA 95407
Phone: 707-578-7188
Fax: 707-578-7995

E-mail: amy@amyskitchen.net
Website: www.amyskitchen.com

Beantree Organics
Website: www.beantreeorganics.com
Organic whole foods, herbs, and spices.

Cascadian Farms
Consumer Services
719 Metcalf Street
Sedro-Woolley, WA 98284
Phone: 800-624-4123
Website: www.cascadianfarm.com
*Organic foods, including frozen fruits and
vegetables.*

Diamond Organics
P.O. Box 2159
Freedom, CA 95019
Phone: 888-674-2642
Website: www.diamondorganics.com
*Online organic foods, including fresh
vegetables.*

Earthbound Farm
1721 San Juan Highway
San Juan Bautista, CA 95045
Phone: 888-328-6742
Website: www.ebfarm.com
Organic fruits and vegetables.

**EcoNatural Solutions/
St. Claire's Organic**
6235 Lookout Road, Suite A
Boulder, CO 80301
Phone: 303-527-1554
Website: www.econaturalsolutions.com

Eden Foods
701 Tecumseh Road
Clinton, MI 49236
Phone: 517-456-7424, 888-424-EDEN
Fax: 517-456-7854
Website: www.edenfoods.com
Variety of organic foods.

Horizon Organic
P.O. Box 17577
Boulder, CO 80308
Phone: 888-494-3020

Fax: 503-652-1371
Website: www.horizonorganic.com
Organic dairy.

Lotus Foods
921 Richmond Street
El Cerrito, CA 94530
Phone: 510-525-3137
Fax: 510-525-4226
Website: www.lotusfoods.com
Organic grains.

Lundberg Family Farms
P.O. Box 369
Richvale, CA 95974
Phone: 530-882-4551
Fax: 530-882-4500
Website: www.lundberg.com
Organic grains.

Melissa's/World Variety Produce Inc.
P.O. Box 21127
Los Angeles, CA 90021
Phone: 888-588-0151
Fax: 323-584-7385
E-mail: hotline@melissas.com
Website: www.melissas.com
Organic foods and many recipes.

Organic Kingdom
192 West 1480 South
Orem, UT 84058
Phone: 801-426-0604
Fax: 801-426-7627
Website: www.organickingdom.com/
index.html

Organic Planet
231 Sansome Street, #300
San Francisco, CA 94104
Phone: 415-765-5590
Fax: 415-765-5922
Website: www.organic-planet.com

Organic Valley Family of Farms
507 West Main Street
La Farge, WI 54639
Phone: 888-444-6455
Fax: 608-625-2600

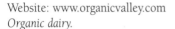

Website: www.organicvalley.com
Organic dairy.

Purely Organic Ltd.
P.O. Box 847
Fairfield, IA 52556
Phone: 641-472-7873
Fax: 641-472-1754
Website: www.purelyorganic.com
*Imported organic condiments, grape juice
from Italy.*

Seeds of Change
3209 Richards Lane
P.O. Box 15700
Santa Fe, NM 87506
Phone: 323-586-3455
Fax: 323-586-3420
Website: www.seedsofchange.com

ShopNatural
350 South Toole Ave.
Tucson, AZ 85701
Phone: 502-884-0745
Website: www.shopnatural.com
Online organic food and products store.

South Pacific Trading Company
22601 East La Palma Ave., Suite 102
Yorba Linda, CA 92887
Phone: 888-505-4439
Fax: 714-692-9681
Website: www.nonipacific.com

Stonyfield Farms
10 Burton Drive
Londonderry, NH 03053
Phone: 800-776-2697
Fax: 603-437-7594
Website: www.stonyfield.com
Organic yogurt.

SunOrganic Farm
411 South Las Posas Road
San Marcos, CA 92069
Phone: 888-269-9888
Fax: 760-510-9996
Website: www.sunorganic.com
Online organic foods, free catalog.

Whole Foods Market, Inc.
700 Lavaca Street, Suite 500
Austin, TX 78701
Phone: 512-477-4455
Website: www.wholefoodsmarket.com

Wild Oats Market, Inc.
3375 Mitchell Lane
Boulder, CO 80301
Phone: 303-440-5220
Website: www.wildoats.com

GARLIC SUPPLEMENTS

**ATTR—National Sustainable
Agriculture Information Service**
P.O. Box 3657
Fayetteville, AR 72702
Phone: 800-346-9140
Websites: www.attra.ncat.org
www.attra.ncat.org   *(search "garlic")*

Enzymatic Therapy
825 Challenger Drive
Green Bay, WI 54311
Phone: 800-783-2286
Fax: 888-570-6460
Website: www.eticonsumer.com

New Chapter
22 High Street
Brattleboro, VT 05301
Phone: 800- 543-7279
Fax: 800-470-0247
E-mail: info@new-chapter.com
Websites: www.new-chapter.com *or*
www.newchapter.info

Kyolic
23501 Madero
Mission Viejo, CA 92691
Phone: 949-855-2776, 800-421-2998
Fax: 949-458-2764
E-mail: info@wakunaga.com
Website: www.kyolic.com

GRAPE SEED EXTRACT

Enzymatic Therapy
825 Challenger Drive

Green Bay, WI 54311
Phone: 800-783-2286
Fax: 888-570-6460
Website: www.eticonsumer.com
Available in Protective Breast Formula
(www.protectivebreast.com / 866-795-3517)

GREEN TEA

Blue Moon Tea
Website: www.bluemoontea.com

Celestial Seasonings
Website: www.celestialseasonings.com/
products/organic/got.php

Choice Organic Teas
Website: www.choiceorganicteas.com

Health to a Tea Natural Products Inc.
Website: www.organicgreenteas.com/tea/
index.php3

HerbalHut.Com
Website: www.herbalhut.com/mfrs/
st_dalfour_teas.htm

Numi Teas and Teasans
Website: www.numitea.com

Stash Tea
Website: www.stashtea.com/w-113082.htm

Traditional Medicinals
Website: www.traditionalmedicinals.com

Xianju Organic Green Tea
Website: www.worldconsortium.com/
tea.htm

Yogi Tea
Website: www.yogitea.com

GREEN TEA SUPPLEMENTS

Enzymatic Therapy
825 Challenger Drive
Green Bay, WI 54311
Phone: 800-783-2286
Fax: 888-570-6460
Website: www.eticonsumer.com

Available in Protective Breast Formula
(www.protectivebreast.com / 1-866-795-3517)

New Chapter
22 High Street
Brattleboro, VT 05301
Phone: 800-543-7279
Fax: 800-470-0247
E-mail: info@new-chapter.com
Websites: www.new-chapter.com *or*
www.newchapter.info

HERBAL ANTI-INFLAMMATORY (ZYFLAMEND)

New Chapter
22 High Street
Brattleboro, VT 05301
Phone: 800-543-7279
Fax: 800-470-0247
E-mail: info@new-chapter.com
Websites: www.new-chapter.com
www.newchapter.info

HERBS

Frontier Natural Products Co-op
P.O. Box 299
3021 78th Street
Norway, IA 52318
Phone: 800-669-3275
Fax: 800-717-4372
Website: www.frontiercoop.com
*World's largest supplier of organic herbs and
spices—available in many stores including
online stores.*

HOME DETOX PROGRAMS

**Enzymatic Therapy Natural
Medicines**
Website: www.eticonsumer.com
Whole Body Cleanse Kit

HealthWorld Online
Website: www.healthy.net/Nutrit/specdiet/
detox/index.asp

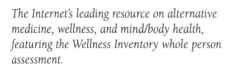

The Internet's leading resource on alternative medicine, wellness, and mind/body health, featuring the Wellness Inventory whole person assessment.

Maharishi Ayurveda
Website: www.mapi.com
Type in "home detox" into search engine to find several articles from past newsletters with instructions and recipes for home detox programs.

Mind Your Body Detoxification & Meditation Programs
Contact: Dr. Maya Nicole Baylac
Website: www.mindyourbody.info/
  programs.html
Personal cleansing and detoxification program in your home.

HOUSEHOLD CLEANING PRODUCTS

Country Save
19704 60th Avenue NE
Arlington, WA 98223
Phone: 360-435-9868
Fax: 360-435-0896
E-mail: info@countrysave.com
Website: countrysave.com/prods.php

Ecover
P.O. Box 9111058
Commerce, CA 90091
Phone: 800-449-4925
Fax: 323-720-5732
Website: www.ecover.com

Earth Friendly
44 Green Bay Road
Winnetka, IL 60093
Phone: 800-335-3267
Fax: 847-446-4437
Website: www.ecos.com

Mountain Green
7956 East Via Costa
Scottsdale, AZ 85258
Phone: 866-686-4733
Fax: 866-686-4732
E-mail: info@mtngreen.com
Website: www.mtngreen.com

Planet, Inc.
2676 Wilfert Road, Suite 201
Victoria, BC V9B 5ZE
Canada
Phone: 250-478-8171
Fax: 250-478-3238
Website: www.planetinc.com

INDOLE-3-CARBINOL SUPPLEMENTS

Enzymatic Therapy
825 Challenger Drive
Green Bay, WI 54311
Phone: 800-783-2286
Fax: 888-570-6460
Website: www.eticonsumer.com
Available in Protective Breast Formula (www.protectivebreast.com / 866-795-3517)

INSECT REPELLENT

All Terrain
P.O. Box 840, 920 Route 11
Sunapee, NH 03782
Phone: 800-246-7328
Website: www.allterrainco.com

Burt's Bees
P.O. Box 13489
Durham, NC 27709
Phone: 800-849-7112
Fax: 800-429-7487
Website: www.burtsbees.com

INSULATION

Building for Health Materials Center
Website: buildingforhealth.com/
  naturalfiber.html

Cellulose
Website: www.cellulose.org

Icynene
Website: www.icynene.com

Nirvana Safe Haven
Website: www.nontoxic.com

Shelter Ecology, Inc.
Website: www.shelterecology.com

LIGNAN SUPPLEMENTS

Brevail
Lignan Research LLC
9921 Carmel Mountain Road, #339
San Diego, CA 92129
Phone: 888-503-8300
Fax: 800-501-6176
E-mail: info@brevail.com
Website: www.brevail.com

LOW-EMF HAIR DRYER

Angelite Hair Dryer
Phone: 877-460-9151
Website: www.lowemf.com

MAHARISHI VEDIC ORGANIC AGRICULTURE

Maharishi Vedic Organic Agriculture Institute
1431 South Pennsylvania Ave., Suite #3
Casper, WY, 82609
Phone: 307-237-1055
Fax: 307-237-5547
E-mail: MVOAI@Maharishi.net
E-mail: Vedicorganicsales@earthlink.net
Website: www.mvoai.org

MAITAKE MUSHROOM SUPPLEMENTS

Diamond Organics
P.O. Box 2159
Freedom, CA 95019
Phone: 888-674-2642
Website: www.diamondorganics.com
Online organic foods, including fresh vegetables.

Enzymatic Therapy
825 Challenger Drive
Green Bay, WI 54311
Phone: 800-783-2286
Fax: 888-570-6460
Website: www.eticonsumer.com
Available in Protective Breast Formula (www.protectivebreast.com / 866-795-3517)

Fungi Perfecti, LLC
P.O. Box 7634
Olympia, WA 98507
Order Line: 800-780-9126
Phone: 360-426-9292
Fax: 360-426-9377
E-mail: mycomedia@aol.com
Website: www.fungi.com

Mycological Natural Products Ltd.
P.O. Box 24940
Eugene, OR 97402
Phone: 888-465-3247
Website: www.mycological.com
Organic dried Maitake mushrooms.

New Chapter
22 High Street
Brattleboro, VT 05301
Phone: 800-543-7279
Fax: 800-470-0247
E-mail: info@new-chapter.com
Websites: www.new-chapter.com
www.newchapter.info

MEAT SUBSTITUTES

Boca Foods
910 Mayer Ave.
Madison, WI 53704
Phone: 847-646-2000
Fax: 847-646-2800
Website: www.bocaburger.com

Light Life
53 Industrial Blvd.
Turners Falls, MA 10376
Phone: 800-SOYEASY (769-3279)
Website: www.lightlife.com

Morningstar Farms
One Kellogg Square
Battle Creek, MI 49016
Phone: 269-961-2001
Fax: 269-961-6286
Website: www.morningstarfarms.com
Made with organic ingredients.

Veat Inc.
20318 Gramercy Place
Torrance, CA 90501
Phone: 310-320-8611
Fax: 310-320-8805
Website: www.vanswaffles.com

MUSHROOMS, DRIED

Solutions Unlimited
871 Engleville Road
Sharon Springs, NY 13459
Phone: 518-284-2203
Fax: 303-568-2465
Website: www.flushitsolutions.com/
dried_mushrooms.htm

NONALCOHOLIC WINES AND JUICES

Purely Organic Ltd.
P.O. Box 847
Fairfield, IA 52556
Phone: 641-472-7873
Fax: 641-472-1754
Website: www.purelyorganic.com
Imported organic condiments, grape juice from Italy.

Ariel
P.O. Box 3437
Napa, CA 94558
Phone: 800-456-9473
E-mail: info@arielvineyards.com
Website: www.arielvineyards.com
Nonalcoholic wines.

Walnut Acres
An Acirca Inc. Company
A division of The Hain Celestial Group, Inc.
One Ranado Plaza, Floor 7
New Rochelle, NY 10801

Phone: 866-492-5688
Website: www.walnutacres.com
Organic fruit and vegetable juices.

Santa Cruz
Phone: 530-899-5010
E-mail: info@scojuice.com
Website: www.scojuice.com
Organic fruit and vegetable juices.

PAINTS, STAINS, WALL COVERINGS, AND CLEANERS

American Formulating and Manufacturing
Website: www.afmsafecoat.com
Phone: 800-239-0321

Bioshield Paint
Phone: 800-621-2591
E-mail: info@bioshieldpaint.com
Website: www.bioshieldpaint.com

Auro Organic Paints
Unit 2, Pamphillions Farm
Purton End, Debden
Saffron Walden, Essex, CB11 3JT
UK
Phone: +44-01799-543-077

Maya Romanoff
1730 West Greenleaf
Chicago, IL 60626
Phone: 773-465-6909
Fax: 773-465-7089
E-mail: customerservice@mayaromanoff.
com

Merco Joint Compound
Website: www.mold-
help.org/pages/submenus/mold_and_
sick_buildings/hiddentoxins.htm

PAPER—TREE-FREE AND RECYCLED

Greenline Paper Company
631 South Pine Street
York, PA 17403
Phone: 800-641-1117
Website: www.greenlinepaper.com

New Leaf
215 Leidesdorff Street, 4th Floor
San Francisco, CA 94111
Phone: 888-989-5323
Website: www.newleafpaper.com

Living Tree Paper Company
1430 Willamette Street, Suite 367
Eugene, OR 97401
Phone: 800-309-2974
Website: www.livingtreepaper.com

PERSONAL-CARE PRODUCTS

Aubrey Organics
4419 North Manhattan Ave.
Tampa, FL 33614
Phone: 800-237-4270
Fax: 813-876-8166
Website: www.aubry-organics.com

Burt's Bees
P.O. Box 13489
Durham, NC 27709
Phone: 800-849-7112
Fax: 800-429-7487
Website: www.burtsbees.com

Natracare, LLC
14901 East Hampden Ave., #190
Aurora, CO 80014
Phone: 303-617-3476
Fax: 303-617-3495
Website: www.natracare.com
Chlorine-free feminine hygiene products.

Tom's of Maine
P.O. Box 710
302 Lafayette Center
Kennebunk, ME 04043
Phone: 800-FOR-TOMS
Fax: 207-985-2196
Website: www.tomsofmaine.com

PEST CONTROL— LAWN AND GARDEN

Arbico Organics
P.O. Box 8910
Tucson, AZ 85738

Phone: 800-827-2847
Fax: 502-825-2038
E-mail: info@arbico.com
Website: www.arbico.com

Garden's Alive! Inc.
5100 Schenley Place, Dept. 4680
Lawrenceburg, IN 47025
Phone: 812-537-8650
Website: www.gardens-alive.com

Peaceful Valley Farm Supply
P.O. Box 2209, #NGP
Grass Valley, CA 95945
Phone: 888-784-1722
Website: www.groworganic.com

PRANAYAMA

The Art of Living Foundation
Phone: 800-420-4193
Website: www.artoflivingAZ.org
E-mail: info@artoflivinngAZ.org

The Pranayama Institute
P.O. Box 1360
East Ellijay, GA 30539-1360
Website: www.pranayama.org

YogaVidya.Com
Website: www.yogavidya.com/yoga-81.html

The Yoga Site
Website: www.yogasite.com/pranayama.htm

PRODUCTS FOR THE HOME

Gaiam
360 Interlocken Blvd., Suite 300
Broomfield, CO 80021
Phone: 800-869-3603
Phone: 800-482-3747
Website: www.gaiam.com
Free catalog: Harmony

Healthy Home
2435 Dr. Martin Luther King Jr. Street North
St. Petersburg, FL 33704
Phone: 800-583-9523
Website: www.HealthyHome.com
Catalog available.

ShopNatural
350 South Toole Avenue
Tucson, AZ 85701
Phone: 502-884-0745
Website: www.shopnatural.com
Online organic food and products store.

Whole Organics Inc.
1488 Sandbridge Road
Virginia Beach, VA 23456
Phone: 757-721-3900
Website: www.wholeorganics.com

PROTECTIVE BREAST FORMULA

Enzymatic Therapy
825 Challenger Drive
Green Bay, WI 54311
Phone: 800-783-2286
Fax: 888-570-6460
Website: www.eticonsumer.com
(www.protectivebreast.com / 866-795-3517)

RAW-FOODS BLENDER

Vita-Mix Corporation
8615 Usher Road
Cleveland, OH 44138
Phone: 887-848-2649
Fax: 440-235-7155
Website: www.ultimateblender.com

RESOURCE ORGANIZATIONS

National Green Pages
Co-op America Business Network
1612 K Street NW, Suite 600
Washington, DC 20006
Phone: 800-58-GREEN
Website: www.greenpages.org
*Directory to socially and environmentally
responsible businesses.*

National Nutritional Foods Association
3931 Macarthur Blvd., Suite 101
Newport Beach, CA 92660
Phone: 949-622-6272
Fax: 949-622-6266
Website: www.nnfa.org

Organic Consumers Association
Phone: 218-226-4164
Website: www.organicconsumers.org

Organic Trade Association
P.O. Box 547
60 Wells Street
Greenfield, MA 01302
Phone: 413-774-7511
Fax: 413-774-6432
Website: www.ota.com

U.S. Green Building Council
1015 18th Street NW
Washington, DC 20036
Phone: 202-828-7422
Fax: 202-828-5110
E-mail: info@usgbc.org
Website: www.usgbc.org

Vegetarian Resource Group
P.O. Box 1463
Baltimore, MD 21203
Phone: 410-366-8343
Website: www.vrg.org

ROSEMARY PRODUCTS

Frontier Natural Products Co-op
30217 78th Street
Norway, IA 52318
Phone: 800-437-3301
Website: www.frontiercoop.com

SELENIUM SUPPLEMENTS

New Chapter
22 High Street
Brattleboro, VT 05301
Phone: 800-543-7279
Fax: 800-470-0247
E-mail: info@new-chapter.com
Websites: www.new-chapter.com
www.newchapter.info

SOCIALLY RESPONSIBLE INVESTING

Calvert Group Ltd.
Phone: 800-771-9436
Website: www.calvert.com

Domini Social Investments
Phone: 800-225-FUND
Website: www.domini.com

Green Century Funds
Phone: 800-93-GREEN
Website: www.greencentury.com

Neuberger Bergman Socially Responsible Fund
Phone: 888-556-8590
Website: www.nbfunds.com

Pax World Funds
Phone: 800-767-1729
Website: www.paxworld.com

Trillium Asset Management
Phone: 800-548-5684
Website: www.Trilliuminvest.com

SOY FOODS

Light Life
153 Industrial Blvd.
Turners Falls, MA 10376
Phone: 800-SOYEASY (769-3279)
Website: www.lightlife.com
Tempeh and large variety of soy meat substitutes.

Morinaga Nutritional Foods, Inc.
2441 West 205th Street, Suite C-102
Torrance, CA 90501
Phone: 310-787-0200
Fax: 310-787-2727
E-mail: healthfoods@morinu.com
Website: www.morinu.com

Sunrise Soya Foods
729 Powell Street
Vancouver, BC V6A-1H5
Canada
Phone: 604-253-2326
Fax: 604-251-1083
Website: www.petestofu.com
Pete's Tofu–flavored tofu meals.

Soyco Foods
A division of Galaxy Nutritional Foods
2441 Viscount Row
Orlando, FL 32809

Phone: 407-855-5500
Website: www.soyco.com
Soy cheese—Veggy Singles.

Vitasoy USA, Inc.
One New England Way
Ayer, MA 01432
Phone: 800-VITASOY
E-mail: info@vitasoy-usa.com
Website: www.nasoya.com

White Wave
1990 North 57th Court
Boulder, CO 80301
Phone: 720-565-2344
Fax: 303-443-3952
Website: www.silkissoy.com
Tofu and soy milk.

WholeSoy
353 Sacramento Street SE, Suite 1120
San Francisco, CA 94111
Phone: 415-495-2870
Fax: 415-495-3060
Website: www.wholesoy.com

SOY NUTS

Mighty Mo Munchies
P.O. Box 335 Highway 111 W
Oregon, MO 64473
Phone: 800-762-1384
Website: www.mightymomunchies.com

STEVIA PRODUCTS

Body Ecology/Stevia.Net
Website: www.stevia.net

HealthWorld Online
Website: www.healthy.net/nutrit/kitchen/
foods/stevia.asp

Wisdom Natural Brands
2546 West Birchwood Ave., #104
Mesa, AZ 85202
Phone: 800-899-9908
Fax: 480-966-3805
E-mail: wisdom@wisdomnaturalbrands.com
Website: www.wisdomherbs.com/
products/sweetleaf/

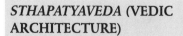

STHAPATYAVEDA (VEDIC ARCHITECTURE)

Maharishi Sthapatya Veda
Website: www.sthapatyaveda.com

TRANSCENDENTAL MEDITATION (TM)

Maharishi Peace Palace
5504 Edson Lane North
Bethesda, MD 20852
Phone: 301-770-5690
Toll-free: 800-LEARNTM
E-mail: info@bethesdapeacepalace.org
Website: www.mvc-
bethesda.org/index.php

TURMERIC PRODUCTS

Enzymatic Therapy
825 Challenger Drive
Green Bay, WI 54311
Phone: 800-783-2286
Fax: 888-570-6460
Website: www.eticonsumer.com
*Available in Protective Breast Formula
(www.protectivebreast.com / 866-795-3517)*

Frontier Natural Products Co-op
P.O. Box 299
3021 78th Street
Norway, IA 52318
Phone: 800-669-3275
Fax: 800-717-4372
Website: www.frontiercoop.com
*World's largest supplier of organic herbs and
spices—available in many stores including
online stores.*

New Chapter
22 High Street
Brattleboro, VT 05301
Phone: 800-543-7279
Fax: 800-470-0247
E-mail: info@new-chapter.com
Websites: www.new-chapter.com
www.newchapter.info

VITAMIN SUPPLEMENTS

Enzymatic Therapy
825 Challenger Drive
Green Bay, WI 54311
Phone: 800-783-2286
Fax: 888-570-6460
Website: www.eticonsumer.com

New Chapter
22 High Street
Brattleboro, VT 05301
Phone: 800-543-7279
Fax: 800-470-0247
E-mail:info@new-chapter.com
Websites: www.new-chapter.com
www.newchapter.info

WAKAME SEAWEED

Eden Foods
701 Tecumseh Road
Clinton, MI 49236
Phone: 517-456-7424, 888-424-EDEN
Fax: 517-456-7854
Website: www.edenfoods.com

WATER-FILTRATION SYSTEMS

Shelter Ecology, Inc.
Website: www.shelterecology.com

Nirvana Safe Haven
Website: www.nontoxic.com

Building for Health Materials Center
Website: buildingforhealth.com

WEDDING PLANNER, ORGANIC

Organic Weddings
365 Boston Post Road, Suite 320
Sudbury, MA 01776
Phone: 888-267-2814
Website: www.organicweddings.com

Recommended Reading

AYURVEDA

Chopra, Deepak, M.D. *Perfect Health.* New York, NY: Harmony Books, 1991.

Dreyer, Ronnie. *Vedic Astrology.* York Beach, ME: Samuel Weiser, 1997.

Hagelin, John, Ph.D. *Manual for a Perfect Government.* Fairfield, IA: Maharishi University Management Press, 1998.

Levacy, William. *Beneath the Vedic Sky.* Carlsbad, CA: Hay House, 1999.

Lonsdorf, Nancy, M.D. *A Women's Best Medicine for Menopause.* New York, NY: Contemporary Books, 2002.

Lonsdorf, Nancy, M.D., Veronica Butler, M.D., and Melaine Brown, Ph.D. *A Woman's Best Medicine.* New York, NY: Putnam, 1995.

O'Connell, David, Ph.D., and Charles Alexander, Ph.D. *Self Recovery: Treating Addictions Using Transcendental Meditation and Maharishi Ayur-Veda.* Binghamton, NY: Harrington Park Press, 1994.

Roth, Robert. *Transcendental Meditation.* New York, NY: Donald Fine, 1994.

Sharma, Hari, M.D. *Freedom from Disease.* Toronto, Canada: Veda Publishing, 1993.

Sharma, Hari, M.D., and Christopher Clark, M.D. *Contemporary Ayurveda.* New York, NY: Churchill Livingstone, 1998.

Tirtha, Swami Sada Shiva. *The Ayurvedic Encyclopedia.* Bayville, NY: Ayurveda Holistic Center Press, 1998.

Wallace, Robert, Ph.D. *The Neurophysiology of Enlightenment.* Fairfield, IA: Maharishi International University Press, 1991.

Wallace, Robert, Ph.D. *The Physiology of Consciousness.* Fairfield, IA: Maharishi International University Press, 1993.

BREAST CANCER

Arnot, Bob, M.D. *The Breast Cancer Prevention Diet.* Boston, MA: Little, Brown & Co., 1998.

Epstein, Samuel, M.D., and David Steinman. *The Breast Cancer Prevention Program.* New York, NY: MacMillan, 1997.

Gaynor, Mitchell, M.D. *Dr. Gaynor's Cancer Prevention Program.* New York, NY: Kensington, 1999.

Gaynor, Mitchell, M.D. *Sounds of Healing.* New York, NY: Broadway Books, 1999.

Keuneke, Robin. *Total Breast Health.* New York, NY: Kensington, 1998.

Lee, John, M.D. *What Your Doctor May Not Tell You About Breast Cancer.* New York, NY: Warner Books, 2002.

Tagliaferri, M., M.D., Isaac Cohen, O.M.D., L.Ac., and Dubu Tripathy, M.D. *Breast Cancer: Beyond Convention.* New York, NY: Atria Books, 2002.

EMOTIONAL AND SPIRITUAL HEALTH

Myss, Carolyn, Ph.D. *Anatomy of the Spirit: The Seven States of Power and Healing.* New York, NY: Harmony Books, 1996.

Myss, Carolyn, Ph.D. *Sacred Contracts.* New York, NY: Three Rivers Press, 2002.

Myss, Carolyn, Ph.D. *Why People Don't Heal and How They Can.* New York, NY: Three Rivers Press, 1997.

Ornish, Dean, M.D. *Love and Survival.* New York, NY: Harper Collins, 1995.

Tipping, Colin. *Radical Forgiveness.* Marietta, GA: Global 13, 2002.

Tolle, Eckhart. *The Power of Now.* Novato, CA: New World Library, 1999.

FLAX COOKBOOKS

Beutler, Jade. *Flax for Life: 101 Delicious Recipes and Tips Featuring Fabulous Flax Oil.* Encinitas, CA: Progressive Health Publishing, 1996.

Magee, Elaine. *The Flax Cookbook: Recipes and Strategies for Getting the Most from the Most Powerful Plant on the Planet.* New York: Marlowe & Co., 2003.

Reinhardt-Martin. *Flax Your Way to Better Health.* Moline, IL: Jane Reinhardt-Martin, 2001.

FOOD AND NUTRITION

Boyens, Ingeborg. *Unnatural Harvest.* Toronto, Canada: Doubleday Canada, 1999.

Cummins, Ronnie, and Ben Lilliston. *Genetically Engineered Food.* New York, NY: Marlowe and Company, 2000.

Garrett, Howard. *J. Howard Garrett's Organic Manual.* Fort Worth, TX: The Summit Group, 1993.

Gastelu, Daniel, and Fred Hatfield, Ph.D. *Dynamic Nutrition for Maximum Performance.* Garden City Park, NY: Avery Publishing Group, 1997.

Hospodar, Miriam. *Heaven's Banquet: Vegetarian Cooking for Life Long Health the Ayurveda Way.* New York, NY: Dutton, 1999.

Johari, Harish. *The Healing Cuisine: India's Art of Ayurvedic Cooking.* Rochester, VT: Healing Arts Press, 1994.

Richard, David, and Dorie Byers. *Taste Of Life! The Organic Choice.* Bloominton, IL: Vital Health Publishing, 1998.

Robbins, John. *The Food Revolution.* Berkeley, CA: Conari Press, 2001.

Schlosser, Eric. *Fast Food Nation.* New York, NY: Houghton Mifflin, 2001.

Steinman, David. *Diet for a Poisoned Planet.* New York, NY: Harmony, 1990.

HERBS AND SUPPLEMENTS

Murray, Michael, N.D. *Encyclopedia of Nutritional Supplements.* Roseville, CA: Prima Publishing, 1996.

Newmark, Thomas M., and Paul Schulick. *Beyond Aspirin: Nature's Challenge to Arthritis, Cancer & Alzheimer's Disease.* Prescott, AZ: Hohm Press, 2000.

NONTOXIC HOME

Harwood, Barbara. *The Healing House.* Carlsbad, CA: Hay House, 1997.

Marinelli, Janet, and Paul Beirman-Lytle. *Your Natural Home.* Boston, MA: Little, Brown & Co., 1995.

Pearson, David. *The Natural House Catalog.* New York, NY: Fireside, 1996.

Pearson, David. *The New Natural House Book.* New York, NY: Fireside, 1998.

QUANTUM PHYSICS

Greene, Brian. *The Elegant Universe.* New York, NY: Vintage Books, 1999.

TOFU COOKBOOKS

Ecookbooks.Com
Website: static.ecookbooks.com/categories/h/healthycookingsoyandtofu/

Greenberg, Patricia. *The Whole Soy Cookbook, 175 Delicious, Nutritious, Easy-to-Prepare Recipes Featuring Tofu, Tempeh, and Various Forms of Nature's Healthiest Bean.* New York: Three Rivers Press, 1998.

Hagler, Louise. *Tofu Cookery.* Summertown, TN: The Book Publishing Co., 1991.

Hagler, Louise. *Tofu Quick and Easy.* Summertown, TN: The Book Publishing Co., 1992.

Landgrebe, Gary. *Everyday Tofu: From Pancakes to Pizza.* Santa Cruz, CA: Crossing Press, 1999.

Madison, Deborah. *This Can't Be Tofu: 75 Recipes to Cook Something You Never Thought You Would—and Love Every Bite.* New York: Broadway Books, 2001.

WOMEN'S HEALTH

Love, Susan, M.D. *Dr. Susan Love's Breast Book.* Reading, MA: Addison-Wesley, 1990.

Love, Susan, M.D. *Dr. Susan Love's Hormone Book.* New York, NY: Times Books, 1998.

Northrup, Christiane, M.D. *Women's Bodies, Women's Wisdom.* Revised edition. New York, NY: Bantam Books, 1998.

Northrup, Christiane, M.D. *The Wisdom of Menopause.* New York, NY: Bantam Books, 2001.

References

Chapter 1: Breast Cancer Epidemic

www.cancer.org

Keyserlink, J.R., P.D. Ahlgren, E. Yu, et al. "Functional infrared imaging of the breast." Journal of IEEE, *Engineering in Medicine & Biology Magazine* Vol. 19. (May/June 2000): 30–41.

Mettlin, C. "Global breast cancer mortality statistics." *CA: A Cancer Journal for Clinicians* Vol. 49. (May/June 1999): 138–144.

Parisky, Y.R., A. Sardi, R. Hamm, et al. "Efficacy of computerized infrared imaging analysis to evaluate mammographically suspicious lesions." *American Journal of Roentgenology* Vol. 180. (Jan 2003): 263–269.

Chapter 2: Rediscovering Ancient Healing

Chopra, Deepak, M.D. *Perfect Health*. New York. NY: Harmony Books, 1991.

Sharma, Hari, M.D., and Christopher Clark, M.D. *Contemporary Ayurveda*. New York, NY: Churchill Livingstone, 1998.

Chapter 3: The Birth of the Beast

Arnot, B. *The Breast Cancer Prevention Diet*. Boston, MA: Little, Brown & Co., 1998.

Almada, A. "Brevail: SDG precision standardized flaxseed extract." *Scientific Research Monograph*. San Diego, CA: Lignan Research, 2003.

Lee, J. *What Your Doctor May Not Tell You About Breast Cancer*. New York, NY: Warner Books, 2002.

Love, Susan, M.D. *Dr. Susan Love's Breast Book*. Reading, MA: Addison-Wesley, 1990.

Chapter 4: Your Inner Healing Intelligence

Sharma, Hari, M.D., and Christopher Clark, M.D. *Contemporary Ayurveda*. New York, NY: Churchill Livingstone, 1998.

Chapter 5: The Intelligence of Plants

Arnot, B. *The Breast Cancer Prevention Diet*. Boston, MA: Little, Brown & Co., 1998.

About organic. Organic Farming Research Foundation www.ofrf.org/about_organic/index.html 1998.

De Santos, Silva I., P. Mangtani, V. McCormack, et al. "Lifelong vegetarianism and risk of breast cancer: a population-based case-control study among South Asian migrant women living in England." *International Journal of Cancer* Vol. 99. (May 10, 2002): 238–244.

Howe, G.R., T. Hirohata, T.G. Hislop, et al. "Dietary factors and risk of breast cancer: combines analysis of 12 case-control studies." *Journal of the National Cancer Institute* Vol. 82. (April 4, 1990): 561–569.

Hulten, K., A.L. Van Kappel, A. Winkvist, et al. "Carotenoids, alpha-tocopherols, and retinol in plasma and breast cancer in northern Sweden." *Cancer Causes Control* Vol. 12. (August 2001): 529–537.

La Marchand, L. "Cancer preventative effects of flavonoids—a review." *Biomedical Pharmacotherapy* Vol. 56. (Aug 2002): 296–301.

Le Vecchia, C., A. Altieri, and A. Tavani. "Vegetables, fruits, antioxidants and cancer: a review of Italian studies." *European Journal of Nutrition* Vol. 40. (Dec 2001): 261–267.

Levi, F., C. Pasche, F. Lucchini, et al. "Dietary intake of selected micronutrients and breast cancer risk." *International Journal of Cancer* Vol. 91. (Jan 15, 2001): 260–263.

McCarty, M.F. "Vegan proteins may reduce risk of cancer, obesity, and cardiovascular disease by promoting increased glucagon activity." *Medical Hypotheses* Vol. 53. (Dec 1999): 459–485.

Peterson, J., P. Lagiou, E. Samoli, et al. "Flavonoid intake and breast cancer risk: a case-controlled study in Greece." *British Journal of Cancer* Vol. 89. (Oct 6, 2003): 1255–1259.

Piernick, E. "The color of health." www.organicfrog.com/pub.article2.asp The Organic Frog Inc., 2002.

Ronco, A., E. De Stefani, P. Boffetta, et al. "Vegetables, fruits, and related nutrients and risk of breast cancer: a case control study in Uruguay." *Nutrition & Cancer* Vol. 35. (Issue 2, 1999): 111–119.

Segasothy, M., and P.A. Phillips. "Vegetarian diet: panacea for modern lifestyle diseases?" *QJM: An International Journal of Medicine* QJM: monthly journal of the Association of Physicians Vol. 92. (Sept 1999): 531–544.

Smith-Warner, S., D. Spiegelman, and S.S. Yaun. "Intake of fruits and vegetables and risk of breast cancer." *Journal of the American Medical Association (JAMA)* Vol. 285. (Feb 14, 2001): 769–776.

Toniolo, P., A.L. Van Kappel, A. Akhmedkhanov, et al. "Serum carotenoids and breast cancer." *American Journal of Epidemiology* Vol. 153. (Jun 15, 2001): 1142–1147.

Worthington, V. "Nutritional quality of organic verses conventional fruits, vegetables, and grains." *Journal of Alternative & Complementary Medicine* Vol. 7. (Issue 2, 2001): 161–173.

Cruciferous Vegetables

Ashok, B.T., Y. Chen, X. Liu, et al. "Abrogation of estrogen-mediated cellular and biochemical effects by indole-3 carbinol." *Nutrition & Cancer* Vol. 41. (Issue 1-2, 2001): 180–187.

Ashok, B.T., Y. Chen, X. Liu, et al. "Multiple molecular targets of indole-3 carbinol, a chemopreventative anti-estrogen in breast cancer." *European Journal of Cancer Prevention* Vol. 11. (Aug 2002; Suppl 2): S86–S93.

Brignall, M.S. "Prevention and treatments of cancer with indole-3 carbinol." *Alternative Medicine Review* Vol. 6. (Dec 2001): 580–589.

Fahey, J.W., Y. Zhang, and P. Talalay. "Broccoli sprouts: an exceptionally rich source of inducers of enzymes that protect against chemical carcinogens." *Proceedings of the National Academy of Science USA* Vol. 94. (Sept 16, 1997): 10367–10372.

Guthrie, C. "Why Eat Your Broccoli?" *Yoga Journal.* (March/April 2002).

Hanausek, M., Ph.D., Z. Walaszek, Ph.D., and T.J. Slaga, Ph.D. "Detoxifying Cancer Causing Agents to Prevent Cancer." *Integrative Cancer Therapies* Vol. 2. (Issue 2, 2003): 139–144.

Lord, R.S., B. Bongiovanni, and J.A. Bralley. "Estrogen metabolism and the diet-cancer connection: rationale for assessing the ratio of urinary hydroxylated estrogen metabolites." *Alternative Medicine Review* Vol. 7. (Apr 2002): 112–129.

Meng, Q., I.D. Goldberg, E.M. Rosen, et al. "Inhibitory effects of Indole-3 carbinol on invasion and migration in human breast cancer cells." *Breast Cancer Research & Treatment* Vol. 63. (Sept 2000): 147–152.

Meng, Q., M. Qi, D.Z. Chen, et al. "Suppression of breast cancer invasion and migration by indole-3 carbinol: associated with up-regulation of the BRCA1 and E-cadherin/catenin complexes." *Journal of Molecular Medicine* Vol. 78. (Issue 3, 2000): 155–165.

Meng, Q., F. Yuan, I.D. Goldberg, et al. "Indole-3 carbinol is a negative regulator of estrogen receptor-alpha signaling in human tumor cells." *Journal of Nutrition* Vol. 12. (Dec 2000): 2927–2931.

Oganesian, A., J.D. Hendricks, and D.E. Williams. "Long term dietary indole-3 carbinol inhibits diethylnitrosamine-initiated hepatocarcinogenesis in the infant mouse." *Cancer Letters* Vol. 18. (Sept 16, 1997): 87–94.

Rahman, K.M., O. Aranha, A. Glazyrin, et al. "Translocation of Bax to mitochondria induces apoptotic cell death in indol-3 carbinol (I3C) treated breast cancer cells." *Oncogene* Vol. 19. (Nov 23, 2000): 5764–5771.

Rahman, K.M., O. Aranha, and F.H. Sarkar. "Indole-3 carbinol induces apoptosis in tumorigenic but not in nontumorigenic breast epithelial cells." *Nutrition & Cancer* Vol. 45. (Issue 1, 2003): 101–112.

Riby, J.E., G.H. Chang, G.L. Firestone, et al. "Lignand-independent activation of estrogen receptor function by 3,3' diindolylmethane in human breast cancer cells." *Biochemical Pharmacology* Vol. 60. (Jul 15, 2000): 167–177.

Riby, J.E., C. Feng, Y.C. Chang, et al. "The major cyclic trimeric product of indole-3 carbinol is a strong agonist of the estrogen receptor signaling pathway." *Biochemistry* Vol. 39. (Feb 8, 2000): 910–918.

Sepkovic, D.W., H.L. Bradlow, and M. Bell. "Quantitative determination of 3,3' diindolylmethane in urine of individuals receiving indole-3 carbinol." *Nutrition & Cancer* Vol. 41. (Issue 1-2, 2001): 57–63.

Stoner, G., B. Casto, S. Ralston, et al. "Development of a multi-organ rat model for evaluation chemoprotective agents: efficacy of indole-3 carbinol." *Carcinogenisis* Vol. 23. (Feb 2002): 265–272.

Telang, N.T., H.L. Bradlow, and M.P. Osborne. "Molecular and endocrine biomarkers in noninvolved breast: relevance to cancer chemoprevention." *Journal of Cellular Biochemistry.* (16G, 1992): 161–169.

"Calcium-D-Gluterate." *Alternative Medicine Review: A Journal of Clinical Therapeutic* Vol. 7. (Aug 2002): 336–339.

Chapter 6: Mother Nature Knows Best

Bernstein, I.L., J. A. Bernstein, M. Miller, et al. "Immune Responses in farm workers after exposure to *Bacillus thuringiensis* pesticides." *Environmental Health Perspectives* Vol. 107. (July 1999): 575–582.

Bradlow, H.L., D.L. Davis, G. Lin, et al. "Effects of pesticides on the ratio of 16 alpha/2-hydroxyestrone: a biologic marker of breast cancer risk." *Environmen-*

tal Health Perspectives Vol. 103 Supplement. (Oct 1995): 147–150.

Cabello, G., A. Juarranz, L.M. Botella, et al. "Organophosphorous pesticides in breast cancer progression." Journal of Submicroscopic Cytology & Pathology Vol. 35. (Jan 2003): 1–9.

Coco, P., N. Kazerouni, and S.H. Zahm. "Cancer mortality and environmental exposure to DDE in the United States." Environmental Health Perspectives Vol. 108. (Jan 2000): 1–4.

Davis, J. "Alleviating political violence through enhancing coherence in collective consciousness: impact assessment amlusis of the Lebanon war." Dissertations & Abstracts International Vol. 49. (Issue 8, 1988): 2381A.

Demers, A., P. Ayotte, J. Brisson, et al. "Risk and aggressiveness of breast cancer in relation to plasma organochlorine concentrations." Cancer Epidemiology, Biomarkers & Prevention Vol. 9. (Feb 2000): 161–166.

"Environmental estrogens and other hormones." Tulane University website: www.tmc.tulane.edu/ecme/eehome/basics/

Epstein, S. "Pesticides and Cancer." Transcript of lecture given in 1993.

Guttes, S., K. Failing, K. Neumann, et al. "Chlororganic pesticides and polychlorinated biphenyls in breast tissue of women with benign and malignant breast disease." Archives of Environmental Contamination and Toxicology Vol. 35. (Jul 1998): 140–147.

Horner, C., M.D. "Organic means pure food." Channelcincinnati.com. June 9, 2001.

Horner, C., M.D. "GE food questioned." Channelcincinnati.com. May 15, 2001.

Horner, C., M.D. "Genetically engineered foods." Channelcincinnati.com. May 17, 2001.

Hoyer, A., T. Jorgensen, P. Grandjean, et al. "Repeated measurements of organochlorine exposure and breast cancer risk (Denmark)." Cancer Causes and Control Vol. 11. (Feb 2000): 177–184.

Hoyer, A.P., P. Grandjean, T. Jorgensen, et al. "Organochlorine compounds and breast cancer—is there a connection between environmental pollution and breast cancer." Ugeskr Laeger Vol. 162. (Feb 14, 2000): 922–926.

Hoyer, A.P., T. Jorgensen, J.W. Brock, et al. "Organochlorine exposure and breast cancer survival." Journal of Clinical Epidemiology Vol. 53. (Mar 2000): 323–330.

Jaga, K., and D. Brosius. "Pesticide exposure: human cancers on the horizon." Reviews on Environmental Health Vol. 14. (Jan-Mar 1999): 39–50.

Jaga, K., and H. Duvvi. "Risk reduction for DDT toxicity and carcinogenesis through dietary modifications." Journal of the Royal Society of Health Vol. 121. (Jun 2001): 107–113.

Mathur, V., P. Bhatnagar, R.G. Sharma, et al. "Breast cancer incidence and exposure to pesticides among women originating from Jaipur." Environment International Vol. 28. (Nov 2002): 331–336.

Moysich, K.B., C.B. Ambrosone, P. Mendola, et al. "Exposures associated with serum organochlorine levels among postmenopausal women from western New York State." American Journal of Industrial Medicine Vol. 41. (Feb 2002): 102–110.

Northwest Coalition for Alternatives to Pesticides (NCAP). "Are pesticides hazardous to our health." Journal of Pesticide Reform Vol. 19. (Issue 2, 1999): 2–3.

Organic trade association website for new organic standards, www.ota.com.

Orme-Johnson, D.W., C.N. Alexander, J.L. Davies, et al. "International peace project in the Middle East: the effects of Maharishi Technology of the Unified Field." Journal of Conflict Resolution Vol. 32. (1988): 776–812.

Worthington, V. "Effects of agriculture methods on nutritional quality: a comparison of organic and conventional crops." Alternative Therapies in Health & Medicine Vol. 4. (Jan 1998): 58–69.

Chapter 7: Fields of Gold

Arts, C.J., C.A. Govers, H. Van den berg, et al. "Effect of wheat bran on excretion of radioactively labeled estradiol-17 beta and estrone-glucuronide injected intravenously in male rats." Journal of Steroid Biochemistry & Molecular Biology Vol. 42. (Mar 1992): 103–111.

Arts, C.J., and J.H. Thijssen. "Effects of wheat bran on blood and tissue hormone levels in adult female rats." Acta Endocrinologica (Copenhagen) Vol. 127. (Sep 1992): 271–278.

Challier, B., J.M. Perarnau, and J.F. Viel. "Garlic, onion, and cereal fiber as protective factors for breast cancer: French case control study." European Journal of Epidemiology Vol. 14. (Dec 1998): 737–747.

Pena-Rosas, J.P., S. Rickard, and S. Cho. "Wheat bran and breast cancer: revisiting the estrogen hypothesis." Archivos Latinoamericanos de Nutricion Vol. 49. (Dec 1999): 309–317.

Slavin, J. "Why whole grains are protective: biological mechanisms." Proceedings of the Nutrition Society Vol. 62. (Feb 2003): 129–134.

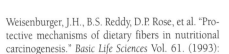 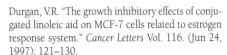

Weisenburger, J.H., B.S. Reddy, D.P. Rose, et al. "Protective mechanisms of dietary fibers in nutritional carcinogenesis." *Basic Life Sciences* Vol. 61. (1993): 45–63.

Chapter 8: Fats—The Good and the Bad

Arnot, B. *The Breast Cancer Prevention Diet.* Boston, MA: Little, Brown & Co., 1998.

Bagga, D. "Dietary modulation of Omega-3/Omega-6 poly-unsaturated fatty acids ratios in patients with breast cancer." *Journal of the National Cancer Institute* Vol. 89. (Issue 15, 1997): 1123–1131.

Barrett-Conner, E., and N.J. Friedlander. "Dietary fat, calories, and the risk of breast cancer in postmenopausal women: a prospective population based study." *Journal of the American College of Nutrition* Vol 12. (Aug 1993): 390–399.

Cho, E., et al. "Premenopausal fat intake and the risk of breast cancer." *Journal of the National Cancer Institute* Vol. 95. (Jul 2003): 1079–1085.

Nettleton, J. "Omega-3s shine at international fatty acid conference." *Holistic Primary Care.* (Oct 15, 2002).

Simopoulos, A.P. "The importance of the ratio of Omega-6/Omega-3 essential fatty acids." *Biomedicine & Pharmacotherapy* Vol. 56. (Oct 2002): 365–379.

Stannard, E. "Depression, brain cells, and essential fatty acids." *Well Being Journal.* (Issue 7, 2000): 8–9.

Stoll, A.L. "The Omega-3 solution fatty acids fight heart disease, arthritis, obesity and more." *Bottom Line Health.* (June 2001).

Stoll, A.L., W.E. Severus, M.P. Freeman, et al. "Omega-3 fatty acids in bipolar disorder: a preliminary double-blind, placebo-controlled trial." *Archive of General Psychiatry* Vol. 56. (May 1999): 407–412.

Conjugated Linoleic Acid (CLA)

Aro, A., S. Mannisto, and I. Salminen. "Inverse association between dietary and serum conjugated linoleic acid and the risk of breast cancer in postmenopausal women." *Nutrition & Cancer* Vol. 38. (Issue 2, 2000): 151–157.

Chajes, V., F. Lavillonniere, and V. Maillard. "Conjugated linoleic acid content in breast adipose tissue of breast cancer patients and the risk of metastasis." *Nutrition & Cancer* Vol. 45. (Issue 1, 2003): 17–23.

Cunningham, D.C., L.Y. Harrison, and T.D. Shultz. "Proliferative response of normal mammary and MCF-& breast cancer cells to linoleic acid, conjugated linoleic acid, and eicosanoid synthesis inhibitors in culture." *Anticancer Research* Vol. 17. (Jan-Feb 1997): 197–203.

Durgan, V.R. "The growth inhibitory effects of conjugated linoleic aid on MCF-7 cells related to estrogen response system." *Cancer Letters* Vol. 116. (Jun 24, 1997): 121–130.

Ip, C., and J.A. Scimeca. "Conjugated linoleic acid and linoleic acid are distinctive modulators of mammary carcinogenesis." *Nutrition & Cancer* Vol. 27. (Issue 2, 1997): 131–135.

Ip, C., S.F. Chin, J.A. Scimeca, et al. "Mammary cancer prevention by conjugated deinoic derivative of linoleic acid." *Cancer Research* Vol 51. (Nov 15, 1991): 6118–6124.

Ip, C., J.A. Scimeca, and H.J. Thompson. "Conjugated linoleic acid. A powerful anticarcinogen from animal fat sources." *Cancer* Vol. 74. (Aug 1, 1994; 3 Suppl): 1050–1054.

Mjumder, B., K.W. Wahle, and S. Moir. "Conjugated linoleic acids (CLAs) regulate the expression of key apoptotic genes in human breast cancer cells." *The FASEB Journal* Vol. 16. (Sep 2002): 1447–1449.

Thompson, H., Z. Zhu, and S. Banni. "Morphological and biochemical status of the mammary gland as influenced by conjugated linoleic acid: implications for a reduction in mammary cancer risk." *Cancer Research* Vol. 15. (Nov 1997): 5067–5072.

Visonneau, S., A. Cesano, S.A. Tepper, et al. "Conjugated linoleic acid suppresses the growth of human breast adenocarcinoma cells in SCID mice." *Anticancer Research* Vol. 17. (Mar-Apr 1997): 969–973.

rBGH

Chen, J., P.M. Starvo, and L.U. Thompson. "Dietary Flaxseed inhibits human breast cancer growth and metastasis and down regulates expression of insulin-like growth factor and epidermal growth factor receptor." *Nutrition & Cancer* Vol. 43. (Issue 2, 2002): 187–192.

Epstein, S. "Monsanto's hormonal milk poses serious risks of breast cancer." *PRNewswire.* (Jun 22, 1998).

Krajcik, R.A., N.D. Borofsky, S. Massardo, et al. "Insulin-like growth factor I (IGF-1), IGF-binding proteins, and breast cancer." *Cancer Epidemiology, Biomarkers & Prevention* Vol. 11. (Dec 2002): 1566–1573.

Larsen, Hans. "Milk and the cancer connection." *International Health News.* (April 1998).

Martin, M.B., and A. Stoica. "Insulin-like growth factor-I and estrogen interactions in breast cancer." *Journal of Nutrition* Vol. 132. (Dec 2002): 3799S–3801S.

Outwater, J.L., A. Nicholson, and N. Barnard. "Dairy products and breast cancer: the IGF-1, estrogen, and rBGH hypothesis." *Medical Hypotheses* Vol. 48. (Jun 1997): 453–461.

Schmitz, K.H., R.L. Ahmed, and D. Yee. "Effects of a 9-month strength training intervention on insulin, insulin-like growth factor (IGF-1), IGF-binding protein (IGFBP)-1, and IGFBP-3 in 30–50 year old women." *Cancer Epidemiology, Biomarkers & Prevention* Vol. 11. (Dec 2002): 1597–1604.

Silva, J., A. Beckedorf, and E. Bieberich. "Osteoblast-derived oxysterol is a migration-inducing factor for human breast cancer cells." *Journal of Biology & Chemistry* (May 6, 2003). www.ncbi.nlm.nih.gov/entrez/query.fcgi?cmd=Retrieve&db=journals&list_uids=4559&dopt=full.

Chapter 9: A Fortress Made of Seeds

Alexander, J.W. "Immunonutrition: the role of Omega-3 fatty acids." *Nutrition* Vol. 14. (Jul-Aug 1998): 627–633.

Almada, A. "Brevail: SDG precision standardized flaxseed extract." *Scientific Research Monograph.* (2003).

Barlean's Organic Oils. "A very important message to women: Lignans reduce risk and spread of malignant disease." *The Breast Cancer Prevention Files: The Doctor's Prescription for Healthy Living* Vol. 4. (Issue 10).

Chajes, V., W. Sattler, A. Stranzl, et al. "Influence of n-3 fatty acids on the growth of human breast cancer cells in vitro: relationship to peroxides and vitamin E." *Breast Cancer Research & Treatment* Vol. 34. (Jun 1995): 199–212.

Chen, J., P.M. Starvo, and L.U. Thompson. "Dietary Flaxseed inhibits human breast cancer growth and metastasis and down regulates expression of insulin-like growth factor and epidermal growth factor receptor." *Nutrition & Cancer* Vol. 43. (Issue 2, 2002): 187–192.

Dabrosin, C., J. Chen, L. Wang, et al. "Flaxseed inhibits metastasis and decreases extracellular vascular endothelial growth factoring human breast cancer xenografts." *Cancer Letters* Vol. 185. (Nov 2002): 31–37.

Fife, B. "The Facts on flax." *Saturated Fats May Save Your Life.* Website: www.Coconut-info.com/facts_on_flax.htm.

Haggens, C.J., A.M. Hutchins, B.A. Olson, et al. "Effects of flaxseed consumption on urinary estrogen metabolites in postmenopausal women." *Nutrition & Cancer* Vol. 33. (Issue 2, 1999): 188–195.

Haggans, C.J., E.J. Travelli, W. Thomas, et al. "The effects of flaxseed and wheat bran consumption on urinary estrogen metabolites in premenopausal women." *Cancer Epidemiology, Biomarkers & Prevention* Vol. 9. (Jul 2000): 719–725.

Horner, C., M.D. "Flax: the food no home should be without." Channelcincinnati.com. (Mar 15, 2001).

Kurzer, M.S., J.W. Lampe, M.C. Martini, et al. "Fecal Lignan and isoflavonoid excretion in premenopausal women consuming flaxseed powder." *Cancer Epidemiology, Biomarkers & Prevention* Vol. 4. (Jun 1995): 353–358.

McCann, S.E., K.B. Moyisch, J.L. Freudenheim, et al. "The risk of breast cancer associated with dietary lignans differs by CYP17 genotype in women." *Journal of Nutrition* Vol. 132. (Oct 2002): 3035–3041.

Phippes, W.R., M.C. Martini, J.W. Lampe, et al. "Effects of flax seed ingestion on the menstrual cycle." *The Journal of Clinical Endocrinology & Metabolism* Vol. 77. (Nov 1993): 1215–1219.

Simopolus, A.P. "Essential fatty acids in health and chronic disease." *American Journal of Clinical Nutrition* Vol. 70. (Sep 1999; 3 Suppl): 560S–569S.

Ward, W.E., F.O. Jiang, and L.U. Thompson. "Exposure to flaxseed or purified lignan during lactation influences rat mammary gland structures." *Nutrition & Cancer* Vol. 37. (Issue 2, 2000): 187–192.

Chapter 10: Asian Defense

Allred, C.D., K.F. Allred, H.J. Young, et al. "Soy processing influences growth of estrogen-dependent breast cancer tumors in mice." *Carcinogenesis* Vol. 25. (Sep 2004): 1649–1657.

Bouker, K.B., and L. Hilakivi-Clarke. "Genistein: does it prevent or promote breast cancer?" *Environmental Health Perspectives* Vol. 108. (Aug 2000): 701–708.

Dai, Q., A.A. Franke, F. Jin, et al. "Urinary excretion of phytoestrogens and risk of breast cancer among Chinese women in Shanghai." *Cancer Epidemiology, Biomarkers & Prevention* Vol. 11. (Issue 9, 2002): 815–821.

"Environmental estrogens and other hormones: phytoestrogens." 2001. Website: www.com.tulane.edu/ecme/eehome/basics/phytoestrogens/.

Ghen, M. "Supplements and alternatives." *International Journal of Integrative Medicine* Vol. 3. (Issue 3, 2001): 37–38.

Hargreaves, D.F., C.S. Potten, C. Harding, et al. "Two-week dietary soy supplementation has an estrogenic effect on normal premenopausal breast." *Journal of Clinical Endocrinology & Metabolism* Vol. 84. (Nov 1999): 4017–4024.

Ingram, D., K. Sanders, M. Kolybaba, et al. "Case-control study of phyto-estrogens and breast cancer." *The Lancet* Vol. 350. (Issue 9083, 1997): 990–994.

Kishida, T., M. Beppu, et al. "Effects of dietary soy isoflavone aglycones on the urinary 16 alpha-to-22 hydroxyestrone ratio in C3H/HeJ mice." *Nutrition & Cancer* Vol. 38. (Issue 2, 2000): 209–214.

Lal, A., S. Warber, and A. Kirakosyan. "Upregulation of isoflavonoids and soluble proteins in edible legumes by light and fungal elicitor treatments." *Journal of Alternative & Complementary Medicine* Vol. 9. (Issue 3, 2003): 371–378.

Low Dog, T., D. Riley, and T. Carter. "Traditional and alternative therapies for breast cancer." *Alternative Therapies in Health & Medicine* Vol. 7. (Issue 3, 2001): 36–47.

Mercola, J. "The trouble with tofu: soy and the brain." Website: www.Mercolacom/2000/sept17/soy_brain. htm.

Peeters, P.H., L. Keinan-Boker, et al. "Phytoestrogens and breast cancer risk. Review of the epidemiological evidence." *Breast Cancer Research & Treatment* Vol. 77. (Jan 2003): 171–183.

Petrakis, N.L., S. Barnes, E.B. King, et al. "Stimulatory influence of soy protein on breast secretion in pre- and postmenopausal women." *Cancer Epidemiology, Biomarkers & Prevention* Vol. 5. (Oct 1996): 785–794.

Schmidl, M. "Soybeans and Nutraceuticals." 1999 lecture.

Stephens, F.O. "Breast cancer: Aetiological factors and associations (a possible protective role of phytoestrogens)." *Australia and New Zealand Journal of Surgery* Vol. 67. (Nov 1997): 755–760.

The Phytochemistry of Herbs Phytochemicals of the Month: November 2002: Phytoestrogens. Website: www.herbalchem.net/introductory.htm.

Weil, A. "CAM and continuing education: the future is now." *Alternative Therapies in Health & Medicine* Vol. 7. (Issue 3, 2001): 32–34.

Yamamoto, S., et al. "Soy, isoflavones, and breast cancer risk in Japan." *Journal of the National Cancer Institute* Vol. 95. (Jul 18, 2003): 906–913.

Zheng, W., Q. Dai, et al. "High isoflavone consumption can mean lower risk of breast cancer." *Cancer Epidemiology, Biomarkers & Prevention* Vol. 8. (Jan 1999): 35–40.

Chapter 11: Magic Mushrooms and More

Maitake Mushrooms

Berry, J. "Maitake." *Natural Health Magazine*. (Aug 2001).

Kidd, P.M. "The use of mushroom glucans and proteoglycans in cancer treatment." *Alternative Medicine Review* Vol. 5. (Feb 2000): 4–27.

Kodama, N., K. Komuta, and H. Nanba. "Can maitake MD-fraction aid cancer patients?" *Alternative Medicine Review* Vol. 7. (Jun 2002): 236–239.

Reishi Mushrooms

Hu, H., N.S. Ahn, X. Yang, et al. "Ganoderma lucidum extract induces cell cycle arrest and apoptosis in MCF-7 human breast cancer cells." *International Journal of Cancer* Vol. 102. (Nov 20, 2002): 250–253.

Lu, Q.Y., M.R. Sartippour, M.N. Brooks, et al. "Ganoderma lucidum spore extract inhibits endothelial and breast cancer cells in vitro." *Oncology Report* Vol. 12. (Sep 2004): 659–662.

Sliva, D. "Ganoderma lucidum (Reishi) in cancer treatment." *Integrative Cancer Therapies* Vol. 2. (Dec 2003): 358–364.

Sliva, D., M. Sedlak, V. Slivova, et al. "Biologic activity of spores and dried powder from Ganoderma lucidum for inhibition of highly invasive human breast and prostate cancer cells." *Journal of Alternative & Complementary Medicine* Vol. 9. (Aug 2003): 491–497.

Sliva, D., C. Labarrere, V. Slivova, et al. "Ganoderma lucidum suppresses motility of highly invasive breast and prostate cancer cells." *Biochemical and Biophysical Research Communications* Vol. 298. (Nov 8, 2002): 603–612.

Green Tea

Fijiki, H., M. Suganuma, S. Okabe, et al. "Mechanistic findings of green tea as a cancer preventative for humans." *Proceedings of the Society for Experimental Biology and Medicine* Vol. 220. (Apr 1999): 225–228.

Hirose, M., T. Hoshiya, K. Akagi, et al. "Inhibition of mammary gland carcinogenesis by green tea catechins and other naturally occurring antioxidants in female Sprague-Dawley rats pretreated with 7,12-dimethylbenz[alpha]anthracene." *Cancer Letters* Vol. 83. (Aug 15, 1994): 149–156.

Horner, C., M.D. "Green Tea: a hot healing beverage." Channelcincinnati.com. (Jan 9, 2001).

Nagata, C., M. Kabuto, and H. Shimizu. "Association of coffee, green tea, and caffeine intake with serum concentrations of estradiol and sex hormone-binding globulin in premenopausal Japanese women." *Nutrition & Cancer* Vol. 30. (Issue 1, 1998): 21–24.

Nakachi, K., K. Suemasu, K. Suga, et al. "Influence of drinking green tea on breast cancer malignancy among Japanese patients." *Japanese Journal of Cancer Research* Vol. 89. (Mar 1998): 254–261.

Sadzuka, Y., Y. Yamashita, and T. Sonobe. "Effect of dihydrokainate on the antitumor activity of doxorubicin." *Cancer Letters* Vol. 179. (May 28, 2002): 157–163.

Sadzuka, Y., T. Sugiyama, and T. Sonobe. "Efficacies of tea components on doxorubicin induced antitumor activity and reversal of multidrug resistance." *Toxicology Letters* Vol. 114. (Apr 3, 2000): 155–162.

Sadzuka, Y., T. Sugiyama, and S. Hirota. "Modulation of cancer chemotherapy by green tea." *Clinical Cancer Research* Vol. 4. (Jan 1998): 153–156.

Sadzuka, Y., T. Sugiyama, A. Miyagishima, et al. "The effects of theanine, as a novel biochemical modulator, on the antitumor activity of Adriamycin." *Cancer Letters* Vol. 105. (Aug 2, 1996): 203–209.

Sugiyama, T., and Y. Sadzuka. "Theanine and glutamate transporter inhibitor enhance the antitumor efficacy of chemotherapeutic agents." *Biochimica et Biophysica Acta* Vol. 1653. (Dec 5, 2003): 47–59.

Sugiyama, T., Y. Sadzuka, et al. "Inhibition of glutamate transporter by theanine enhances the therapeutic efficacy of doxorubicin." *Toxicology Letters* Vol. 121. (Apr 30, 2001): 89–96.

Sugiyama, T., and Y. Sadzuka. "Enhancing effects of green tea components on the antitumor activity of Adriamycin against M5076 ovarian sarcoma." *Cancer Letters* Vol. 133. (Nov 13, 1998): 19–26.

Tanaka, H., M. Hirose, M. Kawabe, et al. "Post-initiation inhibitory effects of green tea catechins on 7,12-dimethylbenz[alpha]anthracene-induced mammary gland carcinogenesis in female Sprauge Dawley rats." *Cancer Letters* Vol. 116. (Jun 1997): 47–52.

Valcic, S., B.N. Timmermann, D.S. Alberts, et al. "Inhibitory effect of six green tea catechins and caffeine on the growth of four selected human tumor cell lines." *Anticancer Drugs* Vol. 7. (Jun 1996): 461–468.

Turmeric

Polasa, K., T.C. Raghuram, T. Krishna, et al. "Effect of turmeric on urinary mutagens in smokers." *Mutagenesis* Vol. 7. (Issue 2, 1992): 107–109.

Ramachandran, C., H.B. Fonseca, and P. Jhabvala. "Curcumin inhibits telomerase activity through human telomerase reverse transcriptase in MCF-7 breast cancer cell lines." *Cancer Letters* Vol. 184. (Oct 8, 2002): 1–6.

Singletary, K., C. MacDonald, M. Iovinelli, et al. "Effect of the beta-diketones diferuloylmethane (curcumin) and dibenzoylmethane on rat mammary DNA adducts and tumor induced by 7,12-dimethylbenz[alpha]anthracene." *Carcinogenesis* Vol. 19. (Jun 1998): 1039–1043.

Verna, S.P., B.R. Goldin, and P.S. Lin. "The inhibition of estrogenic effects of pesticides and environmental chemicals by curcumin and isoflavonoids." *Environmental Health Perspectives* Vol. 106. (Dec 1998): 807–812.

Verma, S.P., E. Salamone, and B. Goldin. "Curcumin and genistein, plant natural products, show synergistic inhibitory effects on the growth of human breast cancer MCF-7 cells induced by estrogenic pesticides." *Biochemical and Biophysical Research Communications* Vol. 233. (Apr 28, 1997): 692–696.

Garlic

Amagase, H., and J. Milner. *The FASEB Journal* Vol. 6. (Issue 4, 1992): 3229.

Amagase, H., and J. Milner. "Impact of various sources of garlic and their constituents on 7-12-dimethylbenz[a]anthracene binding to mammary cell DNA." *Carcinogenesis* Vol. 14. (1993): 1627–1631.

Dong, Y., D. Lisk, E. Block, et al. "Characterization of the biological activity of gamma-glutamyl-Se-methylselesnocysteine:a novel, naturally occurring anticancer agent from garlic." *Cancer Research* Vol. 61. (Apr 1, 2001): 2923–2928.

Gued, L.R., R.D. Thomas, and M. Green. "Diallyl sulfide inhibits diethylstilbestrol-induced lipid peroxidation in breast tissue of female ACI rats: Implications in breast cancer prevention." *Oncology Report* Vol. 10. (May-Jun 2003): 739–743.

Hirsch, K., M. Danilenko, J. Giat, et al. "Effect of purified allicin, the major ingredient of freshly crushed garlic, on cancer cell proliferation." *Nutrition & Cancer* Vol. 38. (Issue 2, 2000): 245–254.

Horner, C., M.D. "Garlic: a common herb with uncommon benefits." Channelcincinnati.com. (2002).

Ip, C., D.J. Lisk, and H.J. Thompson. "Selenium-enriched garlic inhibits the early stage but not the late stage of mammary carcinogenesis." *Carcinogenesis* Vol. 17. (Sep 1996): 1979–1982.

Lin, J., J. Milner, et al. *Carcinogenesis* Vol. 13. (1992a): 1847–1851.

Milner, J., J. Liu. First World Congress on the Health Significance of Garlic and Garlic Constituents. (1990): 25.

Nakagawa, H., K. Tsuta, K. Kiuchi, et al. "Growth inhibitory effects of diallyl disulfide on human breast cancer cell lines." *Carcinogenesis* Vol. 22. (Jun 2001): 891–897.

Pinto, J.T., and R.S. Rivlin. "Antiproliferative effects of allium derivatives from garlic." *Journal of Nutrition* Vol. 131. (Mar 2001): 1058S–1060S.

Pinto, J., and R. Rivlin. "Recent Advances on the nutritional benefits accompanying the use of garlic as a supplement." Newport Beach, CA: Nov 15-17, 1998.

Tiwari, R., J. Pinto, et al. *Breast Cancer Research & Treatment* Vol. 27. (Issue 1-2, 1993): 80.

Seaweed

Cann, S.A., J.P. van Netten, and C. van Netten. "Hypothesis: iodine, selenium and the development of breast cancer." *Cancer Causes and Control* Vol. 11. (Feb 2000): 121–127.

Funahashi, H., T. Imai, T. Mase, et al. "Seaweed prevents breast cancer?" *Japanese Journal of Cancer Research* Vol. 92. (May 2001): 483–487.

Kilbane, M.T., R.A. Ajjan, A.P. Weetman, et al. "Tissue iodine content and serum mediated 125I uptake-blocking activity in breast cancer." *Journal of Clinical Endocrinology & Metabolism* Vol. 85. (Mar 2000): 1245–1250.

Smyth, P.P. "The thyroid and breast cancer: a significant association?" *Annals of Medicine* Vol. 29. (Jun 1997): 189–191.

Tasebay, U.H., I.L. Wapnir, O. Levy, et al. "The mammary gland iodine transporter is expressed during lactation and in breast cancer." *Natural Medicine* Vol. 6. (Aug 2000): 871–878.

Updhyay, G., R. Singh, G. Agarwal, et al. "Functional expression of sodium iodide symporter (NIS) in human breast cancer tissue." *Breast Cancer Research & Treatment* Vol. 77. (Jan 2003): 157–165.

Rosemary, Licorice, Black Cohosh, Vitex, Hops, and Chinese Herbs

Amato, P., S. Christophe, and P.L. Mellon. "Estrogenic activity of herbs commonly used as remedies for menopausal symptoms." *Menopause* Vol. 9. (Mar-Apr 2002): 145–150.

Bodinet, C., and J. Freudenstein. "Influence of marketed herbal menopause preparations on MCF-7 cell proliferation." *Menopause* Vol. 11. (May-Jun 2004): 281–289.

Campbell, M.J., B. Hamilton, M. Shoemaker, et al. "Antiproliferative activity of Chinese medicinal herbs on breast cancer cells in vitro." *Anticancer Research* Vol. 22. (Nov-Dec 2002): 3843–3852.

Dixon-Shanies, D., and N. Shaikh. "Growth inhibition of human breast cancer cells by herbs and phytoestrogens." *Oncology Report* Vol. 6. (Nov-Dec 1999): 1383–1387.

Duda, R.B., B. Taback, B. Kessel, et al. "pS2 expression induced by American ginseng in MCF-7 breast cancer cells." *Annals of Surgical Oncology* Vol. 3. (Nov 1996): 515–520.

Duda, R.B., Y. Zhong, V. Navas, et al. "American ginseng and breast cancer therapeutic agents synergistically inhibit MCF-7 breast cancer cell growth." *Journal of Surgical Oncology* Vol. 72. (Dec 1999): 230–239.

Duda, R.B., S. Kang, S.Y. Archer, et al. "American ginseng transcriptionally activiates p21 mRNA in breast cancer cell lines." *Journal of Korean Medical Science* Vol. 16 Suppl. (Dec 2001): S54–S60.

Einbond, L.S., M. Shimizu, D. Xiao, et al. "Growth inhibitory activity of extract and purified components of black cohosh on human breast cancer cells." *Breast Cancer Research & Treatment* Vol. 83. (Feb 2004): 221–231.

Hostanska, K., T. Nisslein, J. Freudenstein, et al. "Cimicifuga racemosa extract inhibits proliferation of estrogen receptor-positive and negative human breast carcinoma cell line by induction of apoptosis." *Breast Cancer Research & Treatment* Vol. 84. (Mar 2004): 151–160.

Jo, E.H., H.D. Hong, N.C. Ahn, et al. "Modulation of the Bcl-2/Bax family were involved in the chemopreventative effects of licorice root (Glycyrrhiza uralensis Fisch) in MCF-7 human breast cancer cell." *Journal of Agricultural and Food Chemistry* Vol. 52. (Mar 24, 2004): 1715–1719.

Lee, Y.J., Y.R. Jin, W.C. Lim, et al. "Ginsenoside-Rb1 acts as a weak phytoestrogen in MCF-7 human breast cancer cells." *Archives of Pharmaceutical Research* Vol. 26. (Jan 2003): 58–63.

Li, X.K., M. Motwani, W. Tong, et al. "Huanglian, A Chinese herbal extract, inhibits cell growth by suppressing the expression of cyclin B1 and inhibiting CDC2 kinase activity in human cancer cells." *Molecular Pharmacology* Vol. 58. (Dec 2000): 1287–1293.

Lupu, R., I. Mehmi, E. Atlas, et al. "Black cohosh, a menopausal remedy, does not have estrogenic activity and does not promote breast cancer cell growth." *International Journal of Oncology* Vol. 23. (Nov 2003): 1407–1412.

Maggiolini, M., G. Statti, A. Vivacqua, et al. "Estrogenic and antiproliferative activities of isoliquiritigenin in MCF7 breast cancer cells." *Journal of Steroid Biochemistry & Molecular Biology* Vol. 82. (Nov 2002): 315–322.

Miranda, C.L., J.F. Stevens, A. Helmrich, et al. "Antiproliferative and cytotoxic effects of prenylated flavonoids from hops (Humulus lupulus) in human cancer cell lines." *Food and Chemical Toxicology* Vol. 37. (Apr 1999): 271–285.

Oh, M.S., Y.H. Choi, H.Y. Chung, et al. "Anti-proliferative effects of ginsenoside RH2 on MCF-7 human breast cancer cells." *International Journal of Oncology* Vol. 14. (May 1999): 869–875.

Plouzek, C.A., H.P. Ciolino, R. Clarke, et al. "Inhibition of P-glycoprotein activity and reversal of multidrug resistance by in vitro rosemary extract." *Euro-*

pean Journal of Cancer Vol. 35. (Oct 1999): 1541–1545.

Rong, H., T. Boterberg, J. Maubach, et al. "8-Prenyl-naringenin, the phytoestrogen in hops and beer, up-regulates the function of E-cadherin/catenin complex in human mammary carcinoma cells." European Journal of Cell Biology Vol. 80. (Sep 2001): 580–585.

Singletary, K., C. MacDonald, and M. Wallig. "Inhibition of rosemary and carnosol of 7,12-dimethyl-benz[a] anthracene (DMBA)-induced rat mammary tumorigenesis and in vivo DMBA-DNA adduct formation." Cancer Letters Vol. 104. (Jun 24, 1996): 43–48.

Singletary, K., et al. "Inhibition of 7,12-dimethyl-benz[a] anthracene (DMBA)-induced mammary tumorigenesis and in vivo formation of mammary DM-BA-DNA adduct by rosemary extract." Cancer Letters Vol. 60. (Nov 1991): 169–175.

Sliva, D., M. Sedlak, V. Slivova, et al. "Biologic activity of spores and dried powder from Ganoderma lucidum for inhibition of highly invasive breast and prostate cancer cells." Journal of Alternative & Complementary Medicine Vol. 9. (Aug 2003): 491–497.

Tagliaferri, M., M.D., I. Cohen, O.M.D., L.Ac., D. Tripathy, M.D. Breast Cancer: Beyond Convention. New York: Atria Books, 2002.

Tamir, S., M. Eizenberg, D. Somjen, et al. "Estrogenic and antiproliferative properties of glabridin from licorice in human breast cancer cells." Cancer Research Vol. 60. (Oct 15, 2000): 5704–5709.

Zierau, O., C. Bodinet, S. Kolba, et al. "Antiestrogenic activity of Cimicifuga racemosa extracts." Journal of Steroid Biochemistry & Molecular Biology Vol. 80. (Jan 2002): 125–130.

Chapter 12: Mighty Micronutrients

Folate

Branda, R.F., J.P. O'Neill, D. Jacobson-Kram. "Factors influencing mutation at the hprt locus in T-lymphocytes: studies in normal women and women with benign and malignant breast masses." Environmental and Molecular Mutagenesis Vol. 19. (Issue 4, 1992): 274–281.

Laux, M. "Breast Cancer and Nutritional Supplements." www.ATDonline.org

Shrubsole, M.J., F. Jin, Q. Dai, et al. "Dietary folate intake and breast cancer risk: results from the Shanghi Breast Cancer Study." Cancer Research Vol. 61. (2001): 7136–7141.

Zhang, S., D.J. Hunter, and S.E. Hankinson. "A prospective study of folate intake and the risk of

breast cancer." Journal of the American Medical Association (JAMA) Vol. 281. (May 5, 1999): 1632–1637.

Zhang, S.M., W.C. Willett, J. Selhub, et al. "Plasma folate, vitamin B_6, vitamin B_{12}, homocysteine, and the risk of breast cancer." Journal of the National Cancer Institute Vol. 95. (Mar 5, 2003): 373–380.

Vitamin B_{12}

Choi, S.W. "Vitamin B_{12} deficiency: a new risk factor for breast cancer?" Nutrition Reviews Vol. 57. (1999): 250–253.

Zhang, S.M., W.C. Willett, J. Selhub, et al. "Plasma folate, vitamin B_6, vitamin B_{12}, homocysteine, and the risk of breast cancer." Journal of the National Cancer Institute Vol. 95. (Mar 5, 2003): 373–380.

Vitamin D

Bortman, P., M.A. Folgueira, M.L. Katayama, et al. "Antiproliferative effects of 1,25-dihydrocyvitamin D_3 on breast cells: a mini review." Brazil Journal of Medical & Biological Research Vol. 35. (Jan 2002): 1–9.

Garland, C.F., F.C. Garland, and E.D. Gorham. "Calcium and vitamin D. Their potential roles in colon and breast cancer prevention." Annals of the N Y Academy of Science Vol. 889. (1999): 107–119.

Lipkin, M., and H.L. Newmark. "Vitamin D Calcium and prevention of breast cancer: a review." Journal of the American College of Nutrition Vol. 18. (Oct 1999; 5 Suppl): 392S–397S.

Mehta, R.G., E.A. Hussin, R.R. Mehta, et al. "Chemoprevention of mammary carcinogenesis by 1 alpha-hydrocyvitamin D_5, a synthetic analog of Vitamin D." Mutation Research Vol. 523–524. (Feb-Mar 2003): 253–264.

Shin, M.H., M.D. Holmes, S.E. Hankinson, et al. "Intake of dairy products, calcium, and vitamin D and risk of breast cancer." Journal of the National Cancer Institute Vol. 94. (Sep 4, 2002): 1301–1311.

Vitamin E

Ambrosone, C.B., J.R. Marshall, J.E. Vena, et al. "Interaction of family history of breast cancer and dietary antioxidants with breast cancer risk." Cancer Causes and Control Vol. 6. (Sep 1995): 407–415.

Dabrosin, C., and K. Ollinger. "Protection by alpha-tocopherol but not ascorbic acid from hydrogen peroxide induced cell death in normal human breast epithelial cells in culture." Free Radical Research Vol. 29. (Sep 1998): 227–234.

Malfa, M.P., and L.T. Neitzel. "Vitamin E succinate promotes breast cancer tumor dormancy." Journal of Surgical Research Vol. 93. (Sep 2000): 163–170.

Schwenke, D.C. "Does lack of tocopherols and to-cotrienols put women at increased risk of breast cancer?" *Journal of Nutrition & Biochemistry* Vol. 13. (Jan 2002): 2–10.

Yu, W., M. Simmons-Menchaca, A. Gapor, et al. "Induction of apoptosis in human breast cancer cells by tocopherols and tocotrienols." *Nutrition & Cancer* Vol. 33. (Issue 1, 1999): 26–32.

Chapter 13: Defense Shields

Austin, S. "Antioxidants and chemotherapy-a rebuttal." *Healthnotes Review of Complementary & Integrative Medicine* (HNR) Vol. 6. (Issue 4, 1999): 234–236.

Ching, S., D. Ingram, R. Hahnel, et al. "Serum levels of micronutrients, antioxidants and total antioxidant status predict risk of breast cancer in a case control study." *Journal of Nutrition* Vol. 132. (Feb 2002): 303–306.

Lamson, D.W., and M. Brignall. "Antioxidants in cancer therapy; their actions and interactions with oncologic therapies." *Alternative Medicine Review* Vol. 4. (Issue 5, 1999): 304–329.

Prasad, K.N., A. Kumar, V. Kochupillai, et al. "High dose of multiple antioxidant vitamins: essential ingredient in improving the efficacy of standard cancer therapy." *Journal of the American College of Nutrition* Vol. 18. (Issue 1, 1999): 13–25.

Simon, M.S., Z. Djuric, B. Dunn, et al. "An evaluation of plasma antioxidant levels and the risk of breast cancer: a pilot case control study." *Breast Journal* Vol. 6. (Nov 2000): 388–395.

Selenium

Cann, S.A., J.P. van Netten, and C. van Netten. "Hypothesis: iodine, selenium and the development of breast cancer." *Cancer Causes and Control* Vol. 11. (Feb 2000): 121–127.

Clark, L.C., G.F. Combs, B.W. Turnball, et al. "Effects of selenium supplementation for cancer prevention in patients with carcinoma of the skin. A randomized controlled trial. Nutritional Prevention of Cancer Study Group." *Journal of the American Medical Association* (JAMA) Vol. 276. (Dec 25, 1997): 1957–1963.

Dong, Y., D. Lisk, E. Block, et al. "Characterization of the biological activity of gamma-glutamyl-Se-methylselenocysteine: a novel, naturally occurring anticancer agent from garlic." *Cancer Research* Vol. 61. (Apr 1, 2001): 2923–2928.

Horner, C., M.D. "Trace minerals: selenium." Channelcincinati.com. (Feb 23, 2002).

Ip, C., M. Birringer, E. Block, et al. "Chemical speci-

ation influences comparative activity of selenium-enriched garlic and yeast in mammary cancer prevention." *Journal of Agricultural and Food Chemistry* Vol. 48 (Jun 2000): 2062–2070.

Ip, C., D.J. Lisk, and H.J. Thompson. "Selenium-enriched garlic inhibits the early stage but not the late stage of mammary carcinogenesis." *Carcinogenesis* Vol. 17. (Sep 1996): 1979–1982.

Food Chemistry Vol. 48. (Jun 2000): 2062–2070.

Jiang, C., W. Jiang, C. Ip, et al. "Selenium-induced inhibition of angiogenesis in mammary cancer at chemopreventative levels of uptake." *Molecular Carcinogenesis* Vol. 26. (Dec 1999): 213–225.

Sinha, R., E. Unni, H.E. Ganther, et al. "Methylseleninic acid, a potent growth inhibitor of synchronized mouse mammary epithelial tumor cells in vitro." *Biochemical Pharmacology* Vol. 61. (Feb 1, 2001): 311–317.

Vadgama, J.V., Y. Wu, S. Hsia, et al. "Anti-neoplastic properties of selenium in various cancers." *Proceedings of the American Association of Cancer Research*. (Mar 1999): 40.

Vadgama, J.V., Y. Wu, D. Shen, et al. "Effect of selenium in combination with Adriamycin and Taxol on several different cancer cells." *Anticancer Research* Vol. 20. (May-Jun 2000): 1391–1414.

Vitamin E

Ambrosone, C.B., J.R. Marshall, J.E. Vena, et al. "Interaction of family history of breast cancer and dietary antioxidants with breast cancer risk." *Cancer Causes and Control* Vol. 6. (Sep 1995): 407–415.

Dabrosin, C., and K. Ollinger. "Protection by alpha-tocopherol but not ascorbic acid from hydrogen peroxide induced cell death in normal human breast epithelial cells in culture." *Free Radical Research* Vol. 29. (Sep 1998): 227–234.

Malfa, M.P., and L.T. Neitzel. "Vitamin E succinate promotes breast cancer tumor dormancy." *Journal of Surgical Research* Vol. 93. (Sep 2000): 163–170.

Schwenke, D.C. "Does lack of tocopherols and to-cotrienols put women at increased risk of breast cancer?" *The Journal of Nutritional Biochemistry* Vol. 13. (Jan 2002): 2–10.

Yu, W., M. Simmons-Menchaca, A. Gapor, et al. "Induction of apoptosis in human breast cancer cells by tocopherols and tocotrienols." *Nutrition & Cancer* Vol. 33. (Issue 1, 1999): 26–32.

CoQ$_{10}$

Folkers, K., A. Osterborg, M. Nylander, et al. "Activities of vitamin Q$_{10}$ in animal models and a serious deficiency in patients with cancer." *Biochemical and Biophysical Research Communications* Vol. 234. (May 19, 1997): 296–299.

Horner, C., M.D. "CoQ$_{10}$." Channelcincinnati.com. (Apr 5, 2001).

Lockwood, K., S. Moesgaard, T. Yamamoto, et el. "Progress on therapy of breast cancer with vitamin Q$_{10}$ and the regression of metastases." *Biochemical and Biophysical Research Communications* Vol. 212. (Jul 6, 1995): 172–177.

Lockwood, K., S. Moesgaard, and K. Folkers. "Apparent partial remission of breast cancer in 'high risk' patients supplemented with nutritional antioxidants, essential fatty acids and coenzyme Q$_{10}$." *Molecular Aspects of Medicine* Vol. 15. (1994; Suppl): S231–S240.

Lockwood, K., S. Moesgaard, and K. Folkers. "Partial and complete regression of breast cancer in patients in relation to dosage of coenzyme Q$_{10}$." *Biochemical and Biophysical Research Communications* Vol. 199. (Mar 30, 1994): 1504–1508.

Portakal, O., O. Ozkaya, et al. "Coenzyme Q$_{10}$ concentrations and antioxidant status in tissues of breast cancer patients." *Clinical Biochemistry* Vol. 33. (Issue 4, 2000): 279–284.

Amrit Kalash

Dileepan, K.N., S.T. Varghese, et al. "Enhanced lymphoproliferative response, macrophage mediated tumor cell killing and nitric oxide production after ingestion of an Ayurvedic drug." *Biochemistry Archives* Vol. 9. (1993): 365–374.

Horner, C., M.D. "Amrit Kalash." Channelcincinnati.com. (Mar 24, 2001).

Misra, N.C., H.M. Sharma, A. Chaturvedi, et al. "Antioxidant adjuvant therapy using a natural herbal mixture (MAK) during intensive chemotherapy: reduction in toxicity." *Proceedings of the XVI International Cancer Congress, Italy.* (1994): 3099–3102.

Sharma, H., D. Chandradhar, B. Satter, et al. "Antineoplastic properties of Maharishi Amrit Kalash, an Ayurvedic food supplement against 7,12- dimethylbenz[a]anthracene-induced mammary tumors in a rat." *Journal of Research & Education in Indian Medicine* Vol. 3. (Jul-Sep 1991): 1–8.

Sharma, H., B. Dwivedi, C. Satter, et al. "Antineoplastic properties of Maharishi-4 against DMBA-induced mammary tumors in rats." *Pharmacology, Biochemistry, and Behavior* Vol. 35. (1990): 767–773.

Srivastava, A., V. Samiya, P. Taranikanti, et al. "Maharishi Amrit (MAK) reduces chemotherapy toxicity in breast cancer patients." The *FASEB Journal* Vol. 14. (Issue 4, 2000; Abstract): A720.

Chapter 14: Smothering the Flames

Abou-Issa, H.M., G.A. Alshafie, K. Seibert, et al. "Dose-response effects of the COX-2 inhibitor, celecoxib, on the chemoprevention of mammary carcinogenesis." *Anticancer Research* Vol. 21. (Sep-Oct 2001): 3425–3432.

Badawi, A.F., and M.Z. Badr. "Chemoprevention of breast cancer by targeting cyclooxygenase-2 and peroxisome proliferators-activated receptor-gamma (Review)." *International Journal of Oncology* Vol. 20. (Jun 2002): 1109–1122.

Badawi, A.F., and M.Z. Badr. "Expression of cyclooxygenase-2 and peroxisome proliferator-activated receptor-gamma and levels of prostaglandin E2 and 15-deoxy-elta 12,14-prostaglandin J2 in human breast cancer and metastasis." *International Journal of Cancer* Vol. 103. (Jan 1, 2003): 84–90.

Bing, R.J., M. Miyataka, K.A. Rich, et al. "Nitric oxide, prostanoids, Cyclooxygenase, and angiogenesis in colon and breast cancer." *Clinical Cancer Research* Vol. 7. (Nov 2001): 3385–3392.

Costa, C., R. Soares, J.S. Reis-Filho, et al. "Cyclo-oxygenase 2 expression is associated with angiogenesis and lymph node metastasis in human breast cancer." *Journal of Clinical Pathology* Vol. 55. (Jun 2002): 429–434.

Davies, G., L.A. Martin, N. Sacks, et al. "Cyclooxygenase-2 (COX-2), aromatase and breast cancer: a possible role for COX-2 inhibitors in breast cancer chemoprevention." *Annals of Oncology* Vol 13. (May 2002): 669–678.

Howe, L.R., and A.J. Dannenberg. "A role for cyclooxygense-2 inhibitors in the prevention and treatments of cancer." *Seminars in Oncology* Vol. 29. (Jun 2002; Suppl 11): 111–119.

Kryzystyniak, K.L. "Current strategies for anticancer chemoprevention and chemoprotection." *Acta poloniae Pharmaceutica* Vol. 59. (Nov-Dec 2002): 473–478.

Kundu, N., M.J. Smyth, L. Samsel, et al. "Cyclooxygenase inhibitors block cell growth, increase ceramind and inhibit cell cycle." *Breast Cancer Research & Treatment* Vol. 76. (Nov 2002): 57–64.

Lu, S., X. Zhang, A.F. Badawi, et al. "Cyclooxygenase-2 inhibitor celecoxib inhibits promotion of mammary tumorigenesis in rats fed a high fat diet rich in n-polyunsaturated fatty acids." *Cancer Letters* Vol. 184. (Oct 8, 2002): 7–12.

Michael, M.S., M.Z. Badr, and A.F. Badawi. "Inhibition of cyclooxygense-2 and activation of peroxisome proliferator-activated receptor-gamma synergistically induces apoptosis and inhibits growth in human breast cancer cells." *International Journal of Molecular Medicine* Vol. 11. (Jun 2003): 733–736.

Singh, B., A. Lucci, et al. "Role of Cyclooxygenase-2 in breast cancer." *Journal of Surgical Research* Vol. 108. (Nov 2002): 173–179.

Spizzo, G., G. Gasti, D. Wolf, et al. "Correlation of COX-2 and Ep-CAM overexpression in human invasive breast cancer and its impact on survival." *The British Journal of Cancer* Vol. 88. (Feb 24, 2003): 574–578.

Zyflamend

Bernis, D.L., K.A. Kozakowski, B.C. Anastasiadis, et al. "Zyflamend, an herbal COX-2 inhibitor with *in vitro* anti-prostate cancer activity." Center for Holistic Urology Columbia University. (2003).

Weil, A. "Breast Cancer: beating the odds?" www.Dr-Weil.com. (2003).

Barberry

Fukuda, K., Y. Hibiya, M. Mutoh, et al. "Inhibition by berberine of Cyclooxygenase-2 transcriptional activity in human colon cancer cells." *Journal of Ethnopharmacology* Vol. 66. (Aug 1999): 227–233.

Feverfew

Hwang, D., N. Fischer, B. Jang, et al. "Inhibition of the expression of inducible Cyclooxygenase and pro-inflammatory cytokines by sesquiterpene lactones in macrophages correlates with inhibition of MAP kinase." *Biochemical and Biophysical Research Communications* Vol. 226. (1996; article 1433): 810–818.

Ginger

Liang, Y.C., Y.T. Huang, and S.H. Tsai. "Suppression of inducible cyclooxygenase and inducible nitric oxide synthase by apigenin and related flavonoids in mouse macrophages." *Carcinogenesis* Vol. 20. (Oct 1999): 1945–1952.

Green Tea

Noreen, Y., G. Serrano, P. Perera, et al. "Flavan-3-ols isolated from some medicinal plants inhibiting COX-1 and COX-2 catalysed by prostaglandin biosynthesis." *Planta Medica* Vol. 64. (Aug 1998): 520–524.

Hops

Yamamoto, K., J. Wang, and S. Yamamoto. "Suppression of cyclooxygenase-2 gene transcription by humulon of beer hop extract studied in reference to glucocorticoid." *FEBS Letters* Vol. 465. (Jan 14, 2000): 103–106.

Huzhang

Subbaramaiah, K., W.J. Chung, P. Michaluart, et al. "Resveratrol inhibits cyclooxygenase-2 transcription and activity in phorbol ester-treated human mammary epithelial cells." *Journal of Biology & Chemistry* Vol. 273. (Aug 21, 1998): 21875–21882.

Holy Basil (Oscimum Sanctum)

Kelm, M.A., M.G. Nair, G.M. Strasburg, et al. "Antioxidant and Cyclooxygenase inhibitory phenolic compounds from Oscimum sanctum." *Phytomedicine* Vol. 7. (Mar 2000): 7–13.

Rosemary

Ringbom, T., L. Segura, Y. Noreen, et al. "Ursolic acid from Plantago major, a selective inhibitor of cyclooxygenase-2 catalyzed prostaglandin biosynthesis." *Journal of Natural Products* Vol. 61. (Oct 1998): 1212–1215.

Scutellariae

Sanchez, T., and J.J. Moreno. "Role of prostaglandin H synthase isoforms in murine ear edema induced by phorbol ester application on skin." *Prostaglandins & Other Lipid Mediators* Vol. 57. (May 1999): 199–231.

Turmeric

Zhang, F., N.K. Altorki, and J.R. Mestre. "Curcumin inhibits cyclooxygenase-2 transcription in bile-acid and phorbol ester-treated human gastrointestinal epithelial cells." *Carcinogenesis* Vol. 20. (Mar 1999): 45–51.

Chapter 15: The Perils of Red Meat

Dai, Q., X.O. Shu, F. Jin, et al. "Consumption of animal foods, cooking methods, and risk of breast cancer." *Cancer Epidemiology, Biomarkers & Prevention* Vol. 11. (Sep 2002): 801–808.

De Stefani, E., A. Ronco, and M. Mendilaharsu. "Meat intake, heterocyclic amines, and the risk of breast cancer: a case-control study in Uruguay." *Cancer Epidemiology, Biomarkers & Prevention* Vol. 6. (Aug 1997): 573–581.

Delfino, R.J., R. Sinha, and C. Smith. "Breast cancer, heterocyclic aromatic amines from meat and N-acetyltransferace 2 genotype." *Carcinogenesis* Vol. 21. (Apr 2000): 607–615.

Herman, S., J. Linseisen, J. Chang-Claude, et al. "Nutrition and breast cancer risk by age 50: a population-based case-control study in Germany." *Nutrition & Cancer* Vol. 44. (Issue 1, 2002): 22–34.

Holmes, M.D., G.A. Colditz, D.J. Hunter, et al. "Meat, fish and egg intake and risk of breast cancer." *International Journal of Cancer* Vol. 140. (Mar 20, 2003): 221–227.

Kulp, K., M. Knize, C. Malfatti, et al. "Identification of urine metabolites of 2-amino-1-methyl-6-phenyl-imidazo[4,5-*b*]pyridine following consumption of a single cooked chicken meal by humans." *Carcinogenesis* Vol. 21. (Nov 2000): 2065–2072.

Shannon, J., L.S. Cook, and J.L. Stanford. "Dietary intake and risk of postmenopausal breast cancer (United States)." *Cancer Causes and Control* Vol. 14. (Feb 2003): 19–27.

Zheng, W., A.C. Deitz, D.R. Campbell, et al. "N-acetyltransfrace 1 genetic polymorphism, cigarette smoking, well-done meat intake, and breast cancer risk." *Cancer Epidemiology, Biomarkers & Prevention* Vol. 8. (Mar 1999): 233–239.

Zheng, W., D. Xie, J.R. Cerhan, et al. "Sulfotransferase 1a1 polymorphism, endogenous estrogen exposure, well-done meat intake, and breast cancer risk." *Cancer Epidemiology, Biomarkers & Prevention* Vol. 10. (Feb 2001): 89–94.

Chapter 16: Dangerous Foe in a Sweet Disguise

Hamelers, I.H., and P.H. Steenbergh. "Interactions between estrogen and insulin-like growth factor signaling pathways in human breast tumor cells." *Endocrine-Related Cancer* Vol. 10. (Jun 2003): 331–345.

Michels, K.B., C.G. Solomon, F.B. Hu, et al. "Type 2 diabetes and subsequent incidence of breast cancer in Nurses' Health Study." *Diabetes Care* Vol. 26. (Jun 2003): 1752–1758.

Muti, P., T. Quattrin, B.J. Grant, et al. "Fasting glucose is a risk factor for breast cancer: a prospective study." *Cancer Epidemiology, Biomarkers & Prevention* Vol. 11. (Nov 2002): 1361–1368.

Potischman, N., R.J. Coates, C.A. Swanson, et al. "Increased risk of early-stage breast cancer related to consumption of sweet foods among women less than age 45 in the United States." *Cancer Causes and Control* Vol. 13. (Dec 2002): 937–946.

Stevia

Cardelo, H.M., M.A. Da Silva, and M.H. Famasio. "Measurement of the relative sweetness of Stevia extract, aspartame and cyclamate/saccharin blend as compared to sucrose at different concentrations." *Plant Foods for Human Nutrition (Dordrecht, Netherlands)* Vol. 54. (Issue 2, 1999): 119–130.

Chan, P., B. Tomlinson, Y.J. Chen, et al. "A double-blinded placebo-controlled study of effectiveness and tolerability of oral stevioside in human hypertension." *British Journal of Clinical Pharmacology* Vol. 50. (Sep 2000): 215–220.

Cohen, J. "The effects of different storage temperatures on the taste and chemical composition of Diet Coke." (1997). www.suewidemark.free servers.com/aspartame-formaldehyde.htm.

Curi, R., M. Alveraz, R.B. Bazotte, et al. "Effects of Stevia rebaudiana on glucose tolerance in normal adult humans." *Brazilian Journal of Medical and Biological Research* Vol. 19. (Issue 6, 1986): 771–774.

Horner, C., M.D. "300 times sweeter—a plant from Paraguay." Channelcincinnati.com. (Mar 14, 2002).

Jeppesen, P.B., S. Gregersen, C.R. Poulsen, et al. "Stevioside acts directly on pancreatic beta cells to secrete insulin: actions independent of cyclic adenosine monophosphate and adenosine triphosphate-sensitive K+- channel activity." *Metabolism* Vol. 49. (Feb 2000): 208–214.

Lee, C.N., K.L. Wong, J.C. Liu, et al. "Inhibitory effects of steviocide on calcium influx to produce antihypertension." *Planta Medica* Vol. 67. www.ncbi.nlm.nih.gov/entrez/query.fcgi?cmd=Retrieve&db=journals&list_uids=6480&dopt=full (Dec 2001): 769.

Melis, M.S. "A crude extract of Stevia rebaudiana increases the renal plasma flow of normal and hypertensive rats." *Brazilian Journal of Medical and Biological Research* Vol. 29. (May 1996): 69–75.

Melis, M.S. "Chronic administration of aqueous extract of Stevia rebaudiana in rats: renal effects." *Journal of Ethnopharmacology* Vol. 47. (Jul 28, 1995): 129–134.

Oyama, Y., H. Sakai, T. Arata, et al. "Cytotoxic effect of methanol, formaldehyde, and formate on dissociated rat thrombocytes: a possibility of aspartame toxicity." *Cell Biology & Toxicology* Vol. 18. (Issue 1, 2002): 43–50.

Takahashi, K., M. Matsuda, K. Ohashi, et al. "Analysis of anti-rotavirus activity of extract from Stevia rebaudiana." *Antiviral Research* Vol. 49. (Jan 2001): 15–24.

Tomita, T., N. Sato, T. Arai, et al. "Bacteriocidal activity of a fermented hot-water extract from Stevia rebaudiana Bertoni towards enterohemorrhagic Escherichia coli 0157:H7 and other food-borne pathogenic bacteria." *Microbiology & Immunology* Vol. 41. (Issue 12, 1997): 1005–1009.

Trocho, C., R. Pardo, I. Rafecas, et al. "Formaldehyde derived from dietary aspartame binds to tissue components in vivo." *Life Sciences* Vol. 63. (Issue 5, 1998): 337–349.

Xylitol

Isokangas, P., et al. "Xylitol chewing gum in caries prevention. A field study in children." *Journal of the American Dental Association* Vol. 117. (Aug 1988): 315–320.

Peldyak, J., Makinen, K.K. "Xylitol for caries prevention." *Journal of Dental Hygiene* Vol. 76. (Fall 2002): 276–85.

Pierini, C., "Xylitol: A sweet alternative." Vitamin Research Products website: www.vrp.com/library/735742.html.

Soderling, E., Makinen, K.K., Chen, C-Y., Pape, Jr., H.R., Makinen, P-L. "Effect of sorbitol, xylitol and xylitol/sorbitol chewing gums on dental plaque." *Journal of Dental Research* Vol. 67. (Special Issue, Abstract 1988): 1334.

Svanberg, M., Knuuttila, M. "Dietary xylitol prevents ovariectomy-induced changes of bone inorganic fraction in rats." *Bone and Mineral* Vol. 26. (July 1994): 81–88.

Chapter 17: Losing Your Goddess-Like Figure

Baillie-Hamilton, P. "Chemical toxins: a hypothesis to explain global obesity epidemic." *Journal of Alternative & Complementary Medicine* Vol. 8. (Issue 2, 2002): 185–192.

Flegal, K., M. Carrol, C. Ogdan, et al. "Prevalence and trends in obesity among US adults, 1999–2000." *Journal of the American Medical Association (JAMA)* Vol. 288. (Oct 9, 2002): 1723–1732.

Franceschi, S., A. Favero, C. La Vecchia, et al. "Body size indices and breast cancer risk before and after menopause." *International Journal of Cancer* Vol. 67. (Jul 1996): 181–186.

Frazier, A.L., C.T. Ryan, H. Rockett, et al. "Adolescent diet and risk of breast cancer." *Cancer Causes and Control* Vol. 15. (Feb 2004): 73–82.

Gastelu, Daniel, and Fred Hatfield, Ph.D. *Dynamic Nutrition for Maximum Performance*. Garden City Park, NY: Avery Publishing Group, 1997.

Horner, C., M.D. "300 times as sweet as sugar: the shrub from Paraguay." Channelcincinnati. com. (Mar 14, 2002).

Huang, Z., S.E. Hankinson, G.A. Colditz, et al. "Avoiding adult weight gain helps women reduce breast cancer risk." *Journal of the American Medical Association (JAMA)* Vol. 278. (Nov 5, 1997): 1407–1411.

Jernstrom, H., and E. Barret-Conner. "Obesity, weight change, fasting insulin, proinsulin, C-peptide, and insulin-like growth factor-1 levels in women with and without breast cancer: the Rancho Bernardo Study." *Journal of Women's Health & Gender Based Medicine* Vol. 8. (Dec 1999): 1265–1272.

Lahmann, P.H., L. Lissner, B. Gullberg, et al. "A prospective study of adiposity and postmenopausal breast cancer: the Malmo Diet and Cancer Study." *International Journal of Cancer* Vol. 103. (Jan 10, 2003): 246–252.

McTiernan, A. "Behavioral risk factors in breast cancer: can risk be modified?" *Oncologist* Vol. 8. (Issue 4, 2003): 326–334.

Mokdad, A., E. Ford, B. Bowman, et al. "Prevalence of obesity, diabetes, and obesity-related risk factors, 2001." *Journal of the American Medical Association (JAMA)* Vol. 289. (Jan 2003): 75–79.

Mokdad, A., E. Ford, B. Bowman, et al. "The continuing epidemic of obesity and diabetes in the United States." *Journal of the American Medical Association (JAMA)* Vol. 286. (Sep 12, 2001): 1195–1200.

Steohensin, G.D., and D.P. Rose. "Breast cancer and obesity: an update." *Nutrition & Cancer* Vol. 45. (Issue 1, 2003): 1–16.

Chapter 18: A Drink Not to Drink

Chen, W.Y., G.A. Colditz, and B. Rosner. "Use of postmenopausal hormones, alcohol, and risk for invasive breast cancer." *Annals of Internal Medicine* Vol. 137. (Nov 19, 2002): 798–804.

Dorgan, J.F., D.J. Baer, and P.S. Albert. "Serum Hormones and the alcohol-breast cancer association in postmenopausal women." *Journal of the National Cancer Institute* Vol. 93. (May 2, 2001): 710–715.

Eng, E.T., J. Ye, D. Williams, et al. "Suppression of estrogen biosynthesis by procyanidin dimers in red wine and grape seeds." *Cancer Research* Vol. 63. (Dec 1, 2003): 8516–8522.

Friedenreich, C.M., G.R. Howe, A.B. Miller, et al. "A cohort study of alcohol consumption and risk of breast cancer." *American Journal of Epidemiology* Vol. 137. (Mar 1, 1993): 512–520.

Gaspstur, S.M., J.D. Potter, C. Dinkard, et al. "Synergistic effects between alcohol and estrogen replacement therapy on the risk of breast cancer differ by estrogen/progesterone receptor status in the Iowa Women's Health Study." *Cancer Epidemiology, Biomarkers & Prevention* Vol. 4. (Issue 4, 1995): 313–318.

Hamajima, N., K. Hirose, K. Tajima, et al. "Alcohol, tobacco, and breast cancer—collaborative reanalysis of individual data from 53 epidemiological studies including 58,515 women with breast cancer and 95,067 women without the disease." *The British Journal of Cancer* Vol. 87. (Nov 18, 2002): 1234–1245.

Jain, M.G., R.G. Ferrace, J.T. Rehm, et al. "Alcohol and breast cancer mortality in a cohort study." *Breast Cancer Research & Treatment* Vol. 64. (Nov 2001): 201–209.

Longnecker, M.P. "Alcohol beverage consumption in relation to risk of breast cancer: meta-analysis and review." *Cancer Causes and Control* Vol. 5. (Jan 1994): 73–82.

Muti, P., M. Trevisan, A. Micheli, et al. "Alcohol consumption and total estradiol in premenopausal women." *Cancer Epidemiology, Biomarkers & Prevention* Vol. 7. (Mar 1998): 189–193.

Rohan, T.E., M. Jain, G.R. Howe, et al. "Alcohol consumption and risk of breast cancer: a cohort study." *Cancer Causes and Control* Vol. 11. (Mar 2000): 239–247.

Schatzkin, A., and M.P. Longnecker. "Alcohol and breast cancer: Where are we now and where do we go from here?" *Cancer* Vol. 74. (Aug 1, 1994; Suppl 3): 1101–1111.

Sharma, G., A.K. Tyagi, R.P. Singh, et al. "Synergistic anti-cancer effects of grape seed extract and conventional cytotoxic agent doxorubicin against human breast carcinoma cells." *Breast Cancer Research & Treatment* Vol. 85. (May 2004): 1–12.

Smith-Warner, S.A., D. Spiegelman, S.S. Yaun, et al. "Alcohol and breast cancer in women: a pooled analysis of cohort studies." *Journal of the American Medical Association (JAMA)* Vol. 279. (Feb 18, 1998): 535–540.

Thomas, D.B. "Alcohol as a cause of cancer." *Environmental Health Perspectives* Vol. 103. (Nov 1995; Suppl 8): 153–160.

Ye, X., R.L. Krohn, W. Liu, et al. "The cytotoxic effects of a novel IH636 grape seed proanthocyanidin extract on cultured human cancer cells." *Molecular & Cell Biochemistry* Vol. 196. www.ncbi.nlm.nih.gov/entrez/query.fcgi?cmd=Retrieve&db=journals&list_uids=5915&dopt=full (Jun 1999): 99–108.

"Grape Seed Extract." www.usana-nutritionals.com/research/USNUSUPPINGREDIE_19499. html

Chapter 19: Sir Walter Raleigh's Folly

Band, P.R., N.D. Le, R. Fang, et al. "Carcinogenic and endocrine disrupting effects of cigarette smoke and risk of breast cancer." *The Lancet* Vol. 360. (Oct 5, 2002): 1044–1049.

Chang-Claude, J., S. Kropp, B. Jager, et al. "Differential effect of NAT2 on the association between active and passive smoking exposure and breast cancer risk." *Cancer Epidemiology, Biomarkers & Prevention* Vol. 11. (Aug 2002): 698–704.

Egan, K.M., P.A. Newcomb, L. Titus-Ernstoff, et al. "Association of NAT2 and smoking in relation to breast cancer incidence in a population-based control study (United States)." *Cancer Causes and Control* Vol. 14. (Feb 2003): 43–51.

Hamajima, N., K. Hirose, K. Tajima, et al. "Alcohol, tobacco, and breast cancer—collaborative reanalysis of individual data from 53 epidemiological studies including 58,515 women with breast cancer and 95,067 women without the disease." *The British Journal of Cancer* (Nov 18, 2002): 1234–1245.

Kropp, S., and J. Chang-Claude. "Active and passive smoking and risk of breast cancer by age 50 years among German women." *American Journal of Epidemiology* Vol. 156. (Oct 1, 2002): 616–626.

"List of Smoking-related diseases expanded: surgeon general warns of other cancer, pneumonia, cataracts and more." Associated Press Release. (May 27, 2004).

"New stats show heart diseases still America's No. 1 Killer, stroke No.3." American Heart Association Journal Report. (Jan 1, 2004). www.americanheart.org/presenter.jhtml?identifier=3018015.

Terry, P.D., and T.E. Rohan. "Cigarette smoking and the risk of breast cancer in women: a review of the literature." *Cancer Epidemiology, Biomarkers & Prevention* Vol. 11. (Oct 2002; 10 Pt 1): 953–971.

Chapter 20: Fatally Flawed Pharmaceuticals

The Pill and HRT

Beral, V., et al. "Breast cancer and hormone-replacement therapy in the Million Women Study." *Lancet* Vol. 362. (Aug 9, 2003): 419-27.

Chen, W.Y., G.A. Colditz, and B. Rosner. "Use of postmenopausal hormones, alcohol, and risk for invasive breast cancer." *Annals of Internal Medicine* Vol. 137. (Nov 19, 2002): 798–804.

Chen, W.Y., N. Weiss, and P. Newcomb. "Hormone replacement therapy in relation to breast cancer." *Journal of the American Medical Association (JAMA)* Vol. 287. (Feb 13, 2002): 734–741.

Colcitz, G.A., and B. Rosner. "Cumulative risk of breast cancer to age 70 years according to risk factor status: data from the Nurses' Health Study." *American Journal of Epidemiology* Vol. 152. (Nov 15, 2000): 950–964.

Daling, J.R., K.E. Malone, and D.R. Doody. "Relation of regimens of combines hormone replacement therapy to lobular, ductal, and other histologic types of breast cancer." *Cancer* Vol. 95. (Dec 15, 2002): 2455–2464.

Edan, J. "Progestins and cancer." *American Journal of Obstetrics & Gynecology* Vol. 188. (May 2003): 1123–1131.

Ginsburg, E.S., B.W. Walsh, and B.F. Shea. "Effect of acute ethanol ingestion on prolactin in menopausal women using estradiol replacement." *Gynecologic and Obstetric Investigation* Vol. 39. (Issue 1, 1995): 47–49.

Humphries, K., and S. Gill. "Risks and benefits of hormone replacement therapy: the evidence speaks." *CMAJ: Canadian Medical Association Journal* Vol. 168. (Apr 15, 2003): 1001–1010.

LeBlanc, E., J. Janowsky, and B. Chan. "Hormone replacement therapy and cognition." *Journal of the American Medical Association (JAMA)* Vol. 285. (Mar 2001): 1489–1499.

Leis, H.P., M.M. Black, and S. Sall. "The pill and the breast." *Journal of Reproductive Medicine* Vol. 16. (Jan 1976): 5–9.

Longman, S.M., and G.C. Buehring. "Oral contraceptives and breast cancer. In vitro effect contraceptive steroids on human mammary growth." *Cancer* Vol. 59. (Jan 15, 1987): 281–287.

Li, C.I., B.O. Anderson, and J.R. Daling. "Trends in incidence rates of invasive lobular and ductal breast carcinoma." *Journal of the American Medical Association (JAMA)* Vol. 289. (Mar 19, 2003): 1421–1424.

Nelson, H., L. Humphrey, et al. "Postmenopausal hormone replacement therapy." *Journal of the American Medical Association (JAMA)* Vol. 288. (Aug 21, 2002): 872–881.

Petitti, D. "Hormone replacement therapy for prevention: more evidence, more pessimism." *Journal of the American Medical Association (JAMA)* Vol. 288. (Jul 3, 2002): 99–100.

Porch, J.V., I.M. Lee, and N.R. Cook. "Estrogen-progestin replacement therapy and breast cancer risk: the Women's Health Study (United States)." *Cancer Causes and Control* Vol. 13. (Nov 2002): 847–854.

Rodriguez, C., A. Patel, and E. Calle. "Estrogen Replacement therapy and ovarian cancer mortality in a large prospective study of US women." *Journal of the American Medical Association (JAMA)* Vol. 285. (Mar 2001): 1460–1465.

Writing group WHI investigators. "Risks and benefits of estrogen plus progestin in healthy postmenopausal women." *Journal of the American Medical Association (JAMA)* Vol. 288. (Jul 17, 2002): 321–333.

Antidepressants and Other Pharmaceuticals

Brandes, L.J., R.J. Arron, R.P. Bogdanovic, et al. "Stimulation of malignant growth in rodents by antidepressant drugs at clinically relevant doses." *Cancer Research* Vol. 52. (Jul 1992): 3796–3800.

Cotterchio, M., N. Kreiger, G. Darlington, et al. "Antidepressant medication use and the risk of breast cancer." *American Journal of Epidemiology* Vol. 151. (May 2000): 951–957.

Kurdyak, P.A., W.H. Gnam, and D.L. Streiner. "Antidepressants and the risk of breast cancer." *The Canadian Journal of Psychiatry* Vol. 47. (Dec 2002): 966–970.

Sharpe, C.R., J.P. Collet, E. Beizile, et al. "The effects of tricyclic antidepressants on breast cancer risk." *The British Journal of Cancer* Vol. 86. (Jan 7, 2002): 92–97.

Chapter 21: Portrait of an Assassin

"Are pesticides hazardous to our health." *Journal of Pesticide Reform* Vol. 19. (Issue 2, 1999): 4–5.

Buros, M. "Farmed Salmon is said to contain high PCB levels." *The New York Times.* (July 30, 2003).

Bradlow, H.L., D.L. Davis, G. Lin, et al. "Effects of pesticides on the ratio of 16 alpha/2-hydroxyestrone: a biologic marker of breast cancer risk." *Environmental Health Perspectives* Vol. 103. (Oct 1995; Suppl 7): 147–150.

Brotons, J.A., et al. "Environmental Health Issues." *Environmental Health Prospectives* Vol. 103. (1995): 608-612.

Cebbelo, G., A. Juarranz, et al. "Organophosphorous pesticides in breast cancer progression." *Journal of Submicroscopic Cytology & Pathology* Vol. 35. (Jan 2003): 1–9.

Chang, J.C., R. Fortmann, et al. "Evaluation of low-VOC latex paint." *Indoor Air* Vol. 9. (Dec 1999): 253–258.

Coco, P., N. Kazerouni, and S.H. Zahm. "Cancer mortality and environmental exposure to DDE in the United States." *Environmental Health Perspectives* Vol. 108. (Jan 2000): 1–4.

Demers, A., P. Ayotte, J. Brisson, et al. "Risk and aggressiveness of breast cancer in relation to plasma organochlorine concentrations." *Cancer Epidemiology, Biomarkers & Prevention* Vol. 9. (Feb 2000): 161–166.

"Environmental estrogens and other hormones." Tulane University website. www.tmc.tulane.edu/ecme/eehome/basics/.

Epstein, S. "Pesticides and Cancer." Transcript of lecture given in 1993.

Franklin, P., P. Dingle, et al. "Raised exhaled nitric oxide in healthy children associated with domestic formaldehyde levels." *American Journal of Critical Care Medicine* Vol. 161. (May 2000): 1757–1759.

Guttes, S., K. Failing, K. Neumann, et al. "Chlororganic pesticides and polychlorinated biphenyls in breast tissue of women with benign and malignant breast disease." *Archives of Environmental Contamination & Toxicology* Vol. 35. (Jul 1998): 140–147.

Horner, C., M.D. "Alternatives to chemical pesticides." Channelcincinnati.com. (May 10, 2001).

Horner, C., M.D. "Hidden toxins in plywood and particle board." Channelcincinnati.com. (Jan 5, 2002).

Horner, C., M.D. "Naturally keeping bugs away." Channelcincinnati.com. (May 5, 2001).

Horner, C., M.D. "Nontoxic bedding." Channelcincinnati.com. (Mar 16, 2002).

Horner, C., M.D. "Nontoxic paints." Channelcincinnati.com. (Jun 10, 2002).

Horner, C., M.D. "Toxic air and household products." Channelcincinnati.com. (Jun 21, 2001).

Hoyer, A.P., P. Grandjean, T. Jorgensen, et al. "Organochlorine compounds and breast cancer—is there a connection between environmental pollution and breast cancer." *Ugeskr Laeger* Vol. 162. (Feb 14, 2000): 922–926.

Hoyer, A.P., T. Jorgensen, et al. "Repeated measurements of organochlorine exposure and breast cancer risk (Denmark)." *Cancer Causes and Control* Vol. 11. (Feb 2000): 177–184.

Hoyer, A.P., T. Jorgensen, J.W. Brock, et al. "Organochlorine exposure and breast cancer survival." *Journal of Clinical Epidemiology* Vol. 53. (Mar 2000): 323–330.

Jaga, K., and D. Brosius. "Pesticide exposure: human cancers on the horizon." *Reviews on Environmental Health* Vol. 14. (Jan-Mar 1999): 39–50.

Jaga, K., and H. Duvvi. "Risk reduction for DDT toxicity and carcinogenesis through dietary modifications." *Journal of the Royal Society of Health* Vol. 121. (Jun 2001): 107–113.

Krishnan, A.V., et al. "Bisphenol-A: an estrogenic substance is released from polycarbonate flasks during autoclaving." *Endocrinology* Vol. 132. (1993): 2279-2286.

Martin, B. *The Journal of Nature Medicine.* (Aug 2003).

Mather, V., P. Bhatnagar, R.G. Sharma, et al. "Breast cancer incidence and exposure to pesticides among women originating from Jaipur." *Environment International* Vol. 28. (Nov 2002): 331–336.

Meinhert, R., J. Schuz, et al. "Leukemia and non-Hodgkin's lymphoma I childhood exposure to pesticides: results of a register-based case-control study in Germany." *American Journal of Epidemiology* Vol. 15. (Apr 1, 2000): 639–646.

Moysich, K.B., C.B. Ambrosone, P. Mendola, et al. "Exposures associated with serum organochlorine levels among postmenopausal women from western

New York State." *American Journal of Independent Indian Medicine* Vol. 41. (Feb 2002): 102–110.

Sonnenschein, C., A.M. Soto. "An updated review of environmental estrogen and androgen mimickers and antagonists." *Journal of Steroid Biochemistry and Molecular Biology* Vol. 65. (Apr 1998): 143–50.

Soto, A.M. et al. "p-Nonyl-phenol: an estrogenic xenobiotic released from "modified" polystyrene." *Environmental Health Perspectives* Vol. 92. (1991): 167–73.

Vaughan, T.L., P.A. Stewart, et al. "Occupational exposure to formaldehyde and wood dust and nasopharyngeal carcinoma." *Occupational & Environmental Medicine* Vol. 57. (Jun 2000): 376–384.

Chapter 22: Invite Friends, Not Foes

Harwood, Barbara. *The Healing House.* Carlsbad, CA: Hay House, 1997.

Horner, C., M.D. "Alternatives to chemical pesticides." Channelcincinnati.com. (May 10, 2001).

Horner, C., M.D. "Hidden toxins in plywood and particle board." Channelcincinnati.com. (Jan 5, 2002).

Horner, C., M.D. "Naturally keeping bugs away." Channelcincinnati.com. (May 5, 2001).

Horner, C., M.D. "Nontoxic bedding." Channelcincinnati.com. (Mar 16, 2002).

Horner, C., M.D. "Nontoxic paints." Channelcincinnati.com. (Jun 10, 2002).

Horner, C., M.D. "Toxic air and household products." Channelcincinnati.com. (Jun 21, 2001).

Marinelli, Janet, and Paul Beirman-Lytle. *Your Natural Home.* Boston, MA: Little Brown & Co., 1995.

Pearson, David. *The Natural House Catalog.* New York, NY: Fireside, 1996.

Pearson, David. *The New Natural House Book.* New York, NY: Fireside, 1998.

Many of the solutions listed are discoveries I made from many different sources over the years in my quest to live a nontoxic life.

Chapter 23: Cellular Housecleaning

Heron, B., and J.B. Fagan. "Effects of Maharishi rejuvenation (Panchakarma) in reducing dangerous environmental toxins." *Alternative Therapies in Health & Medicine* Vol. 8. (Sep-Oct 2002): 93–103.

Horner, C., M.D. "Purification through panchakarma." Channelcincinati.com. (Jan 24, 2002).

Schnare, D.W., M. Ben, and M.G. Shields. "Body Burden reductions of PCBs, PBBs, and chlorinated pesticides in human subjects." *Ambio* Vol. 13. (1991): 37.

Schneider, R.H., K.L. Cavanaugh, et al. "Health promotion with a traditional system of natural health care: Maharishi Ayur-Veda." *Journal of Social Behavior and Personality* Vol. 5. (Issue 3, 1990): 1–27.

Sharma, H., and C. Alexander. "Improvements in cardiovascular risk factors through Panchakarma purification procedures." *Journal of Research & Education in Indian Medicine* Vol. 12. (Issue 4, 1993): 2–13.

Sharma, Hari, M.D. *Freedom from Disease*. Toronto, Canada: Veda Publishing, 1993.

Sharma, Hari, M.D., and Christopher Clark, M.D. *Contemporary Ayurveda*. New York, NY: Churchill Livingstone, 1998.

Waldschutz, R. "Influence of Maharishi Ayur-Veda purification treatment on physiological and psychological health." *Erfhrungsheilkunde-Acta medica empirica* Vol. 11. (1988): 720–729.

Chapter 24: Healing Nectars of the Night

Anisimov, V.N. "The role of pineal gland in breast development." *Critical Reviews in Oncology/Hematology* Vol. 46. (Jun 2003); 221–234.

Bizzarri, M., A. Cucina, M.G. Valente, et al. "Melatonin and vitamin D(3) increase TGF-beta(1) release and induce growth inhibition in breast cancer cell cultures." *Journal of Surgical Research* Vol. 110. (Apr 2003): 332–337.

Blask, D. American Association for Cancer Research 94th Annual Meeting. Washington, DC: Jul 11–14, 2003.

Davis, S., D.K. Mirick, and R.G. Stevens. "Night shift work, light at light, and risk of breast cancer." *Journal of the National Cancer Institute* Vol. 93. (Oct 17, 2001): 1557–1562.

Glickman, G., R. Levin, and G.C. Brainard. "Ocular input for human melatonin regulation: relevance to breast cancer." *Neuroendocrinology Letters* Vol. 23. (Jul 2002; Suppl 2): 17–22.

Kiefer, T., P.T. Ram, L. Yuan, et al. "Melatonin inhibits estrogen receptor transactivation and cAMP levels in beast cancer cells." *Breast Cancer Research & Treatment* Vol. 71. (Jan 2002): 37–45.

Krishan, S. "Sleep like a child." *Total Health Magazine*. (2001).

Kubatka, P., K. Kalick, and M. Chamilova. "Nimesulide and melatonin in mammary carcinogenesis prevention in female Sprague–Dawley rats." *Neoplasma* Vol. 49. (Issue 4, 2002): 255–259.

Lemus–Wilson, A., P.A. Kelly, and D.E. Blask. "Melatonin Blocks the stimulatory effects of prolactin on human breast cancer cell growth in culture." *The British Journal of Cancer* Vol. 72. (Dec 1995): 1435–1440.

Lissoni, P., S. Barni, and M. Mandala. "Decreased toxicity and increased efficacy of cancer chemotherapy using pineal hormone melatonin in metastatic solid tumor patients with poor clinical status." *European Journal of Cancer* Vol. 35. (Nov 1999): 1688–1692.

Ram, P.T., J. Dai, and C. Dong. "Involvement of the mtl melatonin receptor in human breast cancer." *Cancer Letters* Vol. 179. (May 28, 2002): 141–150.

Sanchez-Barcelo, E.J., S. Cos, R. Fernandez. "International congress on hormonal steroids and hormones and cancer: Melatonin and mammary cancer: a short review." *Endocrine-Related Cancer* Vol. 10. (Jun 2003): 153–159.

Stevens, R.G., S. Davis, D.K. Mirick, et al. "Alcohol consumption and urinary concentration of 6-sulfatoxymelatonin in healthy women." *Epidemiology* Vol. 11. (Nov 2000): 660–665.

"Stress and Insomnia." *Total Health New Online*. Maharishi Ayurveda Products International. (Mar 1, 2001).

Electromagnetic Fields (EMFs)

Caplan, L.S., E.R. Schoenfeld, E.S. O'Leary, et al. "Breast cancer and electromagnetic fields—a review." *Annals of Epidemiology* Vol. 10. (Jan 2000): 31–44.

Davis, S., W.Y. Kaune, D.K. Mirick, et al. "Residential magnetic fields, light – at-night, and nocturnal urinary 6-sulfatoxymelatonin concentration in women." *American Journal of Epidemiology* Vol. 154. (Oct 1, 2001): 591–600.

Davis, S., D.K. Mirick, and R.G. Stevens. "Residential magnetic fields and the risk of breast cancer." *American Journal of Epidemiology* Vol. 155. (Mar 1, 2002): 446–454.

Fedrowitz, M., J. Westermann, and W. Losher. "Magnetic field exposure increases cell proliferation but does not affect melatonin levels in the mammary gland of female Sprague-Dawley rats." *Cancer Research* Vol. 62. (Mar 2002): 1356–1363.

Mevissen, M., M. Haussler, and W. Loscher. "Alterations in ornithine decarboxylase activity in the rat mammary gland after different periods of 50Hz magnetic field exposure." *Bioelectromagnetics* Vol. 20. (Sep 1999): 338–346.

Stevens, R.G., S. Davis, and D.B. Thomas. "Electric power, pineal function, and the risk of breast cancer." *The FASEB Journal* Vol. 6. (Feb 1, 1992): 853–860.

Chapter 25: The Medicine of Movement

Carpenter, C.L., R.K. Ross, A. Paganini-Hill, et al.

"Effects of family history, obesity, and exercise on breast cancer risk among postmenopausal women." *International Journal of Cancer* Vol. 106. (Aug 10, 2003): 96–102.

Hirose, K., N. Hamajima, T. Takezaki, et al. "Physical exercise reduces risk of breast cancer in Japanese women." *Cancer Science* Vol. 94. (Feb 2003): 193–199.

Horner, C., M.D. "Ayurvedic approaches to exercise." Channelcincinnati.com. (Apr 7, 2001).

Lee, I.M., et al. "Physical Activity and coronary artery disease risk in men: does the duration of exercise episodes predict risk?" *Circulation* Vol. 102. (Aug 29, 2000): 981–986.

Marcus, P. "Exercise/breast cancer connection." *Bottom Line Magazine.* (Jun 15, 1998).

Moradi, T., O. Nyren, M. Zack, et al. "Breast cancer risk and lifetime leisure-time and occupational physical activity (Sweden)." *Cancer Causes and Control* Vol. 11. (Jul 2000): 523–531.

Rockhill, B., W.C. Willett, D.J. Hunter, et al. "A prospective study of recreational physical activity and breast cancer risk." *Archives of Internal Medicine* Vol. 159. (Oct 25, 1999): 2290–2296.

Steindorf, K., M. Schmidt, and S. Kropp. "Case-control study of physical activity and breast cancer risk among premenopausal women in Germany." *American Journal of Epidemiology* Vol. 157. (Jan 15, 2003): 121–130.

Veerloop, J., M.A. Rookus, K. van der Kooy, et al. "Physical activity and breast cancer risk in women aged 20-54 years." *Journal of the National Cancer Institute* Vol. 92. (Jan 19, 2000): 128–135.

Wyrick, K.W., and F.D. Wolinsky. "Physical activity, disability, and the risk of hospitalization for breast cancer among older women." *The Journals of Gerontology. Series A, Biological Sciences and Medical Sciences* Vol. 55. (Jul 2000): M418–M421.

Chapter 26: Emotional Healing

Balick, M., and R. Lee. "The role of laughter in traditional medicine and its relevance to the clinical setting: healing with ha!" *Alternative Therapies in Health & Medicine* Vol. 9. (Jul-Aug 2003): 88–91.

Bennet, M., J. Zeller, and L. Rosenberg. "The effect of mirthful laughter on stress and natural killer cell function." *Alternative Therapies in Health & Medicine* Vol. 9. (Issue 2, 2003): 38–43.

Berk, L.S., D. Felton, S.A. Tan, et al. "Modulations of immune parameters during the eustress of humor associated with mirthful laughter." *Alternative Therapies in Health & Medicine* Vol. 7. (Issue 2, 2001): 62–67.

Berk, L.S., S.A. Tan, W.F. Fry, et al. "Neuroendocrine and stress hormones change during mirthful laughter." *American Journal of Medical Science* Vol. 298. (Issue 6, 1989): 390–396.

Hillhouse, J., et al. "Stress, health, and immunity: a review of the literature and implications for the nursing profession." *Holistic Nursing Practice* Vol. 5. (Jul 1991): 22–31.

Horner, C., M.D. "The healing power of faith." Channelcincinnati.com. (Feb 10, 2001).

Horner, C., M.D. "The power of love and intimacy." Channelcincinnati.com. (Apr 21, 2001).

Myss, Carolyn, Ph.D. *Why People Don't Heal.* New York, NY: Three Rivers Press, 1997.

Ornish, Dean, M.D. *Love and Survival.* New York, NY: Harper Collins, 1995.

Sharma, Hari, M.D., and Christopher Clark, M.D. *Contemporary Ayurveda.* New York, NY: Churchill Livingstone, 1998.

Tipping, Colin. *Radical Forgiveness: Making Room for the Miracle.* Marietta, GA: Global 13 Publications, 1997.

Tolle, Eckhart. *The Power of Now.* Novato, CA: New World Library, 1999.

Pranayama

Bhargava, R., M.G. Gogate, and J.F. Mascarenhas. "Autonomic responses to breath holding and its variations following pranayama." *Indian Journal of Physiology & Pharmacology* Vol. 32. (Oct-Dec 1998): 257–264.

Horner, C., M.D. "Pranayama: using the breathing for health." Channelcincinnati.com. (Apr 26, 2001).

Raghuraj, P., R. Nagarathna, et al. "Pranayama increases grip strength without lateralized effects." *Indian Journal of Physiology & Pharmacology* Vol. 41. (Apr 1997): 129–133.

Raju, P.S., K.A. Kumar, S.S. Reddy, et al. "Effects of yoga on exercise tolerance in normal healthy volunteers." *Indian Journal of Physiology & Pharmacology* Vol. 30. (Apr-Jun 1986): 121–132.

Telles, S., R. Nagarantha, and H.R. Nagendra. "Physiological measures of right nostril breathing." *Journal of Alternative & Complementary Medicine* Vol. 2. (Winter 1996): 479–484.

Telles, S., R. Nagarantha, and H.R. Nagendra. "Breathing through a particular nostril can alter metabolism and autonomic activities." *Indian Journal of Physiology & Pharmacology* Vol. 38. (Apr 1994): 133–137.

Chapter 27: Turning Inward

Alexander, C.N., M.V. Rainforth, and P. Gelderlos. "Transcendental meditation, self-actualization and psychological health: a conceptual overview and statistical meta-analysis." *Journal of Social Behavior and Personality* Vol. 6. (Issue 5, 1991): 189–247.

Alexander, C.N., P. Robinson, et al. "The effects of Transcendental meditation compared to other methods of relaxation and meditation in reducing risk factors, morbidity, and mortality." *Homeostasis* Vol. 35. (1994a): 243–264.

Alexander, C.N., and P. Robinson. "Treating and preventing alcohol, nicotine, and drug abuse through Transcendental meditation: a review and statistical meta-analysis." *Alcohol Treatment Quarterly* Vol. 11. (1994b): 11–84.

Banquet, J.P. "Spectral analysis of the EEG in meditation." *Electroencephalography and Clinical Neurophysiology* Vol. 35. (1973): 145–151.

Dillbeck, M.C., and D.W. Orme-Johnson. "Physiological differences between Transcendental meditation and the rest." *American Physiology* Vol. 42. (1987): 879–881.

Glaser, J.L., J.L. Brind, et al. "Elevated serum dehydroepiandrosterone-sulfate levels in practitioner of the Transcendental mediation (TM) and the TM-sidhi programs." *Journal of Behavioral Medicine* Vol. 15. (1992): 327–341.

Heron, R.E., S.L. Hillis, et al. "Impact of the Transcendental mediation program on government payments to physicians in Quebec." *American Journal of Health Promotion* Vol. 10. (Issue 3, 1996): 208–216.

Horner, C., M.D. "TM and cancer." Channelcincinnati.com. (Apr 27, 2002).

Orme-Johnson, D.W. "EEG coherence during transcendental consciousness. *Electroencephalography and Clinical Neurophysiology* Vol. 43. (Issue 4, 1977): 581–582 E 487 (abstract).

Orme-Johnson, D.W. "Medical utilization and the Transcendental mediation program." *Psychosomatic Medicine* Vol. 49. (1987): 493–507.

Orme-Johnson, D.W., and C.T. Haynes. "EEG phase coherence, pure consciousness, creativity, and the TM-Sidhi experience." *International Journal of Neuroscience* Vol. 113. (1981): 211–219.

Sharma, Hari, M.D., and Christopher Clark, M.D. *Contemporary Ayurveda.* New York, NY: Churchill Livingstone, 1998.

Wallace, R.K., M.C. Dillbeck, et al. "The effects of Transcendental meditation and the TM-Sidhi program on the aging process." *International Journal of Neuroscience* Vol. 16. (1982): 53–58.

Wallace, Robert, Ph.D. *The Neurophysiology of Enlightenment.* Fairfield, IA: Maharishi International University Press, 1991.

Wallace, Robert, Ph.D. *The Physiology of Consciousness.* Fairfield, IA: Maharishi International University Press, 1993.

Index